Beware of Doctors and Hospitals

by
Roy Manganelli

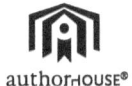

authorHOUSE®

AuthorHouse™
1663 Liberty Drive, Suite 200
Bloomington, IN 47403
www.authorhouse.com
Phone: 1-800-839-8640

First published by AuthorHouse   7/19/2007

ISBN: 978-1-4343-1693-6 (sc)
ISBN: 978-1-4343-1695-0 (hc)

Library of Congress Control Number: 2007904481

Printed in the United States of America
Bloomington, Indiana

This book is printed on acid-free paper.

Table of Contents

WARNING! READ THIS BOOK at your own risk. Upon reading it, some readers may be afraid to visit doctors or hospitals for the rest of their lives. However, other readers might die laughing as they indulge themselves to the variety of the many interesting and scaring subjects that they will read about. If you're planning to visit a doctor or hospital, you should read this book before taking that major step that will probably change your life. If your decision is to go ahead with that visit, let us hope that you don't run into some of the bad doctors and hospitals mentioned in this story. If you ever had any kind of bad experience as a result of visiting a doctor or hospital, or if you ever heard of anyone else who had a bad experience, you should definitely read this book.

This story, although fictional, has been comically exaggerated. However, there is a great deal of reality, and some readers will find it very convincing, especially if they had similar experiences as the ones stated in this book. The story deals with the daily occurrences in certain doctors' offices, as well as certain hospitals in a major metropolitan city in the Northeast of The United States. You will see the worst treatments performed by the worst doctors. However, later on in the story, you will also see the best treatments offered by the best doctors.

The story contains a generous amount of extremely grim occurrences, but it also contains a great deal of generosity and compassion. You will see that there are some people in this story who went out of their way to do the right thing. You will also see that there are numerous people who kept the promises that they made to others when they were in need.

There are many surprises in this story. Therefore, while reading this book, you may find some events, which you may think are not clearly explained, and you may also think that such events don't seem to come to a conclusion – well, there are explanations or conversations later on in the story that will give you a clear picture of everything that you thought needed clarification – just read on, and in due time, you'll see what happens. It is very unlikely that after you read the entire book, you will still think that there are any loose ends.

The names used in this story have been chosen by the author as a description of each person or place involved. Actual names were not used in order to protect the innocent – and the guilty. It may take some readers a little time to accept the names, but after they have accepted them, they will find the story extremely enjoyable and very interesting. Some readers may find it to be a very valuable and educational account of situations that they should avoid.

If this story changes the life of only one person for the better, even for a brief moment, then it was worth writing this book.

Colon Cancer

IT WAS A BEAUTIFUL MONDAY morning in a major city in the Northeast of The United States – the name of the city is not important in this story, but it was in the state of New York. James Syckcolun was sitting at his kitchen table eating breakfast with his wife, Elizabeth. James recently retired, and Elizabeth made a career as a Domestic Engineer. As any other red-blooded American couple, they made sure that they had a thorough medical examination once or twice a year. They were still in great physical and mental condition, and were both very distinguished-looking for their age, so they wanted to enjoy the rest of their lives in good health. They recently had a medical checkup at Kuttemopen Hospital.

As they finished their breakfast, the mailman approached their house to deliver their daily mail. Elizabeth stepped outside to retrieve it. She noticed that one of the letters was from Doctor Manypewlatar at the same hospital. Once inside, Elizabeth quickly opened the letter and read it to James, out loud, "Mr. Syckcolun, your ex-rays show a slight possibility of the onset of colon cancer. I hereby strongly urge you to call my office as soon as possible to make an emergency appointment for exploratory surgery. Sincerely, Doctor Manypewlatar."

James and Elizabeth were totally devastated as she read the letter, and they thought that James should do exactly as Doctor Manypewlatar had instructed him to do. All of a sudden, Elizabeth was very concerned about her husband's well-being, "Do you feel any pain, Honey?"

James answered with confidence, "No, Dear, I don't feel anything at all. I feel as strong as a horse." They called the hospital right away to make an appointment, and it was scheduled for Wednesday, which was two days away. After making the appointment, James and Elizabeth started talking to many people about the situation, and they were given positive and negative advice by many of their friends and family members.

Later on, that same afternoon, James was at home talking to his good friend and neighbor, Wayne Sqaptikal, who thought that he had some very valuable advice for James, "I wouldn't let them cut me open if I were in your shoes."

James acted very confused and asked, "Well, what can I do? They sent me a letter saying that I may be getting colon cancer, and I have to make sure that if I do have it, they catch it in time and treat it successfully."

Wayne felt doubtful and said, "Okay, James, it's up to you, but I wouldn't let them do it to me. There's no guarantee that you'll come out of the hospital alive."

"Why wouldn't you let them cut you open, Wayne?" asked James.

"I think I have a good reason to convince you not to go, James," Wayne answered. "Have you ever known of anyone who was cut open to have his colon cancer treated, and is still alive today?"

"No, and now you're beginning to scare me," James replied.

"There's your answer!" Wayne went on with plenty of confidence. "I feel good because I guess you won't be going to the hospital now – I hope I convinced you. You might be sorry if you decide to go, but it's up to you. Anyway, I have to take my wife shopping, so I'll see you later, James."

"Okay, bye, Wayne," James concluded. After Wayne left, James was more confused than ever. He was scared, and despite this good advice from Wayne, he decided to go through with the operation to make sure that if he had cancer, they would catch it in time and treat it successfully, as he believed.

On Wednesday morning, Elizabeth accompanied James to the hospital. When he was called into the nurse's triage, Elizabeth was told that she couldn't go inside with him, and she had to stay in the waiting room. Doctor Manypewlatar was there because he had already been notified that James was in the hospital. After the nurse finished with James, the doctor brought him into Doctor Butchar's office. Once they arrived, James was given a number of papers that he had to sign. On the papers, Doctor Butchar covered himself and the hospital against anything that could possibly go wrong, even if the doctors caused it. If Sam died during the operation, the hospital would say that he died of complications. From there, after a massive dose of rigmarole from Doctor Butchar and Doctor Manypewlatar, James was put on a gurney and wheeled away by both Doctors into the operating room for immediate surgery.

A short while later, when they placed James on the operating table, they anesthetized him almost immediately. They then made a mark on him with an ink marker from his left thigh all the way up to the right side of his neck – that was where the incision would be made. They then cut him open and proceeded with the operation.

A while after James was wheeled away, a young and attractive woman walked into the main lobby, and the guard at the door asked, "What is your business here, Miss?"

"My name is Betty Whilling, and I came here to see if this hospital needs a receptionist."

"No," said Curtis Hewgegaard, "they don't, because they told me this morning to tell anyone looking for any kind of clerical work to tell them that there aren't any openings." Betty walked out without either one saying another word.

While Elizabeth waited in the waiting room, a man with a beard approached her and said, "Hello, my name is Doctor Sayahagain. Are you Mrs. Syckcolun?"

"Yes, I am," Elizabeth replied.

"I couldn't help overhearing that your husband is being operated on," Doctor Sayahagain went on. "Is he suffering from anything serious?"

"They found out that he may have cancer," she answered.

"I'm sorry to hear that," said the doctor. "I didn't know what his problem was, but I heard two doctors talking while they were wheeling a patient away and saying that they were taking Mr. James Syckcolun to the operating room for immediate surgery. I happen to be a cancer specialist. When your husband gets out of the hospital, please bring him to my office so I can give him the best of care. Here's my card."

Elizabeth took the card from the doctor and said, "Thank you, Doctor, I certainly will. Are you associated with this hospital, Doctor Sayahagain?"

"No," he answered, "I came here to see a friend of mine, Doctor Butchar, but the guard at the door, Curtis Hewgegaard, told me that Doctor Butchar is very busy now, so I went upstairs and talked to other doctors that I know – that's when I learned about Mr. Syckcolun. Coincidentally, one of the doctors who were wheeling your husband away was Doctor Butchar, but I didn't want to disturb him, and he didn't even see me there." Right after he said that, the doctor walked away.

Shortly after that, a seemingly middle-aged woman went to the information desk and spoke with the receptionist. She then took a seat next to Elizabeth who looked at her and said, "Hi, my name is Elizabeth Syckcolun, and I'm here because my husband, James, is being operated on right now. Do you have a family member here in this hospital, Miss?"

"No," the woman replied, "My name is Anna Lyphesayvar, and I came here to see if they have any openings for a job in the hospital's cafeteria because I have three children to support, and I need a job." Anna and Elizabeth continued talking for a while until Anna was called by the receptionist to tell her that they didn't have any openings. As she stood up to leave the hospital, Anna said, "I think there's a psychiatric hospital not too far from here – I'll go there and try to get a job."

As soon as Anna walked out, a man sat next to Elizabeth and said, "Hi, my name is Reverend Stoomaykar. I overheard you talking to that lady who just walked out. I'm sorry to hear that your husband is being operated on. If you need some honest prayers, come to my congregation. Here's my card."

Elizabeth took his card and said, "Thank you. My name is Elizabeth Syckcolun. Are you on religious business here at this time, Reverend?"

"No," he replied, "I came here because I met a fellow by the name of Peter Emppostar the other day at a diner, and he told me that he has seen a lot of old people coming in and out of this hospital. I want to talk to the director of the hospital about a proposition that I have, and…."

"Excuse me," Doctor Manypewlatar interrupted as he approached them, "are you Reverend Stoomaykar?"

"Yes I am," the minister answered.

"I am here to bring you to Doctor Butchar," said the doctor.

"Yes, okay," said the reverend. "Mrs. Syckcolun, don't forget to give me a call, because I want you to become a member of my congregation."

"Okay," Elizabeth replied as the reverend and the doctor started walking away.

When Reverend Stoomaykar and Doctor Manypewlatar arrived at Doctor Butchar's office, Doctor Butchar had already completed his part of James' operation, and was there alone. They talked for a few minutes, and then Doctor Butchar sent for Doctor Oargandeelar. In a few minutes, after Doctor Oargandeelar arrived, the three doctors started talking with the reverend. After a while, they ended the conversation, and Reverend Stoomaykar left with a big smile on his face. From there, Doctor Manypewlatar went back to the operating room to finish with James Syckcolun.

About an hour later, a young doctor named Doctor Guddok entered the hospital to apply for a job as a general practitioner. After his interview, Doctor Butchar wasn't happy with what he heard from Doctor Guddok, so he dismissed him. The young doctor wasn't happy either with what he heard from Doctor Butchar, so if he had been offered a job there, he wouldn't have accepted it. Doctor Guddok then went to a local hospital called Gud Hospital and was hired on the spot by Doctor Honnastt, the head physician.

Four hours later, back at Kuttemopen Hospital, Doctor Manypewlatar personally went to the waiting room to talk to Elizabeth. When he arrived, he saw her sitting in a chair next to a window. "Mrs. Syckcolun," he said, "I personally assisted Doctor Butchar and other doctors as they operated on your husband. The operation was a success, and your husband is a very lucky man because we were able to…"

Elizabeth abruptly interrupted the doctor and said, "Oh, thank God! I'm glad to hear that, Doctor Manypewlatar."

"Please, let me finish, Mrs. Syckcolun," said the doctor. "I was saying that he's a very lucky man because we were able to salvage his left kidney, his heart and his lungs, but we had to remove his right kidney, his entire colon, half of his small intestine, his prostate and three quarters of his stomach. While we were at it, we also removed his scalp and his right ear, just to make sure, in case they were also infected."

Elizabeth started crying after hearing the bad news, and after a few minutes, she finally managed to speak between sobs. "Oh my God!" she said in a loud voice. "Was it that bad, Doctor?"

"Well, we caught it in time," Doctor Manypewlatar answered, "and we had to make sure that it wouldn't spread. Can you imagine what would have happened if it had spread to other parts of his body?"

"Yes, but I can only imagine, and I wouldn't know what would have happened for sure," Elizabeth replied.

"Mrs. Syckcolun," the doctor continued, "I don't think your husband will be ready for you to see him before visiting hours are over – you can come back tomorrow to see him. Okay, Mrs. Syckcolun, I have to go back to the operating room now. Bye."

"Bye, Doctor Manypewlatar, and thank you for everything," Elizabeth concluded.

After the operation, it took James several hours to come to. He was in horrible pain all over his body. Elizabeth wasn't allowed to see him because visiting hours were over, as Doctor Manypewlatar had told her, so she went home.

The following day, during visiting hours, Elizabeth went back to the hospital to see James. When she entered his room, she saw that he was a total mess – he had a bandage covering his entire head, except his face and his left ear. He was hardly able to move, and his speech was slurred. Elizabeth started crying when she saw him, and they weren't able to start a conversation due to his condition. Instead, Elizabeth cried while she was there. After visiting hours were over, she went home again.

Several days passed, and by then, James was able to talk, but he was still in terrible pain. They were getting ready to discharge him so he could begin his convalescence at home. Early one morning, Elizabeth returned to the hospital during visiting hours. The doctors and nurses at the hospital briefed James and Elizabeth – they were thoroughly informed as far as what they were to expect in the days that followed. They were also told what they had to do at home during James' convalescence. The hospital also assigned a nurse to provide nursing care for James at his home. That same day, the hospital presented James with a whopping bill of $587,578.03. After Elizabeth paid the bill, James was finally discharged, but he was hardly able to stand up because his pain was too severe. They had to put him in a wheelchair to take him home.

As soon as James was brought home, he was put in bed because he was in agonizing pain all over his body – he was and felt useless. A strong and robust man was reduced to a frail and cadaverous-looking man.

Meanwhile, shortly after Doctor Guddok started working at Gud Hospital, he learned that Doctor Honnastt was probably the best doctor that he had ever met. He also learned that her top MRI technician was Joe Besttek, and he was the best at reading MRI reports – if there was anything abnormal, he would surely find it. During his numerous conversations with doctors and other hospital employees, Doctor Guddok heard that Kuttemopen Hospital didn't have a good reputation. He was then even more relieved that he wasn't offered a job when he went there for an interview.

As the days and weeks passed, James' condition worsened, and he was making almost daily trips back and forth to the hospital. His medical bills were piling up. On the sixth week after James' operation, Elizabeth received another bill from the hospital for an additional $317,411.81 for services provided during his frequent visits to the emergency room, plus the visiting nurse.

One day, on the fifty sixth day after the operation, James was taken to the hospital because he was having difficulty breathing. He was admitted because his condition wasn't improving. Elizabeth was told to wait in the waiting room. Later that same day, James expired. He lived totally incapacitated and in terrible pain ever since the day that he was cut open.

If James had only listened to his friend, Wayne! A second opinion probably would have saved his life, but of course, the second opinion doctor should have been totally disassociated with Kuttemopen Hospital, and have known absolutely nothing about the first opinion.

Shortly after James passed away, Doctor Oargandeelar went to the waiting room to talk to Elizabeth. Since he was a man of low stature, and lacked self esteem when he was around strangers, he approached her very timidly. "Mrs. Syckcolun," he said while he trembled, "I am Doctor Oargandeelar. I'm sorry to have to inform you that your husband has passed away."

Elizabeth instantly burst into a loud and uncontrollable cry, accompanied by heavy tears. After a few minutes, she finally spoke to the doctor. "Oh my God!" she said. "What should I do now Doctor Oargandeelar?"

The doctor knew exactly what he wanted Elizabeth to do, but he needed assistance because of his lack of courage. "Let me go get another doctor to help you with your misery, Mrs. Syckcolun," he replied. "I'll be right back." A few minutes later, Doctor Oargandeelar returned with an assistant and approached Elizabeth. "Mrs. Syckcolun," he said, "I think that you have already met him, but this is Doctor Manypewlatar, and he will assist you during this critical time in your life."

"Yes, I did meet him," she replied, "and thank you for bringing him here, if he's going to help me."

The conniver, Doctor Manypewlatar, then started his manipulation to convince Elizabeth to do what Doctor Oargandeelar wanted her to do. Doctor Manypewlatar was also a man of low stature, but he had plenty of courage, determination and a great ability to manipulate people. He put his hand on her shoulder and said, "Mrs. Syckcolun, it is always my recommendation that when a loved one goes to the world beyond, his next of kin should have him as close to her heart as possible. Therefore, I strongly suggest that you have his body cremated so that you can have James with you forever, instead of discarding him into the cruel and merciless ground. It is also a much cheaper and easier way to handle the matter."

Elizabeth was immediately convinced that the doctor was right, based on the mention of James' body being discarded into the cruel and merciless ground. "Yes, Doctor Manypewlatar," she replied, "I agree with you, but how do I go about cremating James?"

"Okay, if you don't know anyone, then we can help you with that," Doctor Manypewlatar replied. "Do you have a cremator, Mrs.

Syckcolun?" Of course, Doctor Manypewlatar knew very well that Elizabeth didn't have a cremator – who in the world has a cremator?

Elizabeth foolishly fell into the trap and said, "No, I don't have a cremator. Would you please help me with that?"

Doctor Manypewlatar heard exactly what he wanted to hear, but he pretended that it was a burden for him. "Okay," he lied, "we don't really want to get involved, but, because you're so desperate, we'll make an exception this time, and we will help you."

"Oh, thank you, I appreciate your help tremendously," said Elizabeth. She then went home, leaving everything up to Doctor Oargandeelar and Doctor Manypewlatar.

A few days later, Doctor Oargandeelar phoned Elizabeth. He told her to go to the hospital and pick up an urn containing James' ashes. Elizabeth took the urn home and placed it on her mantelpiece. She was happy that she had James' remains there with her – or at least she thought that she had James' remains. The following day, Elizabeth invited her friends and relatives over to her house to conduct a symbolic wake and funeral for James. That same day, Elizabeth received a final bill for an additional $279,203.67 for nursing services rendered at home, James' last day in the hospital and the cremation of his body.

After what happened to James, Elizabeth was afraid to even go to the doctor. However, as time passed, her fear had almost totally disappeared, and she continued getting her examinations at Kuttemopen Hospital, but only annually, instead of semi-annually.

One day, a week after her annual physical exam, Elizabeth was at home having breakfast alone. She saw the mailman delivering the mail. She stopped her breakfast for a moment to go outside and get it. Again, she saw a letter from Doctor Manypewlatar at Kuttemopen Hospital. A few minutes later, Elizabeth was back at the table finishing her breakfast. She nervously opened Doctor Manypewlatar's letter and read it, "Mrs. Syckcolun, your test results came back from our laboratory. I'm sorry to inform you that they revealed that you have colon cancer. It is very advanced and it has spread to other parts of your body. It is our sincere recommendation that you call us right away to make an emergency appointment for surgery so we can save your life."

Elizabeth was totally devastated when she read the letter – she went through one cancer calamity already, and then she received such horrible news. She really didn't know what to do from fear of what had happened to her husband, James. Even though he was getting semi-annual checkups, and they caught his cancer in time, he still died. What's more, he died in terrible pain, and was unable to do anything at all following his operation. Not to mention that their life savings were almost depleted. Elizabeth didn't jump from her chair to make that phone call to the hospital. Instead, she consulted everyone that she knew and told them what happened – as in James' case, she was hearing positive and negative feedback from several people. Elizabeth then remembered that she met a doctor named Doctor Sayahagain in the waiting room at Kuttemopen Hospital, and he told her that he was a cancer specialist. She was going to go to his office for treatment, but then she decided to wait a while before going.

Several days passed, and she was still feeling fine and had no pain whatsoever. She hadn't even called the hospital yet. Then one day, late in the afternoon, Elizabeth was sitting at her kitchen table, having dinner, when she started thinking, almost out loud, "Why should I go to the hospital to get an operation, and then be in terrible pain like James was? He died anyway, and the same thing could happen to me if I'm operated on. No! I'm not going. Let the cancer eat me if it wants to, but I'm not going through what James went through. Besides, I don't have enough money to pay for an operation after they ripped us off so badly during James' ordeal."

Several months passed, and Elizabeth was still feeling fine. She hadn't called the hospital yet because she still didn't feel any pain, so she made a final decision not to go at all. She also made a decision not to go see Doctor Sayahagain either. She was determined to stop getting her annual checkups – after all, she had already lived much longer than James did after he was diagnosed with cancer. Besides, she hadn't suffered from physical or financial pain. She concluded that if the cancer wanted to take her life, let it be. Elizabeth even started thinking that maybe she didn't have cancer at all.

Eventually, Elizabeth's fear had almost totally disappeared, and she decided to continue getting her semi-annual examinations, but she decided never to contact Kuttemopen Hospital ever again. Instead, she decided to go to a local doctor. Her new doctor told her that she was in perfectly good health. She was so happy to hear the good news that she practically forgot about her ordeal regarding Kuttemopen Hospital.

The Quest for the Cure

BASED ON THE RAPIDLY growing number of people supposedly dying of cancer every year, the government decided to do something about it – it offered grants to anyone who had the right qualifications and was willing to do research to find the cure for cancer.

One day, five doctors, Doctor Dredfall, Doctor Krooll, Doctor Malishuss, Doctor Theeph and Doctor Wykkedd, walked into the main lobby at Kuttemopen Hospital. After a few minutes of talking to Curtis Hewgegaard, they were escorted to Doctor Butchar's office. When they arrived, they told Doctor Butchar that they had just graduated from medical school and were cancer specialists. They wanted to apply to work there, but Doctor Butchar didn't trust them and dismissed them after a short interview. They left the hospital and decided to try elsewhere, but they wanted to stay together as a team. Shortly after they failed to get jobs at Kuttemopen Hospital, they heard about the government grant program and decided to participate in it. They arranged a meeting with a government agent named Wallace Koropted to discuss the necessary requirements to begin doing cancer research. When they finally met Wallace, after listening to him for a few minutes, Doctor Dredfall realized that Wallace was a sleazy character and probably easily persuaded to cooperate with them if they compensated him financially.

After a few days, they completed the submission of all the paperwork that was required. They were soon awarded with a grant of $20,000,000 to begin their work. They put themselves on the payroll immediately with a starting salary of $500,000 annually each. The day after they had the money in the bank, they decided to get together at a local eatery called "Gudphood Diner" to start planning their venture. Gudphood Diner was located across the road from a major hospital. Although it was called a diner, it was a full-service restaurant and very spacious. It was a single-story building with a very large parking lot. The lot was surrounded by a tall fence with rose bushes all along it. When the five doctors arrived at the diner, they went into a private booth. Doctor Dredfall was the shortest and the loudest of all five. What he lacked in height, he made up for in self confidence. He was the unofficial and self-appointed leader of the group. "Now that we have the grant money in the bank," he began, "and we're giving ourselves weekly paychecks, we don't have to rush into finding a place to start working right away. We have $20,000,000 in the bank. Even if we don't get any more grant money, we can pay ourselves the same salary for eight years – maybe nine years with the interest – so why rush?"

"True," Doctor Theeph agreed, "but we have to report to them quarterly, and we have to make it look good."

"Well, yes, that's true," Doctor Krooll also agreed. "You're both right. Anyway, our kids just started their summer vacation, so now is the perfect time to go away. Let's go to The Bahamas and take a vacation and call it a 'Research Trip.' We'll bring our entire families and use grant money to pay for the trip. We can have a great time there."

"That sounds great!" Doctor Malishuss added. "I agree with all of you. We can stay in The Bahamas almost three months and come back just before it's time to report to the government, which is about the same time that our children have to go back to school. When we return, we can tell them at the government that we made a lot of progress while on the research trip. If they ask us what the progress was, we can tell them that we found out why the red-dotted ladybugs of The Bahamas don't get sick, but we have to go back and do more research on them to see if we can come up with the cure for cancer. This way, we can leave the doors open to take another wonderful government-paid vacation in The Bahamas at a later time."

Doctor Wykkedd was the complete opposite of Doctor Dredfall. He was not only the tallest, but he also lacked self confidence, so it took him a while to finally pitch in and contribute to the conversation, "Is there such a thing as a red-dotted ladybug of The Bahamas? If so, is it true that it doesn't get sick?"

"I don't know if there's such a thing," Doctor Malishuss replied, "but I doubt it – I just made it up, but who cares? Neither the government nor the public will know the difference anyway."

"I totally agree with everyone," Doctor Wykkedd added, "so let's go to The Bahamas – what are we waiting for?"

Following their mutual agreement, they went home. Later that same day, Doctor Dredfall phoned Wallace Koropted to tell him to alert the media. After that, everyone packed their bags and went to Paradise, as the doctors called it, to spend a glorious time there at the expense of the hard-working taxpayers. Of course, Uncle Sam didn't know what the doctors were up to. As soon as they left, Wallace told the media that five medical giants went on a trip to The Bahamas because they were on the verge of finding the cure for cancer. The media gobbled up the story and anxiously waited for their return.

The doctors and their families finally arrived at the place they called "Paradise." They had absolutely no worries of any kind. They spent money as if there were no end to it. Every cent that they spent was entered into the records as a research expense.

Some major news networks even sent reporters to The Bahamas to get ahead of the others and find out as much as they could about the cancer research. Since the doctors were only there to have a good time, no one was able to find them because there was no evidence of anyone doing any research. The reporters then concluded that the doctors were incognito to safeguard their findings, so they abandoned their quest and returned home.

After nearly three months, the doctors eventually got bored and tired of spending money. It was almost time to report to the government, and for their children to return to school, so they packed their bags and flew back home.

As soon as they returned, the five doctors were surrounded by reporters everywhere they went. They were plastered all over the media as giants who were about to discover the coveted cure for cancer. They reported to the government grant program administrators, under the leadership of Wallace Koropted, and told them exactly the story that they had planned to tell them. They also presented the government with a whopping expense bill of $1,653,578.03, which was deducted from the grant money that they had already received.

When the doctors saw the attention that they were getting, they took the opportunity to apply for additional funds from the grant program. They told the administrators that because they were so close to finding the cure, they needed to improve their plans by opening a much larger and better research center than they had originally planned to open. Within days, they received an additional $20,000,000. With that extra money, they still had over $38,000,000 after they deducted the trip expenses plus their weekly salaries. Immediately after receiving the money, they increased their salaries to $600,000 annually each. From that day on, the doctors started creating a special relationship with Wallace Koropted.

The five doctors eventually started talking about making up a name for their cancer research facility. During one of their many meetings at Gudphood Diner, Doctor Dredfall came up with a name and suggested it to the others. "Hey!" he said. "I've got an idea for the name of our research facility – let's call it 'Ghetrychkwik Cancer Research Center.' What do you guys think about this name?" The other four doctors had no objections and went along with this name.

Shortly after the name was registered, donations in the millions started pouring in from all over the world into a Post Office Box address that they had to use until they found a location for their center. The doctors then took a few weeks off, but stayed in town. After a while, they decided that it was time to really begin working, because they were getting bored, so they started searching for a good location to set up their operation. They had to submit quarterly reports to the government, and the next two documents that they submitted, three months apart, were the same – that they were still looking for an ideal location.

A few weeks later they finally found that ideal location for their operation. They purchased a commercial building for a whopping $12,000,000. Their grant funds were getting somewhat low, and they still had to renovate the building and buy all the necessary research equipment, so they presented a proposal to the government. Upon approval, they asked for an additional $30,000,000. A few days later, they had the money in the bank. The first thing that they did was to buy themselves brand new and expensive automobiles because they figured that their vehicles would be business expenses, so why not use grant money? They went a step further – they also bought similar automobiles for all the adult members of their families – they deemed those vehicles to be business expenses also because their families often delivered lunch and personal mail to them. They really had found an easy way to rip off Uncle Sam.

As time passed, and several quarterly reports later, they finally had the facility ready. They started working immediately. Ghetrychkwik Cancer Research Center was then in full operation. The five doctors were honestly trying to find the cure for cancer. They knew that they had a long road ahead of them because after all, others had tried it before and no one had found it yet, or at least, if they did find it, it was kept a secret.

Government inspectors frequented the center and were pleased with the way that the research center was set up. They were also pleased with the activities that they saw. The center was superbly equipped and staffed, and the Government inspectors found the facility to be operating in good faith. The five doctors were very busy and actively engaged in honest and legitimate cancer research. Their funds weren't getting low yet, but they felt that they had to really try to accomplish something in order to continue receiving funds from the grant program, as well as donations from the public. At the facility, they tried their experiments on everything that they could think of, but they still weren't anywhere even near finding the cure. They tried testing on every kind of animal possible, including fish and insects, but after several months of tests, they still didn't have the cure.

One day, Doctor Theeph was at his work table working very hard when he took a moment off to talk to the others. "Wow!" he said. "We have tried everything, and we still have nothing to show for all the hard work that we have done. There must be something that we haven't tried that will do it for us."

"I agree," said Doctor Krooll, "but what is it?"

"We've tried just about everything," Doctor Malishuss added, "and we don't have it yet. I hate to say it, but I wonder if we should just give up! I really can't think of anything else."

"Wait a minute," Doctor Wykkedd disagreed, "first of all, we can't give up. Secondly, I've got an idea – we haven't tried insects from other countries – wouldn't it be ironic if we go back to The Bahamas and try the red-dotted ladybug, if there is such a thing, and it works?"

After hearing what Doctor Wykkedd said, Doctor Dredfall came up with another great money-spending. He suggested it to the other four doctors, "You know, that sounds like a great idea – not the part about trying the ladybug, but the part about taking a vacation again – we need it because we have been working nonstop for a long time. Besides, now is a good time to go because our children just started their Christmas vacation today."

"Well," Doctor Theeph added, "I think that if we do go back to The Bahamas, we might as well try the bug anyway – of course, that's providing that there is such a thing as a red-dotted ladybug. If so, we can bring samples back to the center and do experiments on the animals with the bugs."

Following that, they all agreed and told everyone else in the center to go home and stay away from the facility until the doctors notified them to return to work – the five doctors were able to tell everyone else to stay home because the doctors were the only ones who conducted all the experiments in the facility. They didn't have any other doctors employed by the center, and all their employees would have nothing to do while the doctors were gone. Thus, Ghetrychkwik Cancer Research Center was completely idle every time that the doctors were away from it. Of course the employees loved it when the doctors went away because they continued getting a weekly paycheck even though they didn't work. The doctors always gave their accountant a very generous bonus for having to work by issuing weekly checks to all the employees when the doctors were away. After the doctors told their employees to go home and not to return until they told them to, they left the center to go home as well. When the doctors got home, they told their families their plan, and everyone packed their bags again and left the following morning.

Late in the afternoon, they arrived at their hotel and booked several rooms – of course, the grant money covered their expenses. They made themselves comfortable and started their money-spending vacation at taxpayers' expense once again. That same evening, they hired several limousines on a full-time basis with private chauffeurs to take them everywhere they went during their entire stay. Later on, they indulged themselves to the best food and shows in town. The next day, they had breakfast brought to their rooms. After breakfast, they went on a luxurious boat ride that lasted until sunset. The following day, they spent most of the day on the beach. Day after day, they were having a wonderful vacation that only the elite could afford – of course they weren't paying for it out of their own pockets because Uncle Sam was paying for all of it.

Eventually, it was almost time for the children to return to school. Everyone wanted to stay longer because they were having a great time, but they had no choice but to leave soon. Before leaving, the five doctors had a meeting and decided to collect some of the red-dotted ladybugs. The doctors hired some local people and told them to go into the woods to collect plenty of red-dotted ladybugs for them. The local people didn't ask the doctors any questions – it was then that the doctors thought that maybe there was such a thing as a red-dotted ladybug. Later that afternoon, the bug collectors returned with a basket filled with plenty of what everyone thought were red-dotted ladybugs. The basket was lined with a sheet. The sheet was tied with a knot on top. The doctors didn't even bother to look inside of the sheet to see if the bugs had red dots. They didn't even know whether they were ladybugs or not. For that matter, they didn't even know if the sheet contained bugs at all – they didn't care.

After paying the locals for collecting the bugs, the doctors started planning their return trip. Before leaving, they had to obtain special environmental permission to transport the bugs to their research center – with Uncle Sam's money, anything was possible. The bugs had to be placed in a sealed metal box in order for the permits to be issued. The following morning, right after breakfast, they left their hotel and went to the airport. Later on, early in the afternoon, they boarded a plane and flew back home.

As soon as the doctors arrived at the airport, the media swarmed around them to get as much information as they could about them regarding their research trip, because the whole world had been waiting for that coveted cancer cure. Doctor Dredfall had no choice but to make a short speech. He stood on top of a large suitcase and said, "At this time, we don't have anything that we can tell you, except that we have made a tremendous amount of progress, and we will tell you more in the days to come." With this speech, the media concluded that the doctors had made progress in finding the cure for cancer. As soon as the doctors had a chance, they went back to the center to leave the box containing the bugs there for future experiments. When they entered the center, they noticed a strong smell of rotting flesh all over the facility, but they ignored it and left the box of bugs on a lab table.

During the next several days, there were many headlines all over most of the major publications throughout the world. Here are some examples of the many headlines that were seen by hundreds of millions:

"Hope for Cancer Patients."

"Cancer Cure Almost Found."

"Cancer Deaths Soon to Become a Thing of the Past."

"Medical Giants About to Find the Cure for Cancer."

"Cancer Patients Will End Suffering and Enjoy Healthy Lives."

There were many more, but too numerous to mention here. With such hopeful headlines all over the world, the doctors were receiving millions of letters from people of all walks of life. Here are some passages in the letters that the doctors were happy to read:

"Please, hurry up. My little girl doesn't have long to live if you don't find the cure soon."

"I don't need the cure at this time, but you'll never know when I'll need it. Please find it fast."

"My daddy died of cancer the other day. Please hurry up with the cure so we can bring him back."

"You guys are doing a great job. Keep up the good work."

"You doctors are angels. Please don't give up."

"We had been waiting for a miracle. You have been sent by God to deliver that miracle to us. Thank you."

There were thousands of letters that the doctors enjoyed reading, but in spite of all the positive feedback from thousands, the doctors were also receiving letters containing plenty of negative reactions from many others. Here are some passages in the letters that the doctors didn't like to see:

"You guys better stop what you're doing, or else I'll make you stop."

"If you find the cure, you won't live to enjoy it."

"Leave well-enough alone, or else you'll regret it."

"I'm a cancer specialist. If you guys find the cure, I'll be out of business. Stop your research right now, or else I'll sue you."

"I've had it with you guys. Many of my cancer patients have stopped coming to my clinic for their treatment because they decided to wait for the cure. Don't find it, or I'll do something that you will definitely regret."

The number of letters that the doctors didn't like to read was in the thousands. After receiving several death threats, the doctors hired numerous body guards for themselves, as well as all the members of their families – of course, the body guards were paid with Uncle Sam's money. With such an overwhelming amount of correspondence, the doctors had to set up a new department in the research center to handle the volume. They had to hire several new people to staff the newly created department to work exclusively on the massive amount of correspondence that they received on a daily basis – Uncle Sam picked up the tab for that also.

With such a huge amount of attention, the doctors applied for additional funds from the grant program. Within days, they were awarded with an additional $40,000,000. The first thing that they did was to give themselves another raise. Donations were still pouring in from all over the world into Ghetrychkwik Cancer Research Center. After the doctors returned from their second trip to The Bahamas, the donations were pouring in much more rapidly. Most of the donations were received by check, but a great amount was also received in cash. The five doctors running the center had several safety deposit boxes, and they were renting more and more boxes as the donations kept pouring in. The doctors made almost daily trips to the bank, carrying full brown paper bags. They entered the bank and went into the safety deposit box rooms. When they came out of the bank, they were carrying empty brown paper bags – we can only wonder what was in those paper bags when they were full! We can also wonder where the contents came from!

Several weeks after they returned, the doctors decided to go back to work. The first thing they did was to inform all their employees to return to the center the following Monday at eight in the morning. By that time, the bugs had died, rotted and were covered with mold. Even though the box containing the bugs was sealed, the stench was all over the facility – not only from the dead bugs, but also from all the animals that were left in the center, which had died from starvation. When the doctors arrived, before anyone else was there, they turned on the ventilation system, but it wasn't enough to clear the air, so they had to open all the windows and doors and go outside until the stench was somewhat tolerable.

After a while, everyone had arrived at the center, but no one was able to go inside due to the horrible smell. One of their employees suggested hiring some day laborers to dispose of all the dead animals. Doctor Dredfall gave him a bonus and told him to go ahead and handle the hiring and supervise the entire matter. After the day laborers got rid of all the dead animals, it was safe to go back in, and the doctors started their day on the job by once again making honest efforts into finding the cure for cancer. Later that day, they bought a variety of laboratory animals to replace the ones that had died. The doctors finally opened the box containing the bugs, and untied the knot on the sheet. They immediately smelled a very strong stench coming from the dead bugs. They looked at the bugs for the first time, but they didn't see any red dots on them – actually, they were so moldy that they were fuzzy and brownish in color, and the doctors couldn't tell if they were ladybugs. They took the moldy bugs and extracted a murky and smelly juice out of them. They took the juice and started experimenting with it.

As the days passed, the doctors made several futile attempts to kill cancer cells from infected mice by injecting bug juice into them. They also made equally futile attempts to kill cancer cells from all the other infected animals.

Sometime later, the doctors were almost on the verge of giving up on the red-dotted ladybug juice idea. By that time the media attention was winding down, causing donations to decrease, but they were still coming in by the millions of dollars every month.

After several days of getting nowhere, the five doctors got together at a conference table at the facility to try to come up with a plan while they had their lunch. Doctor Dredfall began the conversation by talking about making more money, "We have to come up with another idea to boost our donations by letting the media know that we're up to something."

The other four doctors agreed, and Doctor Wykkedd said that he had to go to the men's room. He stepped away from the table, but instead of going to the bathroom, he headed towards the main laboratory. When he got to one of the experiment rooms, he started filling a cup with some of the bug juice. He had the intention of bringing it back to the conference table to play a joke on the rest of the doctors. As he continued filling the cup, he accidentally spilled some of the bug juice on several of the animals in the cages. He then left the room to return to the table. In a few minutes, Doctor Wykkedd sat at the table again and proceeded with his joke, "I have some delicious bug juice here in this cup. I'm going to drink it with my lunch, but I'll put some sugar in it before I drink it." He then put two spoonfuls of sugar into the cup containing the bug juice.

As Doctor Wykkedd was stirring his ladybug juice, Doctor Dredfall said, "If you drink that sweetened bug juice, you'll get cancer for sure – there's no doubt in my mind. Then we'll definitely have to find the cure right away." After that, they all started laughing, and the discussions continued.

Several minutes passed as they were talking and eating at the same time. All of a sudden, the sweetened bug juice started foaming and overflowing out of the cup. Doctor Theeph looked at it and said in a very loud voice, "Oh my God! Look at that bug juice go!"

"Hey," said Doctor Krooll, "it looks like some chemical reaction took place with the sugar."

"Yeah, we should try it now," Doctor Malishuss added.

"Try to drink it?" Doctor Wykkedd asked. "No way, not me! If you want to drink it, you go ahead and do it, but not me!"

Doctor Malishuss then went on, "No, I didn't mean that we should try to drink it – I meant that we should try it for our research." They all agreed that Doctor Malishuss was right, and they should try it – after all, they had tried hundreds of different things, so why not try one more thing?

Shortly after that, they finished their lunch and headed back to the main laboratory. When they got back, they noticed that many of the animals had died of cancer. They also noticed that some of the animals, dead or alive, had lost a great deal of hair on several spots on their bodies. Doctor Wykkedd then realized why some animals lost some hair. "Wow, look at all those bald spots on some of those critters!" he exclaimed. "Some bug juice accidentally spilled all over the cages and on some of the animals when I came here before to get some juice to play a joke on you guys."

After the doctors realized what happened, they conducted numerous tests on the live animals that had lost some of their hair, and they found out that the animals had absolutely no side effects, other than the loss of hair. The doctors further realized that they had come up with a formula that removed hair permanently, because there were no signs of any possibility of the hair ever growing back on the bald spots. It was a formula far better and more effective than any other in existence. It was definitely a very simple formula because it only had one ingredient – red-dotted ladybug juice, or so they thought. They dropped everything and decided to make their findings public in an effort to increase the flow of donations. They told the media that they had inadvertently found a hair-removing drug while experimenting with animals to try to find the cure for cancer – it was the absolute truth for a change, and probably the first and only thing that they had ever said that was true. However, they didn't tell anyone what the formula was, but they did say that it contained hundreds of different ingredients. They also told the media that the ratio of each ingredient was the key to the formula.

Over the next few weeks, the doctors had achieved their goal – donations were pouring in faster than ever. The most important thing was that they had bought additional time. Following the attention that the doctors were getting after discovering that ladybug juice removed hair, they applied for additional grant money. Within days, they had the money in the bank – of course, they gave themselves another big raise. By that time, it was Easter vacation for their children, so it was a good time to get away again. They told everyone at the center to stay home again until they were told to return to work. They thought that it was time for another Bahamas vacation. They then packed their bags. As they were leaving, they told the media that they were going back to The Bahamas for additional work on their cancer research.

When they arrived at their destination, the doctors had no worries about doing any work, and they had no intention of doing any research whatsoever because they were under no pressure that time. After spending plenty of money, the doctors had the most wonderful time ever, but they couldn't stay any longer because Easter vacation was almost over, and their kids had to go back to school in two days, so they decided to go home.

When the doctors returned, the media surrounded them again because they were expecting another miracle. The doctors told the media that they had made additional progress, but they needed more time to experiment before making any statements. The doctors were still under no pressure after finding the hair-removing formula – it was such a huge discovery, that the media focused their attention on the formula, and the cancer cure quest was put on hold for the time being. By that time, they had established an even closer relationship with the government grant program Head Administrator, Wallace Koropted. He made sure that the government inspections on the research center were stopped, thus, giving the doctors more freedom to do what they wanted. Wallace also made it unnecessary for the doctors to submit quarterly reports. Wallace was also making frequent trips to different banks with brown paper bags filled with something – the doctors seemed to have found a way to make sure that the grant program kept giving them money for a very long time.

After a few weeks of loafing around, the doctors decided that it was time to go back to their research. They decided to continue experimenting with the bug juice after they discovered that sugar caused it to bubble. They told everyone to go back to the center to begin working. When they returned to the center, the bug juice had an absolutely putrid stench, and there was a horrible smell all over the facility – again, not only from the rotten bug juice, but also from all the animals that were left in the center, which had died from starvation. The smell was so strong, that the ventilation system didn't help at all, so they had to open all the windows and doors again, but that time, they had to leave them open for an entire day before anyone could even go inside. At the end of the day, they closed the doors, but they left the ventilating system on and the windows open.

They following day, the smell was almost totally gone, but they had to hire some more day laborers to dispose of all the dead animals again. They also had to order more laboratory animals. They then continued their research and infected several animals with cancer again. Many of the animals died on a daily basis. After several of the infected animals were injected with sweetened bug juice, the doctors noticed that several days had passed without one single death among the animals that they treated. They were astonished with the possibility that they had finally found the cure for cancer. They decided to investigate further.

After conducting several tests on the infected animals that they had injected with the sweetened bug juice, they found absolutely no evidence of cancer in any of them. There was also no evidence of any kind of side effects. The doctors were overwhelmed with their findings. They had finally found the coveted cure for cancer. At that point, the doctors had a good reason to celebrate because they were truly giants in the medical profession. They decided to take their experiment a step further – they had only infected the animals with colon cancer, so they had to see if their discovery was good for any other kind of cancer. Brain cancer, breast cancer, lung cancer and prostate cancer had been four major causes of death throughout the world for a long time. The doctors infected one group of animals with Brain cancer, another group with breast cancer, another group with lung cancer and a fourth group with prostate cancer. After injecting the infected animals with a single dosage of sweetened bug juice, the cancer was completely eradicated from all the groups of animals – the results were astonishing again.

After such a great achievement, they wanted to put their formula through various other tests before going public. They infected other animals with many other types of cancer. Test after test, the results were all the same – the cancer was completely eradicated from all the animals with one dose of the sweetened bug juice. When they ran out of types of cancer, they concluded that their job was done, and it was done far better than anyone had ever expected. The doctors then felt that they were ready for the media, but they decided to take a few days off before going public. They gave everyone time off as long as they themselves were away from the center.

Two weeks later, the doctors decided to get together at a very nice restaurant to discuss the situation over dinner. As soon as they arrived at the restaurant, Doctor Dredfall showed some concern about divulging their findings to the public. "You know," he began, "I'm not quite sure that we should go public. As soon as we do, the whole world will know that the cure for cancer has been found, and we'll be out of a job. Of course, we'll become very famous celebrities, but eventually the issue will be put to sleep. After a while, we'll become has-beens – that wouldn't make us any more money. Besides, when we started, we got several threats from people who don't want the cure to be found. Maybe they'll live up to the threats they made if we reveal the cure. In my opinion, it's better to continue doing what we're doing, and keep the formula a secret."

"That's very true," Doctor Theeph agreed. "I hadn't thought about that. If we do tell them, then our Bahamas vacations would have to be paid with money out of our own pockets."

"That's for sure," Doctor Krooll also agreed. "It makes no sense to report our findings. We have Wallace Koropted under control, and he'll continue giving us grant money for us to keep on running the center, even if we don't do anything else."

Doctor Malishuss also agreed, but he added a little of his own maliciousness to their scheme, "Okay, but if we don't reveal the cure, and continue operating, then we'll have to do something to make believe that we're still trying to find the cure. I think that we shouldn't be too hasty to try to make a decision right now. We should go home and think about what's best for us. Let's think about different options over the next few days." The other four doctors agreed, and they all decided to meet again in another week to continue their discussion. They concluded their conversation and left after allowing Uncle Sam to pay for their dinner as a business expense.

A week later, they met for dinner at the same restaurant. As they were waiting for their dinner, they continued their discussion. Doctor Wykkedd started the dialogue with a big dose of wickedness, "After our discussion last week, I remain even more convinced that we should keep the cure a secret. There are plenty of reasons not to reveal it – if we do, all cancer doctors would be out of business, not to mention the fact that other cancer research organizations will also be out of business. Hospitals that specialize in treating people with cancer will also suffer catastrophic financial losses. The negative impact would be tremendous."

"Yes, that's very true," Doctor Dredfall added, "but we must keep the formula for us, so we can use it for our families in case the need ever arises."

Doctor Theeph accepted Doctor Dredfall's idea, "That's right, and I think that we have come to a good conclusion. Tomorrow we can call Wallace Koropted to see if it's possible to continue receiving grant money forever without any further pressure from Uncle Sam."

"That's a great idea!" Doctor Malishuss added. "After all, Wallace is still young and has no intention of leaving such a lucrative position. As long as he continues giving us money, we can continue washing his hands – there's no reason why he shouldn't continue cooperating with us."

Doctor Krooll put his head down and said, "I just remembered something, Dredfall said that we should keep the formula for us – well, that's very true, but we're not sure that we even know the main ingredient in the formula."

"Rotten red-dotted ladybug juice," Doctor Malishuss replied, "with sugar in it."

Doctor Krooll wasn't satisfied with Doctor Malishuss' answer. "How do we know that we used red-dotted ladybugs?" he asked. "When we finally opened the box, we didn't see any red dots on them. They were moldy, fuzzy and brownish all over, and we don't even know if they were really ladybugs." All the other doctors agreed with Doctor Krooll, and they concluded that they should do something about it – they planned to return to The Bahamas and collect some more bugs to make sure.

While they were still in the restaurant, it finally occurred to Doctor Dredfall that they had to do something about the smell in the center every time they returned after being away. After a few minutes of discussions, they concluded that they would dispose of all their animals before going away, and then buy more when they returned – they figured that that would solve the stink problem permanently. They came to this conclusion not because they cared about the poor animals starving to death, but because they didn't want the smell of rotting carcasses in the facility again.

After several hours, they finished their discussion and decided to keep the cancer cure a secret. Shortly after that, as always, the doctors allowed Uncle Sam to pay for their meals, and then left the restaurant. From there, they went to the center, and called some day laborers to dispose of all the animals, whether they were dead or alive.

Shortly after that, the doctors went back to The Bahamas for a worry-free vacation. After they ended their vacation, they found some of the same locals who had collected the bugs for them before. They told them to go back into the woods and collect a few more, but to make sure that they collected the same kind again. When the locals returned with the bugs, the doctors looked at them and found out that they weren't ladybugs at all, but actually a species of stinkbugs that had some brownish dots on them. They then realized why the stench was so strong when the bugs died in the center.

When the doctors returned to the center, they didn't have to deal with the stench of rotting flesh anymore because they had found a solution to this problem before they left, and didn't leave the animals there to die. They then bought some more animals and started experimenting to make sure that they had brought back the same kind of bugs that they had used before. After numerous experiments, they were satisfied that the bugs were the same because they killed all kinds of cancer using the same method again. They had to rewrite all the entries that they had made on their secret logs and change the name from "Ladybug" to "Stinkbug." They also realized that the bug juice didn't have to be rotten to cure cancer, because they didn't wait for the bugs to even die before they started experimenting with them. Right after that, they once again decided to keep the cancer cure a secret from everyone, except Wallace Koropted, so he would be aware of it and wouldn't let anyone from the government pressure the doctors into rushing to find the cure. This way, he would continue giving them grant money, and they would continue washing his hands with cash.

Shortly after the doctors concluded their cancer research, they had to make sure that no one knew that the cure for cancer was stinkbug juice and sugar. They called a short press conference and told them that they had experimented extensively with ladybugs and found no evidence that they did any good towards curing cancer. They went a step further and told them that they tried thousands of other bug species and found the same results – that they had absolutely no medicinal value. This was to make sure that no one would try to use the stinkbug to do cancer research. Besides, the doctors thought that perhaps the stinkbug wasn't the only bug that cured cancer. Although they had tried numerous other species before they tried the stinkbug, they didn't try all bug species. Besides, they didn't sweeten the other bugs, as they had sweetened the stinkbugs.

They also had to figure out a way to keep all their employees on the payroll to make believe that they were still working on finding the cure. After numerous discussions about the situation, they decided to hire five other doctors. They carefully screened them, and made sure that they had no prior experience with cancer – this way the five bad doctors thought that the new doctors wouldn't have a chance of finding the cure. After they hired them, they told them to go to work on finding the cure for cancer. Of course, they kept their original findings a secret from the newly hired doctors. The bad doctors also told them not to try any bugs in their research because they themselves had tried them all – the real reason was that they didn't want the cure to be found. All the other employees weren't very happy about the hiring of the new doctors because it meant that they wouldn't be given time off anymore. After the new doctors started working, the five bad doctors made frequent visits to the center to make a good impression, but they very rarely stayed longer than a brief moment.

Product Studies

As TIME PASSED, THE five doctors were getting bored of doing nothing with their time. On a Sunday afternoon, shortly after arriving home from a government-paid vacation in sunny Puerto Rico, Doctor Dredfall started thinking about new ways to increase their already tremendous wealth. He phoned his colleagues to arrange a meeting to discuss the possibility of making more money, and they agreed to meet at Gudphood Diner.

Later that day, they arrived at the diner and went into one of the private booths. They ordered dinner and started talking about ways to improve the flow of donations into Ghetrychkwik Cancer Research Center. Doctor Dredfall started the conversation. "Perhaps we can conduct fake studies on anything that comes to our minds to boost people's willingness to donate big bucks to us," he suggested.

Doctor Wykkedd totally agreed, "Sure we can do that! After the great success that we've had in getting grant money from our rich uncle, and donations from unsuspecting people, they'll believe anything that we tell them."

A few minutes later, diner was served, and they continued their dishonest conversation to figure out another plan to swindle the population out of their hard-earned dollars. While they were eating, Doctor Theeph came up with the first idea and suggested doing something completely different, "Maybe we should conduct a study on the digestive system of the red ants of Madagascar. After all, we made a big killing with bugs before, so let's go look at some more bugs."

"That's funny," said Doctor Krooll as he laughed, "what do people care about that? They wouldn't send us any donations for us to study ants."

"Okay," Doctor Theeph replied, "I guess you're right, but I was thinking more about taking a government-paid vacation to Madagascar, rather than conducting any study whatsoever."

After the doctors spent several hours trying to figure out what they should do next, Doctor Malishuss came up with a great idea. "Aha!" he exclaimed. "I've got it! We'll do research on the effects of drinking coffee. At least we'll tell them that this is what we're going to do. This way, we can give ourselves a nice vacation in Colombia at Uncle Sam's expense. We can call it a research trip."

"That's a fantastic idea!" Doctor Wykkedd agreed. "I can't wait to go to Columbia. We don't even have to do anything – we'll just go there and have a wonderful time. After we return, we can tell them anything that they want to hear in order to get money out of their pockets and into our pockets." Following that, they all agreed to proceed with that plan. By then it was getting late, and the doctors decided to call it a day and return to the diner the following morning to continue their discussions over breakfast.

The day after, they returned to the diner, where they continued their despicable plan as soon as they were seated while waiting for their breakfast to be served. Doctor Dredfall had something on his mind that was bothering him. "Before we begin," he said, "I'd like to point something out – I thought of it last night as I was going to bed, and it has been bothering me ever since then – what about our cancer research?"

"We have already found the cure," Doctor Theeph answered, "and there's nothing else for us to do with that."

"Yeah," Doctor Dredfall went on, "WE know that, but THEY don't, and I'm not happy with it because this means that we still have to pretend that we're working on it."

"Don't you know that people forget very quickly and easily?" Doctor Krooll asked.

"That's right," Doctor Malishuss added, "and by the time we make our plans public, there will be nothing else said about the search for the cancer cure. As we all know, that's exactly what happens in our society – people forget about what goes on around them, and fall victims to those who are trying to rip them off – namely, us. Besides, we can still say that we're doing research on cancer anyway, as we pretend that we're conducting our product studies."

Doctor Wykkedd again agreed, "That's true, and we also know that people devour whatever they hear from the media, and when there's nothing else coming from the media, then the issue is completely forgotten. Besides, we still have those five imbecile doctors at the center trying to find the cure – which they never will. Okay, my vote is to proceed with the product studies."

"Okay," said Doctor Dredfall, "now that we have come to an understanding, I'm all for it, but I think that we can enhance our dreadful plan somewhat. I believe that we should take our coffee study a little further to make even more money. Before we make our bogus findings public, we can invest in coffee companies and coffee futures in the commodities markets. Then we'll say something great about coffee, and the price of our investments will go through the roof. We'll make sure that the media keeps talking about our phony research for a long time. Then, when we don't have anything else to say, we'll sell everything we bought and make huge profits. After that, the stock market will take care of itself, as far as coffee companies are concerned."

"I like the idea about playing the stock market," said Doctor Krooll. "After we reveal our bogus coffee study, and sell our coffee investments, we'll let some time pass. Then we'll tell them that we have to make sure that our initial findings were correct. Then we'll invest against coffee companies and against coffee commodities before we say anything else.

After we do this, we'll say something negative about coffee, and watch our investments skyrocket again when the price of coffee plummets. Then we'll sell our investments at a profit again."

"That sounds reasonable to me, so let's do it," said Doctor Wykkedd. By then, it was time to go home again, and the five doctors decided to go back to the diner in two days to continue their sinful plans. They again, very humbly, allowed Uncle Sam to pay for their dinner.

When they met again, Doctor Wykkedd started the conversation by talking about an idea that came to his mind the night before, "So far, the plan that we previously discussed sounds great. We can continue on and on by doing the same thing with other products, such as aspirin, orange juice, soybean, sugar, oil, etc. There will be no end in sight to our moneymaking scheme."

After they spent a few hours planning their scheme, they ended their discussion with a sense of satisfaction that they had accomplished their goal – which at that point was only the planning of their evil and dishonest plot. From here, they went to Ghetrychkwik Cancer Research Center to phone Wallace Koropted to ask him for additional grant funds to conduct a lengthy study on coffee. After Wallace agreed to send them more money, they phoned their stock brokers to instruct them to invest as much money in coffee as their accounts could handle.

Within days, they had the grant money in the bank without any red tape whatsoever. Doctor Dredfall looked at the center's bank account and noticed that they had a fortune in it. He then wrote five separate checks – one to each doctor – and he called them "Bonus Payments." Each check was in the tens of millions. After the checks were issued, they went to the bank and deposited the checks into their own personal accounts. Once they had that money in the bank, no one could touch it or take it away from them – it was an easy and legal way to steal money from the government, because there is no law regulating bonuses issued to employees of an organization. Each doctor then took his share of the money and invested it in coffee.

They always arranged to go away when their children had time off from school. Since summer had just started, and their kids had just finished school, they went home, packed their bags and left for Colombia.

While they were in Colombia, there wasn't a single word mentioned by anyone about doing any kind of research, let alone doing anything about conducting any study. They remained in Colombia for over two months, and after they got tired of being there, they decided to pack their bags and return home. Before leaving Colombia, they phoned Wallace again to tell him to notify the media and tell them that the doctors were returning with good news about their cancer research.

When the doctors returned, the media waited for them at the airport. As soon as they stepped out of the plain, Doctor Dredfall delivered a prepared speech, "We have found something fantastic that every coffee drinker should know, but we will not say what it is now. Instead, we can tell you to keep drinking coffee, because it's good for you. Those people who don't drink coffee should start drinking as much of it as they can and as soon as possible. We intend to return to Colombia to confirm that our findings are correct. At this point, we're only ninety nine percent sure. I'm sorry, that's all we can say right now, except, once again, drink as much coffee as you can – it's good for you. We'll tell you more about it in the near future."

The following day, they presented Uncle Sam with a whopping expense bill of $2,768,002.67 – all in the name of research. Later that day, they watched their coffee investments skyrocket, but not as much as they had anticipated. It was then that they decided to act very quickly before the media's thirst was quenched, so they called a press conference. As soon as all the members of the media arrived, Doctor Dredfall explained to them why the doctors had asked them to be there, "We made tremendous advances in our cancer research when we went to Colombia in the search for the cure. We found a very strong possibility that the answer lies somewhere in the jungles of that coffee-producing country – we believe that coffee may reveal the cure. We'll be leaving again in about a month to continue our studies. Thank you all for being here, and we'll keep you informed as we continue our efforts. Once again, keep drinking coffee, because it's good for you."

Following the press conference, the doctors watched their investments go through the roof, and they immediately called their brokers to instruct them to sell their entire interest in coffee. When their coffee investments were sold, they each made millions of dollars in profits. At the same time, the doctors told their brokers to invest against coffee.

A month later, the five doctors packed their bags once again and left their homes for another government-paid vacation to Colombia. That time, they were unable to bring all their families because their children were in school. On their way to their destination, they made several stops along the way to enjoy their vacation even further.

While in Colombia, the doctors thoroughly discussed what their next step would be. After their vacation became monotonous, they decided to return home. Before leaving, they phoned Wallace Koropted to tell him to alert the media once again. They then packed their bags for their return trip and left Colombia.

As on their first trip, when they arrived, they were swarmed by the media as soon as they exited their plane. Doctor Dredfall delivered a prepared speech to the reporters, "We have once again made tremendous progress in our research. However, we have bad news for every coffee drinker. We won't say anymore at this time, except that coffee is bad for you. Stop drinking it, because it can kill you. We'll tell you more about it in the days to come when we're absolutely sure."

The following day, they presented Uncle Sam with a whopping expense bill, but that time, it was much higher – it was over three million dollars, again, all in the name of research. Later on, they saw their investments skyrocket, because the stock plummeted, but they wanted to make another announcement before selling them.

The day after, they called another press conference, and Doctor Wykkedd delivered a rehearsed speech that Doctor Dredfall had given him, "We have made tremendous scientific advances once again, and this time, we have something bad to report to you. We told you before that the answer for the cure for cancer may have been found in coffee – well, what we discovered, after several very strenuous weeks of research, was that coffee actually causes cancer, instead of preventing it. Therefore, it is our strong recommendation that everyone in the world should stop drinking coffee immediately. We'll be leaving again very soon to continue our studies on other products to see if we can find the cure for cancer. We believe that we're on the verge of finding it. It's just a matter of time, and it won't be long before we find it – you'll see. We intend to study the effects that aspirin has on the human immune system, to see if it has anything to do with cancer – this will be our next product to study. Thank you all once again for being here. We'll keep you informed as we continue our Good-Samaritan efforts to wipe out this malignant disease. Don't forget, stop drinking coffee right away, because it can kill you."

As soon as the doctors stepped out of the spotlight, they saw their investments skyrocket even further. They phoned their stock brokers to instruct them to liquidate all their coffee investments. When everything was sold, they each made millions of dollars in profits again. Afterwards, they decided to take a rest for a while without being in the spotlight. They stayed home for some time while making frequent trips to the research center – simply to make a good impression and to make believe that they were still working.

After a few months, the doctors decided to get the ball rolling again to get the next phase of their scheme into action. They convened at the center almost every day to talk about their low-life plans. Aspirin was the next topic on their long list of bogus product studies. During one of their many meetings in the center, they decided to take another trip, but they hadn't yet chosen a destination, so they started discussing what they were going to do next, and where to go.

One day, while they met at the center, Doctor Theeph chose their next destination. "I'd like to go to Hawaii," he said, "and have a wonderful government-paid vacation on the beautiful beaches there."

Doctor Dredfall was all excited when he heard Doctor Theeph talk about going to Hawaii. "Well, in that case, there's no need to say anything else," he suggested. "Let's pack our bags and go to Hawaii, but let's not say that we're going there to do research on aspirin. Instead, let's tell them that we're going there to study coconut oil, and we can do aspirin next." The other four doctors agreed with Doctor Dredfall. It was a perfect time for them to get away because it was during their children's winter vacation. Besides, it was cold in New York, and Hawaii was very nice and warm during that time of the year, so they immediately left with their families.

They finally arrived at that wonderful paradise, as they called it, and had a worry-free and fantastic vacation for nearly two weeks. After their vacation, they had to leave Hawaii so their children could go back to school. When they returned, they did exactly as they had done with the coffee scheme, and again made huge profits in the stock market.

Following the coconut oil scheme, the doctors went to Australia to conduct their bogus aspirin study because they told the media that they found a very strong resemblance between humans and koala bears. They planned to experiment on those creatures. After aspirin, they reported doing research on numerous other products at many other paradises throughout the world. The bottom line of each bogus report was that they each made millions of dollars in profits in the stock market for each study that they claimed to have conducted – in some cases, they profited tens of millions of dollars each on a single phony study.

As time passed, the doctors had become billionaires – all in the name of research. Of course, no one else, other than the five doctors and Wallace Koropted, ever benefited in any way from the cancer research or the product studies. Uncle Sam, unsuspecting stock market investors and the general public were spending billions of dollars – all for the benefit of six people and their families.

The Abduction

ON A NICE AND sunny morning, a short distance away from where the five doctors conducted their bogus product studies, there lived a man named Peter Emppostar – he was the same man who once told Reverend Stoomaykar that he had seen a lot of old people coming in and out of Kuttemopen Hospital. Although he was originally from the West Coast, Peter lived in the same city in the state of New York. Peter was between jobs, but he had substantial savings, which kept him afloat for a long time. Since he lived alone in a one-room studio, and his expenses were very low, he wasn't worried about being unemployed at that point yet. After Peter showered, shaved and got dressed, he left his studio and went to his usual diner to have his breakfast. When he arrived, he found out that the diner was closed and being renovated to be turned into a Chinese takeout. Peter then remembered that he had been to Gudphood Diner before, but only a few times because it was farther from his home than his usual diner. He then walked the few extra blocks and went there.

As Peter entered the restaurant, he noticed a man who appeared to be a doctor because he was wearing a white robe over his clothes. The man also had a stethoscope partially protruding from his robe pocket. He was sitting at a table at the rear of the dining area eating his breakfast alone. Peter noticed a great similarity between the man and himself. Due to his natural ability to persuade people into at least hearing what he had to say, Peter decided to approach the man. He walked over to his table and said, "Good morning, Doc."

The man was surprised when he heard Peter talk to him. "Good morning, Sir, do I know you?" he asked.

"No, Doc," Peter replied, "I don't know you, and I guess you don't know me, but I simply wanted to be friendly, so here I am, and I hope I haven't offended you. If I have, please accept my apologies."

"No, it's quite all right, Sir, you haven't offended me at all," said the man.

"What's your name, Doc?" asked Peter.

"I am Doctor Ryppemuff," he answered, "and what is your name, Sir?"

"Peter Emppostar, but please call me Peter. Doc, do you mind if I sit at your table?" he asked.

"Not at all, Peter, please do," the doctor answered.

Peter took a seat and made himself comfortable. As soon as he sat, he ordered his breakfast. He was dying to continue his inquisitive conversation with the doctor. Before long, while eating, they were having a very friendly chat. "You work around here, Doc?" Peter asked.

"I'm currently practicing across the road at Deprivayshun Psychiatric Hospital," the doctor replied. "I am the Director and Head Psychiatrist there."

"Oh," Peter exclaimed, "Deprivayshun Psychiatric Hospital! That's the hospital that has a lot of crazy people inside. That's one of a few things that I know about that hospital."

"Yes, that's the one, Peter," Doctor Ryppemuff replied.

"I proofread a medical document once that was written by someone named Melissa Jernolrytar," said Peter. "I don't recall reading anything about Deprivayshun Psychiatric Hospital in the document, but I do know some things about it. Is it true, Doc, that that hospital owns thousands of acres of land right behind it?"

"Not really," the doctor answered, "only a few hundred."

"Is it true that the hospital keeps expanding endlessly?" Peter asked.

"Yes, that's quite true, Peter," Doctor Ryppemuff answered.

"Why does it keep expanding?" asked Peter.

"That's because the number of insane people in our society keeps increasing very rapidly," the doctor responded.

"Does the hospital really have thousands of wards, and they keep making new ones every day, Doc?" asked Peter.

"Well, that's an exaggeration, Peter," Doctor Ryppemuff replied. "It doesn't quite have thousands of wards yet, and they don't make new ones on a daily basis, but they do make quite a few on a yearly basis. Eventually the hospital will have thousands of wards I guess."

"Is it true that the hospital also has old people living there, Doc?" Peter asked.

"Yes, Peter," the doctor answered, "that's true. We have a senior citizens home there as well, and we have to keep expanding because the number of senior citizens keeps growing very fast."

"And these old folks live in the hospital, too?" Peter asked.

"No, Peter," the doctor replied, "the senior citizens live in a different area called 'Diebroak Senior Citizens Home,' but it's in the same building as the hospital. By the way Peter, what do you do for a living?"

"I'm currently between jobs," Peter answered. "My last job was as a proofreader for a book publisher, but I got tired of doing that."

While Doctor Ryppemuff and Peter Emppostar were eating and talking, a man named Anthony Lissenzwel walked into the diner with his wife, Annette and their son, Gene. They were there to celebrate Gene's entry into his last year of law school the following day. Gene was a very bright young man and had big ambitions. The entire family was looking forward to Gene's graduation and hoped that he would become a good lawyer. They stayed in the diner for more than an hour. All during that time, they never noticed Peter and the doctor, who didn't notice the Lissenzwel family either.

As the minutes passed, while at the diner, Peter made tremendous progress in gaining the doctor's confidence. As they continued their conversation, Peter kept noticing that they looked alike and were of almost identical height and weight. They were both about six feet tall and weighed about one hundred and eighty pounds. They both had shiny and wavy hair, and about the same amount of gray hair, which could only be seen on their sideburns. Peter also noticed that even their deep and debonair voices were very similar. The biggest difference between them was that the doctor had a mustache. After a while, they both agreed that they could pass as twins. It was then that Peter Emppostar started thinking about an idea that came to his mind when he realized that they were almost identical. He thought that with a little refining, he could sound and act exactly like Doctor Ryppemuff. Coincidentally, the doctor also thought of an idea of his own. He then tried to learn as much as he could about Peter.

They eventually finished eating their breakfast and continued talking for a few minutes longer. The doctor didn't want to leave without finding out how to meet Peter again. He wanted to give him his card, but didn't want to make his intentions seem too obvious. He decided instead to simply hope that Peter would return to the diner in the future. Peter felt the same way because he also wanted to see the doctor again, so he asked, "Do you come here often, Doc?"

"As a matter of fact, I do, Peter,' the doctor answered with curiosity. "I'm here almost every day. If you ever need my professional services, my fees are very reasonable or nothing at all, depending on your ability to pay. You can find me right here almost any day you need me, but only in the mornings. You can also find me in the hospital, but please, don't go there unless it is an absolute emergency."

After a few more minutes of inquisitive questioning coming from both sides, they finished their breakfast. Shortly after that, they both decided to leave the diner. "Okay, Doc," said Peter, "it was nice meeting and talking to you. Maybe I'll see you here tomorrow. Okay, have a nice day."

"Bye, Peter," Doctor Ryppemuff replied. "The pleasure was all mine. I definitely hope to see you again." They then left the diner. From there, the doctor went to work, and Peter went home. Shortly after the doctor and Peter left the diner, Anthony Lissenzwel and his family also left.

When Doctor Ryppemuff arrived at the hospital, he started thinking of a plan to lure Peter into it, one way or another.

Peter Emppostar went home and started working on the idea that he had thought about while he was at the diner with Doctor Ryppemuff. Peter started growing a mustache from that day on. The following day, he went to a local electronics store and bought two voice-activated mini cassette recorders. From there, he went to the building department to try to find as much information as he could about the layout of the hospital where the doctor worked. Following that, he went to the public library and took out several books related to doctors and medicine.

The day after, first thing in the morning, Peter put one of the cassette recorders in his shirt pocket and left his house to go back to the same diner. When he arrived, he didn't see the doctor right away. After waiting for a few minutes, he decided to ask a waitress if the doctor visited the diner every day at the same time. The waitress told him that Doctor Ryppemuff had his breakfast at the diner at different times during the morning, but some days he didn't show up at all. Peter then ordered his breakfast and took his time eating it. After he finished, he ordered more coffee. After he had five or six cups, he decided to leave because he didn't think that the doctor would show up.

The following morning, Peter Emppostar went back to the diner earlier than the day before. When he arrived, he noticed that the doctor wasn't there that morning either. As he did the day before, he ordered his breakfast and decided to wait for the doctor as long as necessary. Just as the waitress walked away after taking Peter's breakfast order, the doctor walked into the diner. He didn't notice Peter and sat at an empty table at the rear of the dining area. Peter, however, saw him right away when the doctor sat at a table not too far from where he was. He then called out, "Hey, Doc, I'm here. Come over and join me at my table."

"Oh, hi, Peter," Doctor Ryppemuff replied as he stood up and started walking towards Peter's table, "and thank you for asking me to join you." The waitress saw the doctor walking, so she turned back and took his breakfast order after he sat down and greeted Peter again with a handshake. "Hey, Peter, are you growing a mustache?" asked the doctor after the waitress left.

"Sure, Doc! I admire you so much, that I want to look just like you," Peter answered.

"How can you admire me, Peter," asked the doctor, "if you just met me a couple of days ago, and we only spent a little while together, and only here in the diner?"

"That's because you're a very likable person, Doc," Peter replied. "You're an overall nice guy, and I noticed that in you right away!"

"I hope you mean that, Peter," the doctor added, "because you don't know me well-enough to admire me, but I'm flattered, and I thank you. You're also a very nice guy."

"Gee, thanks, Doc," said Peter, "that means a lot to me."

After a few minutes of chatting, their breakfast was served together, and they started eating it. While they were eating, Peter Emppostar asked Doctor Ryppemuff numerous questions about everything that he could think of, but he was very careful not to get the doctor upset. He asked him many questions about medical terms and about the hospital. The doctor didn't mind answering any of Peter's questions as long as the questions didn't get too personal. During their conversation, Peter learned that Doctor Ryppemuff's receptionist's name was Mary Ohnowear, was twenty three years old and had long reddish hair.

What Peter didn't know was that the doctor was also thinking about some kind of plan of his own. The doctor also asked Peter numerous questions about himself and his activities. He learned that Peter was all alone in the East Coast because all of his relatives were in the West

Coast. He also learned that Peter didn't communicate with any of his relatives at all – at least not within the last ten years or so.

After about an hour, they ended their conversation with the doctor paying for Peter's breakfast. They both agreed that they would meet again in the diner whenever possible. Following that, they left the diner – Peter went home and the doctor went to the hospital.

As time passed, and after numerous encounters with Doctor Ryppemuff in the diner, Peter Emppostar had obtained as many medical publications as he could from various sources. He was at a point where he thought that he was able to pass for a doctor because of the massive amount of information that he had absorbed.

Peter visited the diner every single day. Some days the doctor didn't show up at all, and Peter had his breakfast alone while waiting for over two hours. After he was convinced that the doctor wasn't going to be there, he eventually gave up and went home. Every time that the doctor did show up to have his breakfast, the same routine was repeated by the two men.

After a few weeks, Peter had accumulated vast amounts of recordings of his conversations with the doctor. Every night, he went home and listened to the tape and paid close attention to the doctor's voice. He also recorded his own voice on the second recorder, repeating the same things that the doctor had said, and then he listened to both recordings simultaneously to compare the two voices.

Eventually, Peter was satisfied that the two voices sounded identical. He was delighted with the strong voice resemblance. With identical voices, and his fully grown mustache, Peter was convinced that he was a carbon copy of the doctor. One day, Peter and the doctor were having their breakfast at Gudphood Diner when one of the waitresses referred to them as "The Twins." Peter then realized that the recognition by someone else that they looked and sounded alike was enough for him to put his plan to work. Again, Peter didn't know that Doctor Ryppemuff also had his own plan, which he was ready to execute. The doctor thought that he had enough information about Peter to carry out his plan, but he had to find the right opportunity to do it.

The following day, late in the afternoon, Peter decided to meet the doctor in the hospital's parking lot. Since he was very clever, when he entered the lot, he looked all over until he found the sign where the hospital had parking spaces reserved for the doctors. He then looked for the spot with Doctor Ryppemuff's name on it. After he found the doctor's parking space, with a car with MD plates parked in it, he walked away, sat under a tree nearby and waited for the doctor to get out of the hospital.

After a long day at work, Doctor Ryppemuff came out of the hospital and walked towards his car to go home. He didn't see Peter and took the key out of his pocket to open his car door. Peter saw the doctor and stood up. He then started waking towards him because he was ready to carry out his plan. Of course, Peter didn't know that the doctor had his own plan. It was then that Doctor Ryppemuff saw Peter holding a small paper bag in his left hand, but he didn't pay much attention to it because he thought that it wasn't anything significant. However, he also had something in mind, and after seeing Peter there, he thought that that was the perfect time to take action. "Oh, hi, Peter," he said, "I'm so glad to see you here!" Doctor Ryppemuff then began to insert his car key into the keyhole.

"Hi, Doc, how're you doing?" asked Peter.

"Great! And you?" the doctor replied.

"I'm okay, thanks, Doc," Peter answered. "I'm sorry to bother you, but will you please be kind enough to give me a lift over to the other side of the bridge?"

"Sure, hop in, Peter," the doctor responded. Doctor Ryppemuff wanted to make sure that Peter wouldn't get away, so he had to think of something very fast to lure him into the hospital. He made believe that he was struggling to get the key into the keyhole. After a few seconds, he stopped pretending that he was attempting to open the door. He then turned towards Peter and said, "Oh, wait a minute, Peter, before we go, let's go inside of the hospital so I can show you how well we take care of our patients there."

Peter Emppostar became very suspicious of Doctor Ryppemuff because he couldn't believe that a legitimate doctor would want to take an outsider into his hospital to show him anything. He also remembered that the doctor once told him while they were eating breakfast at Gudphood Diner not to go into the hospital unless it was an absolute emergency – Peter didn't see any emergency at that moment, so he felt that he shouldn't go into the hospital at all. Besides, he caught on when the doctor was fumbling with the keys – Peter knew that the doctor was pretending to have trouble opening the door. "No, thanks, Doc," he replied. "I'm in a rush right now, but the next time I see you, I promise I'll go inside with you."

Doctor Ryppemuff didn't want to scare Peter away. He figured that he'd find another way to lure him into the hospital at another time, so he accepted his wish. The doctor then opened the car door without any difficulty at all. Peter noticed, so he was wondering why the doctor did that, but he decided to remain silent about it. The doctor then drove away with Peter sitting next to him.

When they crossed over the bridge, Peter told the doctor to stop under a big tree and let him off there. "Sure! No problem, Peter," the doctor responded. What Doctor Ryppemuff really wanted to do was to turn around and bring Peter back to the hospital so he could carry out his plan. However, he stopped where Peter asked him to because he wanted to make sure that Peter felt at ease so he wouldn't suspect anything. What the doctor didn't realize was that Peter already felt uneasy about the doctor's faked inability to get the key into the keyhole when they were in the parking lot. Of course, after Peter refused to go into the hospital, the doctor had no trouble at all using the key – Peter noticed that also, so he had the upper hand because the doctor didn't suspect Peter in any way. The doctor put his car in Park and then thought of an alternative way to finally carry out his plan. "Wait a minute, Peter," he said, "my robe is stuck. I guess it got caught when I closed the door."

"Okay, Doc, no problem," Peter replied.

Doctor Ryppemuff then twisted his body leftwards to pretend that he was trying to get his robe free, but without opening the door. While the doctor was pretending to free his robe, he took out a syringe from his left robe pocket. He attempted to fill it with the contents of a small bottle that he had in the same pocket. While the doctor was looking away, trying to fill the syringe, Peter took the opportunity to carry out his own plan. He reached into the paper bag that he still had in his left hand and took something out of it. "Okay, Doc, thank you," he said. "Here, just to show you my appreciation, I have something for you."

It was late and beginning to get dark. It was even darker where they were because they were under a tree. Doctor Ryppemuff couldn't see clearly, so he hadn't filled his syringe yet. When he heard Peter talking, he put it back in his pocket together with the little bottle. He then turned around to devote his full attention to Peter, who then took a tranquilizer dart that he had just taken out of the paper bag with his right hand. Peter swiftly plunged the dart into Doctor Ryppemuff's side before the doctor realized what was happening. The doctor moaned in pain as he quickly started to pass out.

Peter Emppostar once worked at an organization that dealt with wild animals. He had experience in the use of syringes, darts, and tranquilizing drugs. While he was making his preparations to carry out his plan against Doctor Ryppemuff, he obtained several darts, syringes and a big bottle of bear tranquilizer, just for that occasion.

After the doctor was completely unconscious, Peter removed the dart from his motionless body. He then removed the doctor's robe and noticed that it wasn't stuck in the door, so he wondered why the doctor lied to him and pretended that the robe was stuck. After a brief moment, he put it on. He also took all the doctor's belongings out of his shirt and pants pockets and put them all in his own pockets. Coincidentally, the doctor's pants and shirt were the same color as Peter's. Therefore, Peter didn't have to remove them from the doctor to put them on. He then took out a razor that he had also put in his paper bag and shaved off the doctor's mustache to make him look somewhat different. He then removed the doctor's shoes. After that, Peter removed his own shoes and put them on the doctor's feet. He then took the doctor's shoes and put them on his own feet. After Peter did everything that he thought he should do, he moved the doctor's motionless body to the passenger side of the car and sat in the driver's seat himself. He then turned the vehicle around and drove back towards the hospital.

A few minutes later, Peter arrived at the hospital's parking lot and got out of the car. He then walked into the hospital. The security guard faced him with a great look of surprise all over his face because he didn't expect to see the doctor there at all after he had left for the day. Because Peter Emppostar ran past him and went towards the receptionist's desk, the guard didn't have time to react verbally to the presence of who he thought was Doctor Ryppemuff.

When Peter arrived, he said to the receptionist, "My brother is not feeling well and I have to take him to my office to examine him. He's in my car. Please get an orderly with a gurney right away. I'll be outside in the parking lot by my car waiting for the orderly."

"Yes, Doctor Ryppemuff, he'll be there just as soon as I find one," said the receptionist, believing that Peter was the doctor.

Peter then started walking back towards the doctor's car. Shortly after that, an orderly with a gurney came out of the hospital and went running to catch up to Peter who was still walking towards the vehicle. When they arrived, they placed Doctor Ryppemuff in the gurney. Peter then realized that he never asked Doctor Ryppemuff where his office was, but he was very clever, so he thought of something very fast. He was somewhat nervous and inadvertently shouted at the orderly, "Quickly, take my brother to my office! I'll follow you!"

When they finally reached Doctor Ryppemuff's office, Peter Emppostar saw a young woman with long reddish hair sitting at a desk right outside of the office. Peter didn't know Doctor Ryppemuff's receptionist, but when he saw the woman there, he felt sure that she was Mary Ohnowear. He already knew her name, age and appearance because of the numerous conversations that he had with Doctor Ryppemuff at Gudphood Diner while eating breakfast there. However, he didn't want to take a chance in case he was wrong, and she was someone else. When Peter and the orderly passed by her, she stood up and said, "Good evening, Doctor Ryppemuff, is everything all right?"

"I'm sorry," Peter replied, "I can't talk now."

"Okay, Doctor, I'm sorry," the woman responded.

After they rushed Doctor Ryppemuff to his own office, Peter closed the door and told the orderly to stick around while he examined his brother. After Peter pretended to examine Doctor Ryppemuff for several minutes, he turned towards the orderly and said, "Please, go outside and get my receptionist, Mary Ohnowear, and tell her that I want to see her." The orderly opened the door and partially stepped outside of the office. He asked the woman who was sitting outside if she was Mary Ohnowear, and she told him that she was. The orderly then told her that the doctor wanted to see her. Mary stood up and started walking towards the office. Peter intervened because he heard the woman say that she was Mary, and that's all he wanted to know. "Never mind, Mary," he said, "I don't need you anymore, and thank you,"

"Okay, Doctor Ryppemuff," Mary replied as she went back to her desk. Peter was delighted to learn that she was indeed Doctor Ryppemuff's receptionist, and also that she was totally fooled by him. The orderly then went back into the office and closed the door. After another minute, Peter told him to take his brother to the nearest room with an available bed. When the orderly started wheeling the gurney away with Doctor Ryppemuff in it, Peter followed him. They took the elevator and headed upstairs, but Peter had no idea where they were going. A few seconds later, they got off the elevator and started walking through a long corridor.

They finally reached Ward Two Seventeen, and an armed guard at the door greeted Peter thinking that he was the doctor, "Good evening, Doctor Ryppemuff."

Peter took a few seconds to realize that the guard was talking to him, and then he replied, "Oh, hi, good evening. I'm sorry, but my mind was somewhere else because I'm worried about my brother. He's very ill."

"Okay, Doc, good luck," said the guard. "Your brother looks just like you, except that he doesn't have a mustache."

"Thank you. Yes, he does look like me," Peter replied. "Well, I don't mean to be rude, but I have to go and take care of my brother now."

The guard closed the door after Peter and the orderly brought Doctor Ryppemuff into a room where there was another patient. She was a young woman who Peter thought was in a state of almost total confusion because she said to him, "Hello, Mr. President, how are things at The White House?" Peter didn't reply. He and the orderly then placed Doctor Ryppemuff in a bed near her.

When Peter was in the ward, he put his hand in his left robe pocket and finally noticed the syringe and the small bottle that Doctor Ryppemuff had put there. He then realized that that's why the doctor lied to him about having his robe caught in the door. He put two and two together and came up with the answer – he concluded that the doctor wanted to inject him, but he didn't know why. Peter then pretended that he was going to inject his brother, so he took the syringe and filled it with some of the contents of the bottle. He then turned towards the orderly, who was still there with the gurney. "You can go now," said Peter, "and take the gurney with you. Thank you very much for your tremendous assistance."

"Okay, Doctor Ryppemuff, you're welcome. Good night," said the orderly as he started walking away.

"Good night," Peter concluded. When the orderly was completely outside of the room, Peter put the full syringe and the small bottle back in his pocket. Then he also left the room and headed downstairs back to Doctor Ryppemuff's office. When he arrived at the receptionist's desk, right outside of the doctor's office, Mary Ohnowear was still there because she had to work overtime to finish some paperwork that the doctor had given her to do earlier that day. Mary didn't suspect anything at all, and at that point, she wasn't aware of the farce about Doctor Ryppemuff bringing his brother there. "Hi, Mary," said Peter, "I'm sorry I couldn't talk before."

"Hello, Doctor Ryppemuff," Mary replied. "That's quite all right, Doctor. I understand."

Peter walked past her and into Doctor Ryppemuff's office. As soon as he sat at the desk, he said, "Mary, will you please come into my office?"

"Of course, Doctor," she said as she got up and went towards the office.

As soon as Mary walked in, Peter said, "Mary, sit down, because what I have to tell you is going to take a little while. How long are you going to be here tonight?"

"I was planning to leave soon because I just finished the work that you gave me to do earlier today," Mary replied.

"Okay, Mary," Peter went on, "there are a few things that I have to tell you, but first, do I have any medical procedures scheduled in the next few days?"

"Yes, Doctor, quite a few," Mary Ohnowear answered.

"Okay," said Peter, "the first thing I want you to do is to assign another doctor to take my place. However, I want to be present at every procedure while another doctor takes care of my duties – you'll know in the next few minutes why I'm doing this."

"Okay, Doctor, no problem," Mary replied.

"Secondly," Peter continued, "the man I had here before is my brother, and he's very sick."

"Oh, I'm sorry to hear that. Is he all right?" asked Mary.

"I hope so," Peter answered, "but he's seemingly in a coma – he's been like that before, but not as long as he has been today."

"Come to think of it, Doctor Ryppemuff," said Mary, "I didn't know that you had a brother."

"I'd rather not talk about it, Mary," Peter responded in a sad tone of voice in an attempt to end that potentially dangerous discussion about his "Brother." Mary didn't say anything else about his brother, and Peter did his best to disguise his difficulty in completely assuming someone else's identity. He then started to adjust to his new life as Doctor Ryppemuff. "Mary," he said, "as I said before, I had to bring my brother here because he's in bad shape. When I had him here in this office a while ago, I examined him. I found him to be in such bad shape, that I decided to place him upstairs in Ward Two Seventeen. He's in a bed next to the young woman who's in a daze and acts like a zombie."

"Oh," said Mary, "that's Miss Martha Innaddayze."

"Okay," Peter continued, "thank you for telling me. I completely forgot, and you'll now find out why. I need your guidance in remembering some things that I'm beginning to forget – it all started when I got home and saw my brother in the condition that he's in. I'm suffering from some kind of temporary memory lapse – I guess it must be because of all the stress that I have been having lately, especially now that he's in his worst condition. He's been sick for quite some time, but he had never been as bad as he is today. That's why I brought him here to the hospital so I can be near him at all times in case he needs emergency medical care."

"Okay, don't worry, Doctor," said Mary, "I'll help you to remember things."

"Thank you, Mary, I appreciate your help," said Peter.

"You're welcome, Doctor, anytime," she replied.

"I'm going to stick around for a few minutes, and then I'm going home," said Peter. "Mary, how come there's an armed guard at the door of Ward Two Seventeen?"

"Oh," Mary answered, "you made it a rule for all the mental wards to be watched by armed guards at all times, because you said that all mental patients here are dangerous and shouldn't be left unwatched – I guess you forgot that because of your memory situation."

"Yes, I did forget. Thank you, Mary," Peter replied. He then took the syringe out of his robe pocket and said, "Another thing I need you to do, Mary, is to take this syringe and have someone analyze it to see what's in it. I found it in my brother's bedroom, and I'm very worried about it – I don't know if he was injecting himself with it."

"Okay," said Mary, "I'll take care of it tomorrow morning as soon as I come in."

"One last thing, Mary," said Peter, 'I wouldn't want the others to think that I'm going senile – please keep this memory problem of mine a secret."

"Sure thing, Doc," Mary replied. "My lips are sealed."

Peter then concluded, "I'll show you my appreciation by giving you some overtime hours every day even if you don't work them – to start, I'm going to put down that you had to work until midnight tonight – just tell me tomorrow morning what I have to do to accomplish that, because I forgot all about it."

"Okay, Doctor, and thank you for the overtime hours. I surely can use the money," Mary also concluded.

After becoming as acquainted as possible with the location of certain areas of the hospital, Peter left for the night. The first thing that he did after he left was to go to Doctor Ryppemuff's house to become familiar with it. As soon as he arrived, before he opened the front door, a neighbor who happened to be outside greeted him using the doctor's title and name. Peter didn't know who the neighbor was, but he felt that he had just hit the jackpot, because he had the neighbor completely fooled as well. After Peter greeted the neighbor back, he opened the front door with the doctor's keys, and an alarm went off. Within a minute, there were several other neighbors there as well, but everyone thought that they recognized the doctor, so everyone concluded that it was a malfunction. Peter then told them that he forgot the code. The police arrived within a few minutes, but after talking to Peter and a few neighbors, they were satisfied when Peter told them that he reset the alarm that morning and had forgotten the new code. He then showed them identification, and one of the officers had to type in the code, which he had written down. While the officer was typing in the code, Peter looked at a slip of paper in the officer's hand. He saw and memorized the code. As soon as the code was typed in, the alarm stopped. The officer then said, "The code was still the same. I guess you meant to change it, but you typed the same code again."

"Oh, really?" asked Peter. "Let's see – let's close the door and open it again," he concluded as he closed and opened the door – the alarm started again. He typed in the code that he had just memorized, and the alarm stopped. The police then left. Shortly after they left, Peter walked into the house and took over the doctor's identity in his home as well. Peter looked all over the house until he found the manual for the alarm system. He then changed the code.

The next day when Peter was at a point where he was satisfied that he had gotten away with his crime, he went to his old place to give up his one-room studio before going back to his new job as a doctor. When he arrived, the month wasn't over yet, so he kept the keys, but gave the landlord notice that he was leaving at the end of the following month – that was perfect, he thought, because in case something went wrong, he would return and keep the studio. After that, he went to Gudphood Diner to have his breakfast and to try to copy the doctor's activities.

A while later when Peter entered the diner he was wearing the doctor's robe over his clothes. He also had a stethoscope partially protruding from his robe pocket in an attempt to imitate the doctor. The waitress greeted Peter using the doctor's title and name. Peter was totally ecstatic when he realized that he had her totally fooled. After he finished his breakfast, Peter left the diner to go to work. From that day on, he impersonated Doctor Ryppemuff in every way. That was surely a perfectly executed case of identity theft – it appeared that Peter Emppostar got away with it.

When Peter arrived at the hospital, the first thing that he did was to go upstairs to Ward Two Seventeen to give Doctor Ryppemuff another injection of bear tranquilizer. He planned to give him a daily dosage from that day on. Later on that same day, he also told a nurse, with Mary Ohnowear's help, to install the necessary equipment to feed Doctor Ryppemuff intravenously.

After Peter went back to his office, Mary told him that she took the syringe that he gave her the day before to the lab to have it analyzed, and they did it while he was upstairs with his brother. She also told him that they found a very powerful anesthetic in the syringe that doctors often used to make people pass out instantly. Peter then realized that Doctor Ryppemuff wanted to sedate him, but he still didn't know why. He then remembered the farce about Doctor Ryppemuff pretending to have trouble opening the car door the day before in the parking lot. Then he realized that he was lucky that he didn't go inside of the hospital when the doctor told him that he wanted to show him how well they took care of the patients there – he realized that the doctor wanted to sedate him. After seeing Martha Innaddayze's condition, Peter started thinking that she was a previous victim, and the doctor wanted to turn him into a zombie-like patient as well.

Peter Emppostar spent his first full day in the hospital doing things very sluggishly. He was present during all the medical procedures that Doctor Ryppemuff was originally scheduled to perform, which were assigned to other doctors. He actually learned a great deal that day.

Because Peter was so clever, before leaving, he told Mary not to schedule any more medical procedures for him ever again, but to make sure that she let him know when other doctors had procedures scheduled, so he could go and supervise them every time he had a chance – that way, he didn't expose himself to any possible blunders that he was sure that he would be making by performing any procedures himself. It was also a very effective way to get first-hand training during those procedures. Peter eventually got through the day, mostly with the help of Doctor Ryppemuff's receptionist, Mary Ohnowear. When his shift was over, he left for the day.

Back at home, it took Peter a while to get to know who his neighbors were. Whenever he was in a tight spot because he didn't know something in front of his neighbors, he used the excuse that his job was getting to him, and that he was beginning to forget things. Doctor Ryppemuff lived alone – for that reason, Peter didn't have to fake anything while he was inside of the doctor's home.

Peter Emppostar had learned from Doctor Ryppemuff at Gudphood Diner that he was the Director and Head Psychiatrist of Deprivayshun Psychiatric Hospital and Diebroak Senior Citizens Home. Therefore, he was able to get away with a great deal while he was making his adjustments. He kept giving Doctor Ryppemuff a daily dosage of bear tranquilizer, and no one ever questioned him about it.

One morning, when Peter had just finished giving Doctor Ryppemuff his daily injection, he saw a nurse walking into Ward Two Seventeen to give Martha Innaddayze some medication. "What is that medicine you're giving Miss Innaddayze, Nurse?" Peter asked.

"That's the medication that you prescribed for her to make sure that she doesn't get worse, Doctor," the nurse replied. She was surprised that Doctor Ryppemuff didn't call her by her name, because he knew who she was, so she thought, but she didn't do or say anything about it. She was also surprised that he asked her what the medication was, because he had prescribed it himself.

"Leave one of those tablets here with me, please," Peter requested.

"Yes, Doctor Ryppemuff," she said as she left a tablet on a small table and walked out. Peter then took the tablet and walked out of the ward as well.

When Peter got back to his office, he gave the tablet to his receptionist so she could have it analyzed. Mary took it to the lab, and on the same day, Peter got the results back – he learned that the medication was a very powerful drug that kept patients under partial memory loss and in a state of almost total confusion. Peter then wondered what Martha's financial position was. "Mary, how is Miss Innaddayze paying for her hospital stay?" he asked.

"Well, Doc," Mary answered, "I guess you forgot that also – we obtained medical insurance for her, as we do for everyone who doesn't have the financial means to pay his bill." Peter then confirmed his own conclusion that Doctor Ryppemuff wanted to turn him into a zombie, as he referred to Martha Innaddayze, and keep him under the same condition that he kept her in, and rip off an unsuspecting insurance company.

A few days later, Peter went back to Gudphood Diner to have his breakfast, as he did almost every morning. As soon as he sat at a table, the waitress walked over towards him and said, "Good morning, Doctor Ryppemuff. What happened to your twin? He usually comes here every single day, and he even gets here long before you do, but I haven't seen him here for a while."

"Oh, my buddy, Peter Emppostar, he's a nice fellow!" Peter replied. "I'm going to miss him dearly. He had a job offer in the West Coast and left after we had our breakfast the last day that we were here together. I don't think he'll ever be back – too bad!"

"Well, I'm sorry to hear that, Doc," said the waitress. "I really liked him, and I agree with you – he was a nice fellow. Okay, let me take your order now, Doc."

Peter thought at that very moment that he had every angle covered. After a while, he finished his breakfast and went back to the hospital.

Later that day, after Peter left the hospital to go home, he went back to his studio, which he had already emptied and cleaned, and gave it up completely because he felt that he wouldn't need it anymore.

There eventually came a time when Peter no longer needed Mary Ohnowear's help anymore in helping him to remember things that he claimed he forgot. He told her that his memory was almost back to normal, but he didn't tell her that he was fully recovered – that was in case there was something else in the future that he didn't know, and needed to ask her about it.

The General Practitioner

A YEAR AFTER THE abduction of Doctor Ryppemuff, late in the afternoon, Anthony, Annette and Gene Lissenzwel arrived at Gudphood Diner to celebrate the day that Gene graduated from law school with high honors. As soon as they sat in a private booth, the waitress took their dinner orders. While they waited, they started a conversation. "I'm sorry that this is all I can do for you, Gene," said Anthony. "I brought you here to this diner. I wish I could do more for you."

"That's quite all right, Dad," Gene replied. "This is really a nice place, and I really appreciate it. The proof that this is a nice place is that you didn't bring us to the restaurant where you work." The Lissenzwel family stayed in the diner for a couple of hours, talking and eating. After they finished, they left. As they were walking out, Gene told his parents that he had an appointment with the Public Defender's Office the following day for a job interview. They wished him luck, and everyone went home.

Meanwhile, not too far from Gudphood Diner, another doctor had placed an ad in one of the major newspapers of the same city. The add read: "A very busy doctor's office needs a bright woman to work as a receptionist and an administrative assistant. We offer great salary and benefits to the right person. Applicant must be an attractive young female and flexible in every way. Apply in person at 1234 Rich Lane."

The doctor who placed the ad had his medical practice in a very modern commercial building in one of the busiest areas of the city. He had a very lucrative business – his fee was $50 per "Ah," plus expenses plus other charges. The doctor's name was Doctor Sayahagain. He was the same doctor who once told Elizabeth Syckcolun at Kuttemopen Hospital that he was a cancer specialist. He was a towering and slender man with a slight lean towards his left side. He was fifty five years old and had a full beard, almost totally gray. He had an exquisite taste for being well-dressed and groomed.

On a Friday morning, on the first day that the ad appeared, there were many applicants waiting outside of the doctor's office. All the applicants were there long before the doctor arrived. There were numerous, seemingly qualified, attractive young females vying for the job. A copy of the ad was taped on the front door. There was also a notice on the door saying that the office was going to be open that day only to the people applying for the job.

The doctor eventually arrived and entered his office through a rear door. After making himself comfortable, he opened the front door to let everyone in. He told them to stay in the same order as they were lining up outside and sit in the waiting room. The group rushed in so fast that it seemed as though their lives depended on getting in as fast as they could. Doctor Sayahagain told everyone to fill out applications, which he had placed on a table in the waiting room the day before when he left the office. There was also a big sign on the same table telling everyone to take an application and fill it out. He then walked into the examining room and waited a few minutes until the applicants had filled out the forms. It was then that he got ready to start personally interviewing all the women, one by one. He then called the first applicant, "The one who was in front of the line, please come in." The first one who entered the examining room was a very beautiful young lady named Nancy Nohwey. Doctor Sayahagain made sure that he closed the door to the examining room so no one in the waiting room could hear anything. The doctor looked at her from head to toe and was pleased with what he saw. He didn't even bother to look at the rest of her application after he saw her name on it.

"I am Doctor Sayahagain," he said. "Do you know, Miss Nohwey, that I, as a doctor, must have a plaything away from home?"

"I don't know what you mean, Doctor," Nancy replied. "I'm totally confused. Please explain it to me."

"I don't like your answer at all," said the doctor. "I was hoping that you would understand me and accept my proposal. Well, if you don't understand, then I guess you're not qualified for this position."

"I really need the job, Doctor Sayahagain. What are the qualifications necessary to work for you?" Nancy asked.

"This is very annoying!" Doctor Sayahagain yelled. "The ad specifically stated that the applicant must be flexible in every way!"

"Well, I still want to get hired," she said. "I am extremely flexible and I can work long hours. I can go anywhere and do anything."

"Okay, in that case, let me get right to the point," said the doctor. "If you're that flexible and you can do anything, then can you please me in some special personal ways, as much as I need to be pleased?"

"No way!" Nancy yelled. "Just a minute, Doctor Sayahagain! Now I'm the one who's getting annoyed! There's no way that I'll let you do that to me! I was referring to doing anything related to my professional duties as a receptionist, not in any personal way with you."

After several more minutes of futilely attempting to convince Nancy to be his toy, the doctor dismissed her as soon as he realized that she wasn't going to give in. He finally said, "I'm sorry, Miss Nohwey, I have many more beautiful women waiting outside to be interviewed. I'll call you. Good bye."

"No!" Nancy yelled again, "Don't call me! I don't want to work here! You're a despicable man! I'm not going to press charges against you only because I don't have any proof of what you said, and you will definitely deny everything! DROP DEAD!" Nancy then left the examining room with a great feeling of disgust that could be seen all over her face. Following that, on her way out, Nancy walked past all the other applicants. They saw the look on her face and thought that she was upset because she wasn't hired, so they didn't pay much attention, but they were glad because they realized that they still had a chance to be hired themselves.

After Nancy walked out, the doctor called the next applicant. She was a woman named Louise Oldenhevi who was about fifty years old and weighed somewhere in the neighborhood of three hundred and fifty pounds. The doctor only glanced at her slightly and didn't look at her or her application, except that he looked at the line where her name was. "Miss Oldenhevi," he said, "I'll call you. Good bye." Louise left in a rage. All the other applicants saw her rushing out of the office with a grim look on her face. Again they thought that she was upset because she wasn't hired, but that time it was true.

The doctor spent more time talking to applicants that were very young and attractive, but he spent very little time talking to the ones who were older and less attractive. A few hours passed without any success by Doctor Sayahagain in hiring anyone. By then, several more women had entered the waiting room to apply for the job, and the room was completely packed.

After dismissing twenty nine unqualified applicants for very similar reasons as the ones the doctor had for dismissing Nancy Nohwey and Louise Oldenhevi, there were still numerous applicants left to be interviewed. Some of the applicants who were dismissed were: Cathy Twophatt, Nicole Twoshoart, Janice Nottpriti, Jacquelyn Twowyze, Jasmine Notteezee, Mary Deecentladie, Olga Posedathret and many more.

After a while, Doctor Sayahagain was starting to get somewhat despondent. He thought that he might never find the right person. "It would be a shame if I can't find a qualified applicant," he thought to himself, "and I have to advertise again. I would hate to spend more money on another ad, not to mention the money that I'm losing today because I'm not ripping off victims while I'm conducting these interviews."

The next applicant was an attractive young female named Betty Whilling. She was the same woman who went to Kuttemopen Hospital to apply for a receptionist job while James Syckcolun was being operated on. She was not only young and attractive, but she was also dressed in a very provocative way – her makeup, tight-fitting clothes and hairdo made her stand out among all the other applicants. The doctor looked at her from head to toe, exactly as he had done with every attractive applicant before her. He then looked at her application simply to see what her name was. As soon as he saw her name, he didn't look at anything else on the form. He introduced himself and asked her the first question that he had asked everyone else who looked physically qualified for the job, "I am Doctor Sayahagain. Do you know, Miss Whilling, that I, as a doctor, must have a plaything away from home?"

"Well, Doctor Sayahagain," Betty accepted his proposal, "I'm willing to do anything in order to get a job as a receptionist for a great doctor, such as you – as long as the pay is good, I'll go along with what you said."

Doctor Sayahagain let out a huge sigh of relief. "Well!" he exclaimed, "It seems like I finally found a great person to take this even greater job! By the way, Miss Whilling, what did you do before you came here to apply for this job?"

"I went to Kuttemopen Hospital a few years ago to…"

The doctor interrupted Betty and said, "Oh, yes, Kuttemopen Hospital. That's the greatest hospital in the entire nation – maybe in the entire world. Please go on, Miss Whilling."

"Okay," Betty went on, "I went to Kuttemopen Hospital a few years ago to apply for a job there, but they didn't have any openings. After that, I tried another two hospitals and a few doctors' offices, but they didn't have any openings anywhere. I finally went to work for an insurance company, but I didn't really like it there. I stayed at my job for a few years because the pay and the benefits were really good. Now

I have some money saved up, and I can go out and take my time finding a job that I really like. I only left last week."

"Miss Whilling," Doctor Sayahagain continued, "the timing was perfect – I just put this ad in the paper two nights ago, and it appeared today for the first time. You're hired! Excuse me one second, I'll be right back." Doctor Sayahagain stood up and walked over to the waiting room where the other applicants were sitting. When he arrived, he told them that the job had just been filled. He then thanked them for coming and told them that they could go home. The numerous remaining women left the doctor's office very disappointed – they didn't know that they were the lucky ones who didn't have to endure his verbal and moral abuses. After they all walked out, the doctor locked the door and removed the employment ad that was taped onto it. He also taped a notice on the door saying that the receptionist job had been filled. Following that, the doctor went back to the examining room and spent several hours briefing Betty Whilling. He told her what her duties would involve and thoroughly explained to her all the procedures with which she would have to become familiar. He also told her that the whole idea of his medical practice was to get as much money as he could from his victims, as he called his patients, and to do as little as possible to make his job as simple as he could make it.

"Betty," said Doctor Sayahagain as he concluded, "when you report to work on your first day and every day after that, don't forget to have all the patients fill out applications when they come in so you'll know who is rich and who is poor. Before you call a victim into my examining room, tell me what his financial status is, so I can rip him off accordingly. When a rich victim fills out an application, let me know right away so I can rip him off before I rip off all the other patients. You see, I'm a master at taking big money out the pockets of rich people, and I don't want to take a chance that one of them may leave because of the waiting time." At the end of the orientation, the doctor gave Betty a set of keys to the office. After giving her the keys, he dismissed her and told her to report back to the office the following Monday at eight in the morning to start working.

On Monday morning, Doctor Sayahagain's new receptionist was the first one to arrive at his office. She unlocked the front door and went inside. After making sure that everything was in order, she sat at her desk to begin her first day on the job. The receptionist's desk was located in such a way that it could be seen from the waiting room, as well as from the examining room, but the doctor couldn't see the waiting room from his position, and the people in the waiting room couldn't see the examining room. The desk was enclosed in a glass partition with a door leading to the waiting room and another door on a different side leading to the examining room – the reason was to make sure that the people in the waiting room didn't hear anything that the receptionist privately discussed with any of the patients. She communicated with the people in the waiting room with a two-way microphone/speaker, which she always turned off when she had someone with her in the enclosure. The enclosure also had a separate two-way microphone/speaker connected to the examining room so the doctor and the receptionist could communicate without the patients in the waiting room hearing them talking.

A few minutes after Betty sat at her desk, there was a room full of unsuspecting patients. The doctor arrived shortly after that and entered his office through a rear door – he preferred to use the back door so that the people in the waiting room couldn't see him as he entered. He greeted his receptionist and walked towards the examining room. He then walked over to a small black curtain on the wall between the examining room and the waiting room and drew the curtain open. Behind it was a two-way mirror. He looked through it into the waiting room, and after he saw the great number of people waiting, he closed the curtain and started walking towards his desk. As soon as he sat, he talked to his receptionist through the microphone. "Oh my God!" he exclaimed. "Betty, Look at all those wonderful victims outside!"

"Yes, Doctor, there are a lot of them there. Is this unusual?" Betty Whilling asked.

The doctor answered as he made himself comfortable, "No, not really, Monday is usually a busy day because I'm closed on weekends."

"Well, is this good or bad, that we have a lot of people, or victims as you call them?" she asked.

"Are you kidding me?" Doctor Sayahagain responded. "This is wonderful! We're going to make a lot of money today – I'll try to get as many 'Ahs' out of them as possible."

"Ahs?" asked, Betty. "What do you mean by that?"

"Oh," the doctor answered while he looked at Betty, "I forgot to tell you – I specialize in making people open their mouths and say, 'Ah' as soon as they sit in the examining room. If they're not very poor, then I tell them to say, 'Ah' again. If they're rich, then I tell them to say, 'Ah' as many times as possible so I can make more money, because I charge them by the ah – $50 per ah."

"Do they actually fall for that, Doctor Sayahagain?" asked Betty as she displayed a confused face.

"Sure," he answered while shrugging, "haven't you ever been told by a doctor to open your mouth and say, 'ah' as soon as you sit in front of him?"

"Yeah," Betty answered, "but only once per visit."

"Well," Doctor Sayahagain went on, "I got the idea from a doctor a long time ago – my mother brought me to his office, and he told me to open my mouth and say, 'Ah.' After I did as he said, he told me to do it again – I imagined that he missed something the first time, so he had to look in my throat again to look for whatever he was looking for. After we walked out of the examining room, my mother paid $50, so I thought that she paid that amount because I said, 'Ah' twice – I thought that the doctor charged $25 per ah. But that was a long time ago, and this is today, so I have to charge them $50 per ah, plus expenses plus other charges because of inflation."

"Well, Doctor Sayahagain," said Betty Whilling, "I'm glad to hear that we're going to make a lot of money. Why don't you get started with your moneymaking day then?"

"That's a great idea, Betty!" he responded. "Call the first victim and make sure that you write enough useless-medicine prescriptions for everyone that we see today – I'm talking about the placebo that we prescribe to all our victims, which will do absolutely nothing for them, but after they take it, they'll think it did when their problems go away due the body's own immune system."

The receptionist then told the doctor that the first patient was very poor, and she told the unfortunate victim to go see the doctor. As soon as he walked in, Doctor Sayahagain told him to have a seat next to him. He didn't ask the patient why he was there. Instead, he told him to open his mouth and say, "Ah." After the patient did exactly as Doctor Sayahagain told him, the doctor turned on his microphone so his receptionist could hear what he was telling his patient regarding his fee and the medication so she could take appropriate action. He then continued his routine to make money as fast as he could, "That'll be $50, plus expenses plus other charges. Go see my receptionist – she'll tell you what the total is and collect the money from you. She'll give you the prescription for your medicine as well. Good bye. Next!"

As soon as the receptionist heard the doctor say, "Next," while the first patient was walking towards her desk, she told Doctor Sayahagain that the next patient was poor, but not as poor as the one who had just walked out of the examining room. The first patient proved that he was a fool by walking over to the receptionist's desk without ever questioning the doctor about his strange way of practicing medicine. The receptionist called the next patient as she totaled the bill for the first patient. The total was $175, and she collected that amount from the patient. She also gave him a prescription that she had personally prewritten and signed. She also told him to go to the pharmacy across the street to get his prescription filled. The patient proved once again that he was a fool by not asking any questions about the medicine or anything else. He walked out after paying his bill and taking the prescription for his placebo medicine.

The pharmacy across the street happened to be owned by Doctor Sayahagain's brother, or at least, that's what the records showed. However, it was believed that the doctor actually owned it because he was there many times with his accountant when they were working on his income taxes. During such times, the pharmacist gave all the pharmacy records to the doctor, who then started going over the papers with his accountant. The pharmacist walked away, as someone who didn't have any interest in what the doctor was doing.

When the next patient walked in, again the doctor did not ask him why he was there. Instead, he told him to open his mouth and say, "Ah." After the patient did as he was told, Doctor Sayahagain told him to open his mouth and say, "Ah" again. After the patient obeyed the doctor for the second time, Doctor Sayahagain turned on his microphone and went on with his usual routine, "That'll be $100, plus expenses plus other charges. Go see my receptionist. Good bye. Next!" The receptionist totaled the second patient's bill, which was $345. The second patient also proved that he was a fool by remaining silent and obedient about everything that he was told to do.

As the hours rolled by, Doctor Sayahagain had collected as many as seven "Ahs" from various easy and unsuspecting victims. Because there weren't any patients waiting at that moment, he decided to take a short break and use the back door to step outside momentarily to get something to eat. Before Doctor Sayahagain returned from his short lunch break, another patient walked in and went to the receptionist's desk. He was a tall and seemingly strong man walking with a cane. The patient moaned as he spoke to the receptionist, "Good afternoon,

Miss. My name is Sam Towhertz. One of my workers, August Hahmerdrawpper, dropped a sledgehammer on my right foot, and my toe is swollen. I need to see the doctor right away." Betty Whilling gave Sam a form and told him to fill it out. After he completed it, she told him to have a seat and wait. While the patient waited in the waiting room, the receptionist read the form that he had just filled out.

Shortly after that, the doctor returned from his lunch break, and Betty told him that the next patient was a very wealthy real estate developer named Sam Towhertz. Sam was called in, and the doctor did not ask him why he was there. Instead, he told him to open his mouth and say, "Ah." After Sam did as the doctor told him, Doctor Sayahagain told him to open his mouth and say, "Ah" again. After the patient did as the doctor told him for the second time, the doctor put him through an additional dozen "Ahs." Doctor Sayahagain noticed that Sam was becoming impatient, so he decided that he shouldn't extract any more "Ahs" from him. He stopped his "Ah" nonsense to collect the fortune that he expected from the rich victim. He then turned on his microphone and said, "That'll be $700, plus expenses plus other charges. Go see my receptionist. Good bye. Next!"

Sam Towhertz became extremely unhappy and disappointed. He definitely had to question the doctor about his unwillingness to treat him properly, "Doctor Sayahagain, you haven't even asked me why I came here to see you – why is that?" Betty heard Sam complaining, so she didn't call the next patient.

"I am the doctor here," Doctor Sayahagain answered, "and I know what I'm doing – that's why!"

"Okay, Doctor," Sam went on, "I am here because one of my workers dropped a sledgehammer on my foot, and my toe hurts. I have excruciating pain all over my left foot because my toe is swollen."

The doctor wanted to get rid of the patient as quickly as possible so he could move on to the next victim. He didn't even hear what Sam told him about his toe, but he finally looked at Sam's form for the first time to see his name. Once he saw Sam's name, he said, "Whatever your problem is, Mr. Towhertz, it's all in your mind." He then looked at the form again to see what Sam was complaining about. When he saw the patient's problem written down, Doctor Sayahagain had to think of a name for his ailment, "I'll tell my receptionist to make an emergency appointment for you to go see a psychiatrist tomorrow morning, because you're probably suffering from Swelosis, and he specializes exclusively in Swelosis. That'll be $900, plus expenses plus other charges. Go see my receptionist. Good bye. Next!"

"No, Sir!" Sam yelled. "You're beginning to annoy me! My problem is not in my mind! My problem is in my foot!" Again Betty heard Sam talking about his foot, so she waited before calling the next patient.

"Mr. Towhertz," said the doctor, "we're spending too much time on this problem. You have to do as I told you because the more you wait, the worse your mental condition will get. Don't worry. Go see the psychiatrist, and you'll see that he'll take good care of you. He's the best there is. When you see him, your problem will go away very fast – I guarantee you that."

Sam was in a rage and said, "No, Sir, Doctor Sayahagain, I don't have any mental condition, and I don't want to go see a psychiatrist because my toe does hurt a lot, not my mind."

"Okay, then," said the doctor, "maybe I missed it. Open your mouth and say, 'Ah' again to see if I find the problem."

"Ah," said Sam as he opened his mouth.

"Aha!" the doctor exclaimed. "I found it – based on what I see in the back of your throat, you're suffering from Aikosis. I'll send you to Doctor Louzi. He's a medical doctor who specializes exclusively in the treatment of Aikosis. Your bill is much higher now because of all this delay – go see my receptionist so she can total it up and give you Doctor Louzi's address. Good bye. Next!"

Sam was somewhat convinced that Doctor Sayahagain knew what he was talking about, and he thought that the doctor actually found some kind of infection due to his swollen toe. He decided to walk towards the receptionist's desk and follow the doctor's instructions. While Sam was walking out of the examining room, Doctor Sayahagain told his receptionist not to call the next victim yet. Instead, he told her to make an emergency appointment with Doctor Louzi for Mr. Towhertz to see him first thing the following morning. He also told her to transfer the call to his desk after she finished making the appointment. The receptionist totaled Sam's bill, which was $1,475. She collected the money from him and gave him instructions for his appointment with Doctor Louzi. When the patient walked out, Betty told the doctor that she had Doctor Louzi on the line. Doctor Sayahagain leaned back in his seat and picked up the phone. He then whispered because his door was still open, "Hey, Louzi, Sayahagain here. How're you doing, Buddy?"

"Great! How about you?" Doctor Louzi replied.

"Okay," Doctor Sayahagain answered. "I'm sending you a big fish. His name is Sam Towhertz and he's got plenty of bucks."

"Okay – Sam Towhertz – got it. When will he be here?" asked Doctor Louzi.

"He'll be there first thing tomorrow morning, Louzi, and don't forget the usual twenty percent referral fee for me," said Doctor Sayahagain.

"You don't have to remind me of that all the time, Sayahagain. When have I ever failed to pay you?" asked Doctor Louzi.

"Well," Doctor Sayahagain responded, "you still owe me for the last six victims that I sent you yesterday."

"That was only yesterday! Geez!" Doctor Louzi exclaimed.

"By the way, Louzi," Doctor Sayahagain went on, "I told him that he's probably suffering from Aikosis."

"Aikosis! I'm confused! What in the world is Aikosis?" asked Doctor Louzi.

"Hmm! I made it up," Doctor Sayahagain answered, "but I'm sure that you have made up many phony names before. Haven't you?"

"Of course!" Doctor Louzi replied. "I've made up some bogus names in the past many times. We all know that, but I never heard of Aikosis – that's a new one. Okay, Aikosis it is. See ya, Sayahagain."

Doctor Sayahagain concluded, "Take care, Louzi, and send me the money you owe me." Later on that day, after all the victims had been very severely ripped off, Doctor Sayahagain felt like calling the pharmacy across the street from his office to remind them about his kickback. When his brother answered, Doctor Sayahagain said, "Bro, don't forget to set aside twenty percent in cash for me on all the victims that I have been sending you for the useless medicine."

"Wow!" the pharmacist replied. "I'm very happy to hear that you're still sending plenty of victims here! We have to buy more Plasseebow Pharmaceutical Corporation stock. After all these prescriptions for the useless medicine are filled, the stock should go through the roof, because we both know that there are thousands of other doctors out there prescribing the same bogus medicine to their victims."

"Okay," said Doctor Sayahagain, "I'll keep sending them to you as long as you keep setting aside that amount to keep it off the books."

"Right on, Bro," said the pharmacist. "I'm going to call my stock broker right now. See you later."

"That's a good idea," said the doctor, "I'll call my broker also. Bye." Shortly after that, Doctor Sayahagain told his receptionist to connect him with his stock broker. When his broker was on the line, the doctor asked him his opinion of the stock of Plasseebow Pharmaceutical Corporation. When he was told that it was a great opportunity to buy some more, the doctor told him to buy as much as he could for him.

The Psychiatrists

THE NEXT MORNING, AT Doctor Louzi's office, his first patient for the day was Sam Towhertz. He still had excruciating pain in his left foot due to a swollen toe. Sam went through the usual first-time steps. After he completed his paperwork, he was called into the examining room. Doctor Louzi was a heavyset man seemingly with little energy. He had difficulty getting around mostly due to his weight. As soon as Sam walked into the examining room, the doctor slowly turned towards him with his disheveled appearance and told him to lie down in the sofa. As soon as Sam lay down, the doctor started his rigmarole by saying, "My name is Doctor Louzi, and I am a psychiatrist. What is your name, Sir?"

"Wait a minute," Sam replied, "I didn't know that you were a psychiatrist, Doctor Louzi. I told Doctor Sayahagain that I didn't want to go see a psychiatrist, and he told me that you were a medical doctor. Why did he send me here then?"

"Doctor Sayahagain probably thought that you were crazy," Doctor Louzi replied. "Just to prove to him that you're not, I will give you a complete mental evaluation now that you're here. Okay, what is your name, Sir?"

"I don't understand why you don't know my name, Doctor Louzi," said Sam, "because the form I filled out is right in front of you. Anyway, my name is Sam Towhertz."

Doctor Louzi wasn't concerned at all about what was written on the patient's form, but as soon as Sam told him his name, the doctor remembered that Sam was the Aikosis victim that Doctor Sayahagain referred to him. He then continued his nonsense, "How are you today, Mr. Towhertz, and what can I do for you?"

"I am very confused, Doctor Louzi," Sam replied, "because you haven't looked at my form at all. If you had looked at it, you wouldn't have to ask me what you can do for me. Well, I am fine, except for the pain in my left foot."

"What's the matter with your foot?" asked the doctor.

Sam was still confused as he replied, "It's all written down on my application, Doctor. Why don't you just look at it so you'll know?"

Doctor Louzi became very obnoxious and said, "Are you telling me how to be a doctor, Mr. Towhertz? What do you know about medicine?"

"No, Sir," Sam answered, "I'm not telling you how to be a doctor, and I don't know anything about medicine. However, I do know that I wrote down a lot of stuff on that paper, and it seems like I wasted my time, because you haven't looked at it at all."

"Okay, Mr. Towhertz," said the doctor, "let me get back to first grade and I'll listen to my teacher – you!" Doctor Louzi then looked at Sam's form for the first time and continued, "What does it say here about a hammer?"

"One of my workers dropped a sledgehammer on my foot," Sam answered. "I have a swollen toe and excruciating pain all over my entire foot. It's beginning to go upwards into my leg."

"Do you remember when you were born, Mr. Towhertz?" asked the doctor as he ignored what Sam told him about his foot.

"I'm getting frustrated, Doctor," Sam went on as he became very upset, "because you're not asking me anything that makes any sense at all."

"Mr. Towhertz!" Doctor Louzi yelled. "I am the doctor here and I know exactly what I'm doing. Based on your answer, I can see that you need help. Now, answer my question and you'll see. Again, do you remember when you were born?"

"Yes, of course I remember when I was born," Sam answered. "Well, I don't remember being born, but I know the date I was born on."

"That was very good, Mr. Towhertz. Now we're getting somewhere," said the doctor as he was about to ask the next question.

"Where are we getting?" Sam interjected. "I don't understand what my date of birth has to do with the pain in my foot."

Doctor Louzi completely ignored Sam's question. As the minutes passed by, he had asked him numerous irrelevant questions. Sam was getting extremely frustrated about the entire situation. After the doctor ran out of idiotic things to say and ask, he decided to render a verdict, "Mr. Towhertz, you're suffering from a very rare and severely debilitating condition called 'Aikosis.' You're in urgent need of attention by a very highly respected specialist who specializes exclusively in the treatment of Aikosis. You have to go see him right away. His name is Doctor Louziar. His office is only down the block from here. His cost is much higher than mine, but he's really good. He's even better than I am. My fee for this visit is only $2,000, plus expenses plus other charges. Go see my receptionist so she can tell you what the total is and collect the money from you. She'll make an emergency appointment for you to go see Doctor Louziar immediately."

"Doctor Louzi, I'm very unhappy so far with the outcome of this visit," said Sam as he showed a great deal of anger. "What about the pain in my foot? You haven't done anything about it, and you seem to be ignoring it."

"Well," Doctor Louziar responded, "if it makes you feel any better, that's precisely what Doctor Louziar is there for. He'll provide you with the best of care – you'll see."

Sam was hoping that the next doctor would finally tend to his foot problem, so he walked out of the examining room and went to see the receptionist. She totaled his bill, which was $2,875. She also collected the money from Sam and gave him instructions for his appointment with Doctor Louziar. After Sam walked out, the receptionist called

Doctor Louziar to tell him that Sam Towhertz would be there shortly. She then transferred the call to Doctor Louzi because she knew that he would want to speak with him. Doctor Louzi picked up the phone and said, "Hey, Louziar, Louzi here, how's it going?"

"Okay, Louzi," Doctor Louziar answered, "just a little slow – I need victims. And how're you doing?"

"Very busy," Doctor Louzi replied, "that's why I'm calling you – I'm sending you another victim. His name is Sam Towhertz, and he's filthy rich."

"I know – your receptionist just told me," Doctor Louziar replied. "When do you think he'll be here?"

"He just walked out. He'll be there shortly," Doctor Louzi answered.

"What's the matter with him?" asked Doctor Louziar.

"Who cares?" Doctor Louzi responded. "Just make sure that you tell him that he has a very serious condition called 'Aikosis.' That's what Sayahagain and I told him that he's suffering from."

"Great!" Doctor Louziar exclaimed. "I'll go along with that. How do you spell that 'Aikosis' that you mentioned?"

"A-i-k-o-s-i-s," Doctor Louzi answered.

"Okay," said Doctor Louziar, "I'll make a notation of the spelling. Keep those victims coming, Louzi – I need as many as you can send me."

"I still have six more victims waiting," Doctor Louzi added, "and I'll send every one of them to you, because you're slow today. Don't forget my usual twenty percent. Okay, talk to you."

"I won't forget, Louzi," Doctor Louziar concluded. "Bye, and thanks."

Sam Towhertz arrived at Doctor Louziar's office shortly after he left Doctor Louzi's office. After filling out all the necessary paperwork, he waited about ten minutes before he was called in to see the doctor. When Sam finally walked into the examining room, he remained standing because the doctor had his coat on the only empty chair that was there. Doctor Louziar was even more disheveled than Doctor Louzi – his face was unshaven, his hair was uncombed, his shirt was only partially tucked into his pants, one of his shoes was untied, two of his shirt buttons were unbuttoned and his shirt was stained with coffee and jelly doughnuts. He was heavier and moved around with more difficulty than Doctor Louzi. At that point, Sam didn't know that Doctor Louziar was a psychiatrist, but he was thinking that perhaps he was because of his appearance. He was also thinking that maybe Doctor Louziar and Doctor Louzi were sitting down too long without doing any strenuous work and they became heavy because of it. He started wondering if their appearance was a psychiatric trait, because he had never been in a psychiatrist's office before he walked into Doctor Louzi's office. Sam was confused again and said, "Doctor Louziar, "don't tell me that you're also a psychiatrist!"

"Well, yes, I am – didn't you know that?" the doctor asked.

"No! I thought I was sent to a medical doctor!" Sam replied.

The doctor started writing something on a chart. When he finished, he removed his coat from the chair and threw it on the floor near a corner of the room. He then very sluggishly turned towards his victim and said, "Please sit in this chair next to me. Let me tell you that I am not cheap, but I am good – I hope you understand that. As a psychiatrist, my fee is measured based on how much I have to talk to you and how much I have to listen to you. For instance, I'll charge you $50 per word that I say to you plus $50 per word that you say to me. Words that have more than five letters count double. Words that have more than eight letters count triple. In addition to those charges, there are other charges – they are: pauses, waiting time, expenses, $100 for the use of the chair in which you're sitting plus other charges. You have to realize that I am here to give you the best evaluation in the world. Therefore, I have to stay healthy so I can do that. In order to stay healthy, I have to eat a lot, and I have to stop whatever I'm doing periodically to eat something to maintain my health for the good of my patients. You'll see me eating several times during our consultation. The time that it takes me to eat will cost you as pauses, which cost $500 per minute. Therefore, counting the ten minutes that you waited outside, plus my expenses while booking your appointment, plus the use of the chair, plus everything that I have told you, plus everything that you have said to me plus other charges, you owe me $13,850 so far. Our automated system here in my office figures it all out – here, take a look at this machine on my desk." The doctor concluded his deceptive explanation as he showed Sam a small monitor screen on his desk.

By the time Doctor Louziar finished his last sentence, Sam was totally amazed, shocked, confused and speechless. He hadn't said anything at all at that point, other than the initial process that he went through before the expected consultation, and he was being charged for talking to the doctor – he definitely couldn't understand that, but he was so shocked that he didn't say anything about it. He even forgot about the comment he made when he thought that Doctor Louzi sent him to a medical doctor.

Following that, Doctor Louziar picked up a newspaper and started reading it. Neither the doctor nor Sam said anything for several minutes. Finally, Sam couldn't stand the silence anymore and had to say something, even though he knew that he was going to be charged for talking, "Doctor Louziar, why are you so quiet? Besides that, why are you reading the newspaper instead of taking care my foot?"

"Well," the doctor answered, "if I keep on talking, then your bill will be much higher – is that what you want, Sir?"

"No, of course not, Doctor!" Sam answered. "I don't want my bill to be higher, but I don't understand why it should be higher if we continue talking, because you said that pauses also cost me money! Am I right?"

Doctor Louziar hesitated momentarily before answering Sam's question, but after a few seconds, he replied, "I'm looking at the monitor again, and I see that now your total is $31,285 and still going up. The reason why your bill would be higher if we continue talking is because as I told you before, pauses only cost you $500 per minute, and I can say a lot more than $500 worth of words in one minute. If I talk instead of pausing, your bill will be very high then. I was simply trying to save you money by pausing while I was reading the newspaper, but I can see that you're impatient, so let us continue. Can you see in the dark?"

"Well, Doctor Louziar, I'm even more confused than ever now – of course I can't see in the dark, but what does seeing in the dark have to do with the pain in my foot?" asked Sam.

"I am the doctor here and I know how to treat my patients," the doctor answered. "There's a certain procedure that has to be followed in order to properly diagnose any disease, so, please, let me continue."

Several minutes into his stupidity, Doctor Louziar decided to finally collect that expected huge fortune from his victim. It was then that Doctor Louziar looked at Sam's paper for the first time just to see his name. When the doctor saw Sam's name on his form, he realized that Sam was the Aikosis victim that Doctor Louzi had sent him. He also remembered that Doctor Louzi told him that Sam was wealthy, so he decided to talk for a while longer to increase his bill. He hesitated for a moment and then said, "Mr. Towhertz, we still have a lot to talk about to see if we can get to the bottom of your problem – which I'm very concerned about."

Doctor Louziar spent several more minutes talking rigmarole with the sole intention of getting Sam even more confused and to increase his bill. He also took a few breaks to eat, during which Sam was extremely frustrated. After a while the doctor finally said, "Your condition is far worse than I thought – you're suffering from a very rare illness called 'Aikosis,' and we have to hospitalize you immediately. Your bill comes to $87,655. Go see my receptionist. She will collect the money from you and make an emergency appointment for you to be admitted to Kuttemopen Hospital for an immediate evaluation. Kuttemopen

Hospital specializes exclusively in the treatment of Aikosis, and there's no other hospital capable of doing that."

Sam realized that Doctor Sayahagain and both psychiatrists had told him the same thing, so he thought that Aikosis was a problem related to the swelling on his toe. He wanted to have his foot looked at, one way or the other, so he decided to cooperate, "Will they take care of my foot there, Doctor Louziar?"

"Mr. Towhertz," Doctor Louziar replied, "they'll give you the best of care there – I can guarantee you that – you'll see."

Sam finally did as he was told. He was then given instructions to go to the hospital. After Sam left the doctor's office, Doctor Louziar personally called his nephew, Doctor Butchar, at Kuttemopen Hospital. When his nephew was on the line, he said, "Hey Neph, it's Louziar. I got a big fish for you, and he should be there any minute. His name is Sam Towhertz, and he's got so much money that he doesn't know what to do with it."

"Oh boy, a wealthy fish!" Doctor Butchar exclaimed as he sighed. "I'm happy to hear that a rich victim will be here soon."

"Rip him off as much as you can, and make sure that I get my twenty percent," Doctor Louziar added.

"Okay Unc, I'll make sure of that," Doctor Butchar concluded.

Unnecessary Surgery

LATER THAT SAME DAY, Sam Towhertz arrived at Kuttemopen Hospital. He reported to the check-in window, and was told to have a seat and wait. After two hours, he was finally called in and brought to Doctor Butchar's office by an orderly. When Sam walked into Doctor Butchar's office, the doctor already had Sam's information on his desk and was ecstatic to see a wealthy victim there. As the doctor turned towards Sam, there was a very strong resemblance between Doctor Butchar and Doctor Louziar. The two most obvious differences were that Doctor Butchar was a little younger and somewhat thinner, but they were very similar in many other ways. "Good afternoon, Mr. Towhertz," said the doctor. "My name is Doctor Butchar, and I am a surgeon."

"Good afternoon, Doctor Butchar," Sam replied.

"You have no idea how extremely happy I am to see you here, Mr. Towhertz" said Doctor Butchar. "Please sit down in this chair next to me,"

Sam was completely fooled by the doctor and said, "Thank you, Doctor Butchar. I'm pleased to see that you knew my name right away, because the other three doctors that I visited before I came here only knew my name when they were ready to end the consultation."

"Oh, no, I'm not like that!" Doctor Butchar exclaimed. "In order to provide the best of care, I have to make sure that I know the names of all my patients right away."

"I'm glad to hear that, Doctor," Sam added. "Maybe I'll finally get some results here."

"You certainly will, Mr. Towhertz," the doctor went on, "you can bet your life on that. You have to understand that it costs a lot of money to run a hospital. Did Doctor Louziar give you a detailed explanation of his fees?"

"Yes, Doctor Louziar did explain it to me, very thoroughly," Sam responded.

"Well," said the butcher as he continued his rigmarole, "we have exactly the same fees here, except that they are five times the amount. In other words, you have to multiply the final cost by five. In addition to that, we also have other fees here that he did not have. Those fees are much higher, and they are called 'Hidden Fees.' Some of the doctors here refer to them as 'Rip-off Fees,' but I am honest because I call them by their proper names – they are called 'Hidden Fees,' and there's no reason to call them by other names. Now, let us proceed. Based on the two hours that you waited in the waiting room, plus everything that we have said, plus expenses, plus hidden fees plus other charges, your bill is $92,775 so far. We also have an automated system here that keeps track of that. It clearly states how much your bill is now. By using this marvelous system, you don't have to take my word for it. Take a look at this wonderful machine here." The doctor concluded his presentation as he showed the monitor to Sam, who was totally speechless again. He was so shocked, that he couldn't find words to express himself. He was completely overwhelmed after hearing the amount that he owed the doctor without any services being provided at all. Sam was wondering what the doctor would do or say next to rip him off even more. He was thinking of getting up and walking away without paying that ridiculously inflated bill, but before he was able to decide what he was going to do, the doctor started talking again and said, "We have to schedule an emergency appointment for immediate surgery. Will ten minutes be good for you?"

"Yes, of course," Sam replied. "I'm relieved to hear that someone will finally do something about my toe. I'd like to get rid of this pain."

"Oh, does it come with pain as well?" asked the doctor.

"Yes," Sam answered, "I thought you knew that, Doctor Butchar – that's the reason why I'm here. I'm surprised that you didn't know that I have foot pains due to a swollen toe, because I have already written that down on four different applications, and I have told several people about it."

"Oh, well, if it comes with pain, it'll cost you $20,000 more," said the doctor with a grin on his face. "I'm looking at the monitor, and I see that your bill is up to $121,345 now."

Sam wanted to get the surgery done on his toe to relieve the pain, but he had no intention of paying that outrageous bill. He thought that he'd go to court and pay a reasonable amount, determined by a judge. He decided to go along with the doctor's game just to get his toe fixed, so he said, "Okay Doctor Butchar, I'm ready for my operation as soon as you're ready."

Sam was then given a number of papers that he had to sign – documents that completely indemnified the doctors and the hospital and made Sam totally responsible for anything that went wrong, even if it was caused by the doctors. Of course, if Sam were to die, the hospital would say that he died of complications, and Doctor Butchar knew that no one would question it. Shortly after Sam signed all the papers, Doctor Butchar said, "There's one more thing I have to ask you, Mr. Towhertz – does anyone know that you came here today?"

"Yes," Sam answered, "Doctor Sayahagain, two other doctors, and their receptionists."

"Well, I didn't mean them," said the doctor, "I meant people that you know – is anyone that you know aware that you came here?"

"No, nobody," Sam answered. Neither Doctor Butchar nor Sam said anything else, and Sam was rushed to the operating room for immediate surgery.

As soon as Sam was placed on the operating table, the surgeon looked at the chart and read it, "Okay, triple bypass, staple the stomach, remove the spleen, remove the prostate, remove half of the colon and drain fluid from the brain. Okay, let's get started."

"Wait a minute!" Sam yelled. "All I wanted was to have my left foot operated on because one of my workers dropped a sledgehammer on it. I have a swollen toe and excruciating pain all over my entire foot. I thought that Doctor Butchar brought me here to operate on my toe. What's that list all about?" At that instant, Sam made a futile attempt to get off the operating table. Even though he was a very big and strong man, he was overpowered at once by five doctors, two assistants and three orderlies.

The surgeon was only interested in getting the operation started, so he said, "He's hallucinating, quickly, apply the anesthesia!" Another doctor instantly anesthetized Sam, and right after that, they proceeded with numerous unnecessary operations.

After several hours, the operation went as planned – Sam had a triple bypass, his stomach stapled, his spleen removed, his prostate removed, half of his colon removed and fluid drained from his brain, simply because one of his workers dropped a sledgehammer on his toe, and his foot was in pain. Sam was rolled away from the operating room and into a recovery room. He remained there for a few days in terrible pain. His foot was totally ignored, and his pain was still there. He wasn't allowed to have any visitors because the hospital claimed that he was a menace to society. No one who knew Sam was aware that he was in the hospital anyway.

After two months of excruciating pain, on a bright and sunny morning, they decided to release Sam. One of the nurses went to his bedside to let him know, "Good morning, Mr. Towhertz. I have good news for you – you're going home today. I hope you feel better."

"I have terrible pains all over my body," Sam replied, "and my original pain in my left foot is still there because they didn't do anything about it."

"Oh," said the nurse, "let me call Doctor Butchar – maybe he can do something for you. I'll be right back."

After a few minutes, the nurse returned with Doctor Butchar, and they walked into Sam's room. The doctor walked over to Sam's bedside and said, "Mr. Towhertz, I understand that you're experiencing pain in your foot."

Sam was fully aware that Doctor Butchar was responsible for his ordeal, but because of his condition, he felt that he had no choice other than to give the doctor his full cooperation. "Yes, that's the reason why I started this whole mess to begin with," he replied.

"Well," said Doctor Butchar, "we had nothing to do with your foot. Why didn't you go to a doctor who specializes in that kind of problem? We'll send you to a very competent and highly recommended doctor who deals in such cases. His name is Doctor Sayahagain at 1234 Rich Lane."

"That's where I started, and look at me now!" Sam yelled.

"Well, it's not our fault that you don't know what you're doing," Doctor Butchar scolded him. "We have no choice but to send you to a psychiatric hospital where they provide the best of care for people like you."

"No!" Sam yelled again. "I'm ready to explode! I don't want to go anywhere else! Just let me go home!"

"No, Mr. Towhertz," the doctor went on, "you're not the doctor here – I am. You signed some papers giving me the right to decide what's best for you, and I have to make the right decision. You're in no physical or mental condition to be released to society. I know exactly where you belong, but YOU don't know that because your state of mind doesn't allow you to see and think clearly! Trust me – we're trying to help you for your own good."

"Yeah, sure, you're trying to help me," Sam replied. "Look at what you have done to me, simply because I came here with a swollen toe. You'll hear from my lawyer. This hospital will be shut down when this case hits the media. You and your cohorts will end up in jail for the rest of your lives."

After hearing Sam's remarks, Doctor Butchar knew that he couldn't let him get in contact with anyone from the outside world. He stepped away to get assistance while yelling at Sam, "Mr. Towhertz, I've had too much of your nonsense! That's all I want to hear from you! I'll be right back."

In a few minutes, Doctor Butchar returned to Sam's room with an assistant to help him deal with Sam's situation. As soon as Doctor Butchar went to Sam's bedside, he said, "Mr. Towhertz, this is Doctor Manypewlatar. He will assist you with your transfer from this wonderful hospital to another hospital, which is twice as wonderful."

Although Doctor Manypewlatar wasn't a very big man, he was very aggressive and an expert in the art of intimidating people with his extremely deep voice and his rapid speech. The hospital administration utilized his abilities very effectively when someone had to be manipulated in any way. Doctor Manypewlatar leaned over Sam with a big smirk on his face, which was one of his permanent features, "Now, Mr. Towhertz, before we begin the transfer procedure, let me tell you what your estimated final bill will be. So far the total is $1,205,767.09. We have estimated that the final total will be about $1,350,000 after we get through with you. Pay us $1,400,000 now, and we will return the overpayment to you if there is any. On the other hand, if you still owe us more, we'll bill you – that's probably what will happen anyway. Don't worry, Mr. Towhertz, we'll debit it from your bank account so you don't have to inconvenience yourself in any way. We're transferring you to Deprivayshun Psychiatric Hospital.

Doctor Ryppemuff, the director of that hospital, will take very good care of you there. We shouldn't waste any more time because your condition is grave. By now, you should be grateful to us for everything that we have done for you."

Before Sam had a chance to reply, he was quickly sedated and transferred to Deprivayshun Psychiatric Hospital. When Sam left Kuttemopen Hospital, Doctor Butchar personally called his cousin, Doctor Ryppemuff, at Deprivayshun Psychiatric Hospital. Doctor Ryppemuff was actually Peter Emppostar, but Doctor Butchar didn't know that. "Hey, Cuz, Butchar here, how's it going?" he said.

Peter, of course, didn't know who Doctor Butchar was, but he was very clever, so he found the way to handle the situation. "Can you hold on a second, Cuz?" he asked.

"Sure, no problem," Doctor Butchar answered.

Peter put the phone on hold and turned towards his receptionist for assistance before talking to Doctor Butchar again. "Mary, I have my cousin, Doctor Butchar, on the line, but the problem is that I don't remember who he is or anything else about him. Can you please refresh my memory?" he asked her.

"Sure, Doctor," Mary replied, "I'll tell you as much as I know. Well, it goes like this…" she began. She then told him all she could about Doctor Butchar, "Anyway, he used to send you a lot patients, but come to think of it, he didn't sent you anyone for about a year – I wonder why! Well, another thing…"

After a few minutes, Peter had asked Mary numerous questions about Doctor Butchar. When Peter knew enough about him, he returned to the phone, but Doctor Butchar wasn't there anymore, so Peter told Mary to dial his number to get him back. As soon as Doctor Butchar was on the line, Peter said, "I'm sorry Cuz, I couldn't talk to you before because something extremely important came up, which I hope is resolved now."

"No problem, Rypp," said the butcher.

"So, Butch, how are things there at Kuttemopen Hospital?" asked Peter.

"Business here is great!" Doctor Butchar answered. "I called you before to tell you that I got the best victim we've ever had. He's being sent to you as we speak. His name is Sam Towhertz and he's very rich. If he's not there already, he should be arriving soon. Give him the usual final treatment."

"Will do," said Peter.

"And make sure that I get my twenty percent," Doctor Butchar went on. "By the way, why haven't you paid me for my referrals in about a year? I was waiting to see how long you would go without paying me, but it's been too long now."

Peter Emppostar didn't know what Doctor Butchar was talking about, and Mary didn't tell him anything about the twenty percent because she had no knowledge of it, but his quick thinking helped him handle the problem. "I'm sorry, Butch," he said, "but I haven't been myself for a while. I was suffering from almost total memory loss a while ago for a long time, but now I'm only suffering from partial memory lapses. Just to show you how bad I have been, I don't even remember how to go about paying you. Anyway, how much do I owe you?"

"I think you owe me about six million dollars by now," Doctor Butchar answered. "I'll go over my records to make sure. When I find out exactly what the total is, I'll go over to you personally and pick up a check. Is that okay, Rypp?"

Peter was shocked to hear the amount that he owed Doctor Butchar, but he felt that he had no choice but to accept it because he didn't want to arouse any suspicion from anyone about his impersonation of Doctor Ryppemuff. Besides, he had already learned that he had ways to earn a fortune on a daily basis at Deprivayshun Psychiatric Hospital. Six million dollars was only a drop in the bucket compared to the amount that he was planning to earn in a month, so he said, "That's fine, and come tomorrow morning. When you get here, stay in the lobby and have them call me so I can go there and give you the check. Is that okay with you?"

"Sure!" Doctor Butchar responded. "That's the way we always did it. Okay, I'll see you tomorrow. Bye."

"I'll be waiting. See you, Butch," Peter concluded.

Doctor Butchar had stopped talking to his "Cousin" about any of the horrible things that went on in his hospital ever since he stopped getting his kickbacks from Doctor Ryppemuff. All their friends had been asking Doctor Butchar about Doctor Ryppemuff because they hadn't spoken with him in about a year – the fact was that Doctor Butchar hadn't spoken with him either during the same time. Doctor Butchar then started thinking that he wasn't going to talk to him anymore about any hospital activities until he found out what was going on.

Unnecessary Hospitalization

UPON HIS ARRIVAL AT Deprivayshun Psychiatric Hospital, Sam was brought into Ward Two Seventeen, which didn't have any windows. There was only one door leading from the room to a cage where there was an armed guard inside. The walls of the cage were made of two sets of heavy steel bars with a thick and shatter-resistant glass wall between the two sets of bars. The door was made of heavy steel and secured with five locks. There was a similar door leading from the cage to the hallways outside. The room had a camera and a microphone connected to the main security station in the main lobby on the ground floor. The patients were in a state of total deprivation – they were not allowed to read any newspapers, magazines, books or any other publications, except for their dinner menus. They didn't have any televisions or radios. They didn't have a telephone in the ward, so there weren't any means of communicating with the outside world whatsoever.

When Sam was brought into the room, he was almost completely recovered from the effects of the sedation. He was doomed to spend the rest of his life there without visitors because he was considered to be a menace to society. He was assigned to a room where there were two other patients in identical positions. One of the patients was a woman named Martha Innaddayze. Although she was a young and attractive woman with long and curly hair, Martha looked somewhat disheveled due to her condition. She had been there for three years without the possibility of ever seeing freedom again. She was in a state of almost total confusion and had partial memory loss. The other patient was the real Doctor Ryppemuff, who was unable to move or speak. He was heavily sedated by the daily injections of bear tranquilizer. He was being fed intravenously. Sam thought that perhaps the patient was paralyzed and in a coma.

Shortly after Sam was brought into the room, he and Martha started to learn some things about each other. Although Martha was in a state of almost total confusion and partial loss of memory, and didn't make much sense most of the times, Sam managed to understand some of the things that she was telling him. He was also able to make her understand many things that he was telling her. One of the first things that Martha told Sam was that all the talking in the room should be whispered and conducted in such a way that they faced away from the camera. Martha also told Sam that she thought that they had brought the comatose man into the room about a year before. She always called Doctor Ryppemuff "The President," and now, she was calling Peter the same way. She told Sam that she thought that the comatose man was the president's brother because they looked alike.

"What president?" asked Sam.

"Oh," Martha answered, "he's the president of The United States. He comes here on a regular basis, even before his brother was brought in."

Sam didn't reply to that remark, but he asked Martha why she was there. She said that she didn't really know why. She remembered vaguely that she had been at Kuttemopen Hospital, but she didn't remember the rest, or how she arrived at Deprivayshun Psychiatric Hospital. She didn't even remember exactly when she was admitted, but she thought that she had been there for three or four years.

About an hour after Sam was brought into the room, Peter went in, and Martha said, "There's the president now."

Neither Sam nor Peter said anything about Martha's remark, and Peter introduced himself, "Mr. Towhertz, I am, and I am a psychiatrist. Welcome to this wonderful place. This is my humble and magnificent domain. I am here to help you. After I finish telling you why I'm here, you will be extremely grateful to me."

When Sam saw Peter, he realized that Doctor Louzi and Doctor Louziar were heavy, sluggish and disheveled, but those features were not psychiatric traits as he originally thought, because Peter wasn't like them at all. Instead, he was in good physical condition and had an excellent appearance. "I don't belong here, Doctor Ryppemuff. I want to go home," said Sam.

"Mr. Towhertz," Peter responded, "there's no reason for you to go home, because we'll take very good care of you here. You have been placed in a very elite room. It's expensive, but it's the best we have in this magnificent hospital, and there's no better place anywhere else in the world. You're extremely lucky to have been carefully selected to be here.

"By the way, Mr. Towhertz, don't be like Miss Innaddayze here – she spends a lot of money every month ordering things that she really doesn't need. This morning she ordered two sodas – she knows very well that they cost $180 each. Yesterday she ordered coffee with her breakfast – she also knows very well that coffee just went up in price three days ago. It's a good thing that we have obtained insurance to pay for her bills.

"Anyway, the basic price for breakfast just went up this morning – it is now $1,123. If you order black coffee with your breakfast, it'll cost you $150 extra. If you order coffee with milk or sugar, it'll cost you $160 extra. If you order coffee with milk and sugar, it'll cost you $170 extra. The basic price of all the other meals for the day is $4,965, but there's an additional charge for extras, and if you order any extras, then the bill will be higher. The use of the menu is $10 – please order it and take your time reading it for more information. You'll see all the prices on it, and then you'll know what the extras are and how much they'll cost you. Here are some examples of the extras: the use of the dining table is $300, the use of the chair is only $150, toothpicks are

$12 each, coffee stirrers are only $7 each, napkins are only $4 each, used napkins are even cheaper and can be as low as $1 each, depending on their condition. We recommend that you keep yourself clean with a weekly 30-second shower. However, to further cut down on the cost we also recommend that you drip dry rather than spend the extra $500.00 for a towel. If you get a headache, baby aspirins are only $600 each, and regular aspirins are only $900 each.

"Mr. Towhertz, you should be ashamed of yourself because you have already spent over $450,000 here, and you were only admitted about an hour ago. You will probably be as big a spender as Miss Innaddayze. Your total for this month will probably be over $5,000,000 if you keep up your big spending tendencies. However, your stay here will be very pleasant because of the wonderful care you'll get. To make life even easier for you, we will take possession of all your bank accounts, so you don't have to inconvenience yourself when your bills are due – this way we can do you a favor and take the money out of your account to pay for your expenses. Otherwise you wouldn't be able to pay your bills. Of course, we have to charge you a fee for doing this for you. If your money ever runs out, don't worry because we can get insurance for you, so you can pay your bills – we do the same for all our patients here. Try to cut down on your spending, so you won't end up with a very high monthly bill as Miss Innaddayze does. I advise you to order used napkins to try to significantly cut down your bill. By the way, Mr. Towhertz, as I said before, you have already spent over $450,000 – why have you spent so much money already, in such a short time?"

Sam couldn't stop thinking about the ridiculous fact that his bill was already over $450,000, when he was there for only a little over an hour. He hadn't ordered anything at all, so how can his bill be significantly cut down by ordering used napkins? As Peter told him, they only cost $3 less than regular napkins? Sam didn't consider $3 to be a significant reduction on a bill that was already over $450,000. He thought that that doctor must have been totally insane he shouldn't be a psychiatrist at all! Even before Peter finished his last sentence, Sam was already shocked and speechless because he hadn't done or ordered anything at all, and his bill was already ridiculously high. He was unable to reply because of the state of shock that he was in.

"That's okay, Mr. Towhertz," Peter continued, "I can understand why you're not answering my question – because you feel guilty about spending so much money. Now that I have told you everything, do you have any questions?"

Sam was still stunned – perhaps more than he was before, and couldn't answer Peter's last question either.

"Well, Mr. Towhertz, I guess you don't have any questions because I was very thorough in explaining everything to you. By now, you should be very grateful to me for everything that I have done for you. Good bye then," Peter concluded and walked out.

When Peter returned to his office, he had already planned to take possession of Sam Towhertz's bank accounts to take money out to pay for his ridiculously high monthly bills. Peter personally knew a fellow by the name of Karl Ondetayke. Karl was one of the clerks at Judge Pharemynded's office. Peter paid him to forge court orders to take over all of Sam's bank accounts. He also planned to do the same to all future patients – that was part of his plan to make a fortune, as he expected, while he ran the hospital as Doctor Ryppemuff. Before Peter went into Ward Two Seventeen, he raised the price of everything in the hospital so he could extort a substantial amount of money from the hospital's accounts on a monthly basis. He had already set up various bank accounts under fictitious names. He used a variety of occupations – such as plumbers, painters, masons, carpenters, electricians, roofers, etc. He formed phony corporations under those names, and opened several accounts. Peter wrote hospital checks and deposited them into those accounts. Every check he wrote was entered into the books as an expense, claiming that work was needed at the various buildings that the hospital owned.

The hospital also employed several architects, contractors and builders who were constantly erecting new structures for expansion. Peter Emppostar found the way to pay them more than what they wanted for their work, and then he would take very large kickbacks from them. Peter was making a fortune, so the six million dollars that he had to pay Doctor Butchar for previous referrals when he took over Deprivayshun Psychiatric Hospital was not significant anymore. Besides, he managed to use a hospital check anyway, and entered it as an expense.

The Medical Examination

ABOUT TWO WEEKS HAD passed since Sam Towhertz was imprisoned at Deprivayshun Psychiatric Hospital. Meanwhile, on a nice and sunny day, late in the afternoon, in one of the ritziest areas of the city, there was an attractive young woman named Carmen Pynkeehertz who was picking roses from her garden. Carmen had stayed home from work that day, and her mother, Joan, had just arrived at home from her job. Joan saw Carmen outside and immediately started helping her. While picking roses, a small thorn pierced the skin on Carmen's left pinky, and she screamed very loudly, "Ouch! A thorn got stuck in my finger! My pinky hurts!" As she jerked her hand away, the thorn broke, and a very small piece of it remained imbedded just below her skin. Carmen and her mother immediately stopped picking roses and went inside to tend to Carmen's injured pinky.

Once indoors, they both wanted to remove the thorn, but when Joan touched Carmen's finger, it hurt her so much that they decided to give up the idea of removing the thorn. At that point, Carmen was afraid to remove it herself or to have her mother remove it. Instead of removing the thorn, Joan applied an ointment and a home-made dressing on Carmen's pinky, and they decided to have a cup of coffee.

Carmen was completely useless after the thorn incident – she thought that she was unable to do anything as long as the thorn was in her finger. Joan suggested that Carmen should have the thorn removed by a professional. Carmen didn't say anything, and they continued drinking their coffee.

Later on that day, Carmen's father, Mike, came home from work. He saw the bandage on Carmen's pinky and immediately became alarmed, "Oh my God! What happened to your finger, Honey?"

"I have a thorn under the skin of my pinky, and it hurts!" Carmen answered.

"Well, let me pull it out," said Mike.

"No way!" Carmen yelled. "It hurts too much! Mom and I both tried, and the thorn won, so we decided that I should go to a professional to have it removed." Mike accepted their decision, and they went on with their daily activities until it was time to go to bed.

The next morning, Mike left their home to go to work, and Joan left shortly after he did. Carmen decided to go to a nearby professional, as she thought, named Doctor Sayahagain, who had his office at 1234 Rich Lane, which wasn't too far from where they lived. She planned to go to her office after she returned from the doctor. About an hour after Joan left, Carmen left her home to go to Doctor Sayahagain's office to have the thorn removed. She didn't leave a note for her parents to tell them that she had gone to the doctor because she thought that she would be back long before they got home from work.

When Carmen arrived at the doctor's office, she walked in with a bandage on her left pinky and showing signs of pain. Upon entering, she walked towards the receptionist's desk and stopped in front of her. She then told the receptionist why she was there. The receptionist gave her a form to fill out. After Carmen finished filling out the form, the receptionist looked at it and noticed that Carmen was a high-fashion model who also owned a large cosmetics company. She told Carmen to be seated and wait. The receptionist then went to the examining room to tell the doctor that Carmen was very wealthy. Doctor Sayahagain told her to skip all the other patients and send Carmen in. When the receptionist went back to her desk, she told Carmen to go in and see the doctor. The other patients waiting complained about Carmen being called right after she walked in. The receptionist told them that Carmen had been poisoned by a snake bite and needed immediate emergency treatment. Otherwise she could die. The other patients understood and agreed that Carmen should go in right away.

When Carmen walked into the examining room, of course the doctor did not ask her why she was there. Instead, he told her to open her mouth and say, "Ah." After Carmen did as the doctor told her, Doctor Sayahagain told her to open her mouth and say, "Ah" again. After Carmen said, "Ah" for the second time, the doctor had other ideas. He made sure that he had his microphone turned off so his receptionist, Betty Whilling, couldn't hear him until he turned it on again. He looked at Carmen's paper for the first time just to see what her name was. He then said, "Miss Pynkeehertz, please take off your clothes."

Carmen couldn't understand why the doctor wanted her naked, simply because she had a small piece of a rose thorn just under the skin in her finger. "But, Doctor Sayahagain," she said, "I'm here because I have a thorn inside of my left pinky!"

"Are you a doctor?" he asked. "How do you know what's wrong with you? How can you diagnose yourself?"

"No, I'm not a doctor, but I do have a thorn under the skin of my left pinky," she answered.

"Well, then, let us proceed. Please, take off your clothes," the doctor insisted.

"Why do I have to take off my clothes, when my problem is with my pinky?" Carmen asked.

"If you're not a doctor, you shouldn't be asking me anything about medical issues," the doctor continued. "I am the doctor here. As a matter of courtesy, I'll answer your question, but your bill will be much higher now. Okay, here's the answer to your question: diseases have a way of spreading throughout the human body, and I, as a good doctor, have to make sure that your illness hasn't spread yet. Now, please disrobe."

Carmen didn't say anything else and decided to do as the doctor told her. After she reluctantly disrobed, the doctor started manually examining her entire body from head to toe, very slowly and thoroughly. He went over certain areas many times and much more slowly than the rest of her body. Carmen felt extremely uncomfortable and started getting nervous. Doctor Sayahagain noticed her reaction and stopped the examination. He then looked at Carmen's paper again to see what she was complaining about, because he didn't pay any attention to anything that she had told him about her finger. The doctor then turned on the microphone and said, "Miss Pynkeehertz, based on what I saw in the back of your throat, you're suffering from Thawrnitis. I could be wrong, but I doubt it because I'm never wrong about these things. I think that you should go for a second opinion, because we have to make sure that my diagnosis is correct. Your bill here comes to $1,870, plus expenses plus other charges. Go pay the receptionist, and she'll make an emergency appointment for you to go see Doctor Byggliar. He specializes exclusively in the treatment of Thawrnitis, and he's just across the street from here, next to the pharmacy."

Doctor Sayahagain would ordinarily send his victims to see Doctor Louzi, but Doctor Byggliar had requested that every time Doctor Sayahagain ripped off an attractive woman, he'd send her to him so he could fondle her as Doctor Sayahagain had done. Doctor Sayahagain also made up phony diagnosis names that ended with "osis" when he sent patients to the psychiatrist, Doctor Louzi. However, he made up names that ended with "itis" when he sent then to the medical doctor, Doctor Byggliar.

"Will Doctor Byggliar fix my finger?" Carmen asked.

"He'll give you the best of care," Doctor Sayahagain answered. "You'll see. I have other patients to take care of, Miss Pynkeehertz. Good bye."

"Good bye, Doctor Sayahagain," said Carmen as she walked out of the examining room. She then paid the receptionist for her astronomically inflated bill, which was $2,715. She took the instructions given to her to go see Doctor Byggliar and then walked out of Doctor Sayahagain's office. She was hoping that the next doctor would get rid of her nagging thorn.

As soon as Carmen walked out, Doctor Sayahagain told Betty to get Doctor Byggliar on the phone. When Betty had him on the line, Doctor Sayahagain picked up the phone and said, "Hey, Bygg, Sayahagain here. How's it going?"

"Okay, Sayah. What's on your mind?" asked Doctor Byggliar.

"I'm sending you Miss Carmen Pynkeehertz," said Doctor Sayahagain. "She's a beauty and very wealthy. Make sure to send me my usual twenty percent."

"You always remind me of that!" Doctor Byggliar shouted. "When have I ever failed to give you your cut?"

"Just to make sure – that's all," Doctor Sayahagain replied in a low voice. "I'm sure that you remind the next doctor down the line about your twenty percent."

"Always!" said Doctor Byggliar as he laughed. "Okay, Sayah, what's wrong with Carmen?"

"Come to think of it – I don't know, but who cares?" Doctor Sayahagain answered as he also laughed. "My diagnosis was Thawrnitis. Make sure you tell her the same thing."

"Is there such a thing as Thawrnitis, or are you making it up?" asked Doctor Byggliar.

"I never heard of it," Doctor Sayahagain answered as he continued laughing.

"Give me the spelling of that Thawrnitis then," said Doctor Byggliar.

"T-h-a-w-r-n-i-t-i-s," Doctor Sayahagain replied.

"Hmm, okay, will do," said Doctor Byggliar. "See ya, Sayah."

"Talk to you later, Bigg," Doctor Sayahagain concluded.

A few minutes later, Carmen arrived at Doctor Byggliar's office. After reporting to the receptionist, Carmen went through the usual first-time steps. She was then called in to see the doctor. As soon as Carmen walked into the examining room, she felt very uncomfortable because of the smirk on the doctor's face, as well as his incessantly winking left eye. The doctor looked at Carmen's records to see her name. That's when he realized that Carmen was the Thawrnitis victim that Doctor Sayahagain mentioned. He then looked at her from head to toe exactly as a hungry dog looks at a dish of delicious food. He then said, "Good morning, Miss Pynkeehertz, how are you?"

Carmen felt even more uncomfortable when she noticed that the doctor was staring at certain parts of her body. However, she didn't want to reveal her uneasiness, so she replied without showing any emotions, "Good morning, Doctor Byggliar, I'm fine, thank you."

"Miss Pynkeehertz, I am a second opinion doctor," said the doctor, "and you're here for me to see what's wrong with you. I am going to ask you what your problem is – just to show you that I am different. Doctor Sayahagain's receptionist called me to make an appointment for you, but she didn't tell me what your problem is, or what Doctor Sayahagain's diagnosis of you was. Okay, what is your problem, and what can I do for you?"

Poor Carmen still felt very uneasy about the doctor, but she cooperated fully. She was very hopeful and answered while uncovering her finger, "My pinky hurts, because I have a thorn stuck in it. The thorn is just under the skin. Here – take a look." Carmen then uncovered her finger.

Doctor Byggliar at least looked at her finger – that was something that Doctor Sayahagain didn't even bother to do. Just to scare Carmen, he yelled, "Aha!"

Carmen became alarmed and asked, "Does it look bad, Doctor?"

"Well," he replied, "we have to make sure that we don't misdiagnose your problem, so please take off your clothes."

Carmen was a little more trusting by then, because the doctor had told her that he was different. Besides, at least, he did look at her finger. However, she decided to ask him a question before disrobing, "Is it necessary to take off my clothes, when all I want is to have this nagging thorn removed from my pinky?"

"Well," the doctor replied, "I have to make sure that your problem hasn't spread to other parts of your body. These things are very peculiar at times. Please disrobe so we can find out."

"That's pretty much what Doctor Sayahagain told me," said Carmen as she started taking off her clothes.

Once Carmen was fully naked, the doctor examined her manually from head to toe, very thoroughly and slowly. As Doctor Sayahagain had done, Doctor Byggliar also went over certain areas of her body several times. Carmen was feeling very uncomfortable throughout the entire examination.

The doctor eventually noticed her reaction and stopped the abuse. He then confirmed Doctor Sayahagain's phony diagnosis, "Miss Pynkeehertz, you have a very acute form of Thawrnitis. However, I have to make sure that that's what you're suffering from. I'm going to send you for an emergency appointment with a very well-known and respected specialist who deals exclusively in Thawrnitis. His name is Doctor Sharlottan. He will give you an excellent evaluation. Your bill here comes to $3,875, plus expenses plus other charges. Please pay the receptionist, and she'll give you instructions for Doctor Sharlottan's appointment. Good bye."

Doctor Sharlottan also wanted a piece of the action – fondling attractive women – so he had also requested from Doctor Byggliar that every time he ripped off an attractive woman, he should send her to him.

Carmen left the examining room, and again paid an astronomically inflated bill, which was $4,715. After Carmen left, Doctor Byggliar told his receptionist to get Doctor Sharlottan on the phone. When she did, Doctor Byggliar told Doctor Sharlottan about Carmen, and also to make sure that the diagnosis was Thawrnitis. Of course, he also reminded Doctor Sharlottan about his twenty percent referral fee.

Carmen arrived at Doctor Sharlottan's office a short while later. She had high expectations and was hoping that someone would finally remove the nagging thorn from her left pinky. When Carmen walked into the examining room, she felt uncomfortable because she was a giant next to the doctor. "Miss Pynkeehertz, I am Doctor Sharlottan," he said. "I am a specialist and a third opinion doctor. How are you?"

"Fine, except for my pinky," she answered.

Doctor Sharlottan then started overemphasizing his qualifications – since he was such a short man, he had to make himself appear big in other ways. "Miss Pynkeehertz," he said as he started his highway robbery, "my fee is somewhat higher than Doctor Byggliar's fee. Your visit here will cost you $10,000, plus expenses, plus my time plus other charges. I am extremely good at what I do, and I do get things done. I have never been dissatisfied with any of my patients – that's how good I am. There's no one better than I am, and there never will be."

Poor Carmen didn't realize that the fact that the doctor had never been dissatisfied with any of his patients didn't mean that he was good – it simply meant that the patients were good – or unsuspecting to say the least! She innocently continued the conversation with the charlatan as she replied to his rigmarole, "Well, I'm glad, Doctor Sharlottan, because until now, after seeing two other doctors, no one has removed my thorn yet."

Doctor Sharlottan totally ignored what Carmen said about her thorn. "I don't know why you're here, Miss Pynkeehertz," he went on, "but it must be because there's something wrong with you, so let us begin – please remove your clothes."

"But, Doctor Sharlottan, I was already examined by Doctor Sayahagain and Doctor Byggliar. Do I have to take my clothes off again?" she asked.

"You're here for me to give you a third opinion," the doctor answered. "I don't know what conclusion the other two doctors came to, but I have to give you an honest and truthful diagnosis. I am the best there is – if I can't find your problem, nobody will. Be patient and cooperative. I will take good care of you. Now, please disrobe."

Carmen reluctantly took off her clothes, and when the doctor saw her naked, he placed his eyesight on a certain area of her body. He remained staring at that area all throughout his examination. He then started examining her entire body very slowly and thoroughly. He went over certain areas of her body several times, exactly as the other two doctors had done before him. After several minutes of repetitive handling by the doctor, Carmen felt extremely uncomfortable and asked, "Doctor Sharlottan, is it necessary to do what you're doing?"

"I don't think that you're a doctor!" he yelled. "Are you?"

"No, I'm not a doctor," poor Carmen replied with a sad face.

"Very well then, and if you want to get better, let me proceed," the cruel doctor insisted. Carmen didn't say anything else, and the doctor continued his thorough examination. A little later, she was about to scream, but the doctor noticed her reaction and stopped instantly. "I don't know what the other two doctors told you," he said, "but you're suffering from a very severe case of Thawrnitis. There is only one place in the world that handles this rare illness. I have to send you to Doctor Butchar at Kuttemopen Hospital, which is only a block away from here. He will give you the best of care there. Your final bill here is $31,750, plus expenses plus other charges. Please pay the receptionist, and she will give you full details. Good bye."

Carmen was satisfied with the bogus Thawrnitis diagnosis because, as she thought, the three doctors independently told her the same thing. She thought that they had found some kind of infection called

"Thawrnitis" in her body caused by the thorn. She then went to see the receptionist, who collected the money from her and gave her instructions regarding Kuttemopen Hospital. After paying her third astronomically inflated bill and receiving the information, Carmen walked out. Shortly after Carmen left, Doctor Sharlottan personally phoned Doctor Butchar at Kuttemopen Hospital to tell him that Carmen was wealthy, and to remind him about the twenty percent referral fee for him.

A few minutes later, Carmen arrived at Kuttemopen Hospital. She reported to the check-in window and was told to wait. After three hours of waiting, Carmen was finally called and brought to Doctor Butchar's office. When poor Carmen entered Doctor Butchar's private office, he immediately started talking to her about the huge amount of money that he was planning to extract from her, "Good afternoon, Miss Pynkeehertz, my name is Doctor Butchar, and I am a surgeon. Have a seat right here next to me. You have to understand, Miss Pynkeehertz, that it costs a lot of money to run a hospital. Did Doctor Sharlottan give you a detailed explanation of his fees?"

"Yes, he did," Carmen answered, "he explained everything to me, but I don't care, I want my finger looked at and fixed."

Doctor Butchar noticed that Carmen was fully cooperating with him, so he went on. Of course he had a famous speech totally memorized. He gave portions of it with slight modifications to different victims as he saw fit. He continued his rigmarole by telling Carmen how badly he was ripping her off, "Well, Miss Pynkeehertz, your bill is now $92,775 and still going up."

"I told you I don't care," Carmen insisted. "All I want to do is to get rid of this nagging thorn in my pinky."

"We have to schedule an appointment for immediate surgery," the doctor continued. "Will twenty minutes be good for you?"

"Yes, of course, I'd like to get rid of this pain," Carmen answered.

"Oh, does it come with pain as well?" he asked.

"Yes, Doctor Butchar, I thought you knew that. That's why I'm here. I wrote it down on my application," said Carmen as she displayed a look of surprise.

"Oh!" Doctor Butchar exclaimed. "Well, if it comes with pain, it'll cost you $20,000 more. Your bill is up to $121,345 now. Anyway, I have some forms for you to sign." Carmen was given the same forms that were given to James Syckcolun and Sam Towhertz. Of course, she signed them without reading them. The forms completely indemnified the doctors and the hospital against any wrongdoing. After all the forms were signed, Doctor Butchar scheduled another doctor to operate on Carmen.

"One last thing, Miss Pynkeehertz," asked Doctor Butchar, "does anyone know that you came here today?"

"Sure," Carmen replied, "Doctor Sayahagain, Doctor Byggliar, Doctor Sharlottan and their receptionists."

"No one else?" asked the doctor.

"No, that's it," she answered. Neither Doctor Butchar nor Carmen said anything else, and she was rushed to the operating room for immediate surgery.

When she entered the operating room, Carmen was told to lie down on the operating table. Doctor Manypewlatar was the anesthesiologist during Carmen's operation, and he had the needle ready to anesthetize her. The surgeon looked at the chart that Doctor Butchar filled out and started reading it, "Liposuction, remove the right big toe, remove the left kidney, remove the right breast, remove half of the colon and drain fluid from the brain. Okay, let's get started."

As soon as Carmen heard the surgeon read the list of procedures that they had planned for her, she made a futile attempt to get off the operating table. "Wait a minute!" she yelled while still struggling to get off the table. "I only came here because I have a thorn in my left pinky, and I want it removed. What's going on here?"

Carmen was quickly overpowered and prevented from getting off the operating table. The surgeon then turned towards the anesthesiologist and said, "She's hallucinating! Quickly, apply the anesthesia!" Doctor Manypewlatar plunged the needle into Carmen's right arm, and she was instantly anesthetized.

After several hours, the operation went as planned – Carmen Pynkeehertz had liposuction, her right big toe removed, her left kidney removed, her right breast removed, half of her colon removed and fluid from her brain was drained, simply because she had a thorn in her left pinky. What's more important, the thorn wasn't removed. Carmen was rolled away from the operating room into a recovery room. After the operation, during all the time that she spent at Kuttemopen Hospital, she was in terrible pain. She wasn't allowed to have any visitors because the hospital claimed that she had a contagious disease, and nobody from the outside should go near her – no one who knew Carmen was aware of her whereabouts anyway, and she didn't tell anyone where she went when she left her house.

After seven extremely difficult weeks, they decided to release Carmen. One of the nurses went to her bedside to give her the news, "Miss Pynkeehertz, I have good news for you, you're going home today. I hope you feel better."

"My entire body is in terrible pain," said Carmen while moaning, "and the original pain in my left pinky is still there, because they didn't remove the thorn."

"Oh, let me call Doctor Butchar, I'll be right back," the nurse replied.

After a few minutes, Doctor Butchar walked into Carmen's room and said, "Miss Pynkeehertz, I understand that you're experiencing pain in your left pinky."

"Yes," Carmen answered, "that was the only reason why I went to the doctor in the first place – because I have a thorn in my pinky and it hurts."

"Well!" Doctor Butchar yelled. "We had nothing to do with your pinky. We'll send you to a very competent doctor who specializes in such cases. His name is Doctor Sayahagain, and his office is at 1234 Rich Lane."

"That was the first doctor that I visited!" Carmen replied in a loud voice. "He sent me to another doctor. The second doctor sent me to still another doctor, and he sent me here. No one has removed the thorn yet!"

"We're very competent professionals here, Miss Pynkeehertz!" Doctor Butchar yelled. "It's not our fault that you don't know what you're doing. We have no choice but to send you to a psychiatric hospital where they have the best of care for people like you." Doctor Butchar walked out of the room before Carmen had a chance to respond. He went out to get another doctor to help him with the transfer. In a minute or two, Doctor Butchar walked back into Carmen's room. He was followed by Doctor Manypewlatar. Doctor Butchar didn't even remember that he had personally assigned Doctor Manypewlatar to be the anesthesiologist during Carmen's operation. "Miss Pynkeehertz," he said, "this is Doctor Manypewlatar. I don't know if you have already met him. He will assist you with your transfer to that wonderful hospital where they'll take very good care of you."

Doctor Manypewlatar then started his delivery of financial and mental cruelty. He also had a memorized speech, which he had used to tell numerous other victims as he was making the necessary arrangements for their transfers to the same doomsday hospital. He made slight changes to the speech so it would fit Carmen's situation. He concluded by telling her how high her bill was, and where she was going, "Miss Pynkeehertz, so far the total of your bill is $807,761.17. We're transferring you to Deprivayshun Psychiatric Hospital, where Doctor Ryppemuff will make sure that you're well taken care of. We shouldn't waste any more time because your condition is extremely grave. By now, you should be very grateful to us for everything that we have done for you."

Before Carmen was able to say anything, she was sedated and transferred to Deprivayshun Psychiatric Hospital for a larger dose of total cruelty. When Carmen left Kuttemopen Hospital, Doctor Butchar again called Peter at Deprivayshun Psychiatric Hospital, thinking that he was his cousin, Doctor Ryppemuff. When Peter was on the phone, Doctor Butchar said, "Hey, Rypp, Butchar again, how're you doing?"

"Okay, what's up, Butch?" Peter asked.

"I got a beautiful one for you. Her name is Miss Carmen Pynkeehertz," Doctor Butchar answered.

"Great! Is she coming now?" asked Peter.

"She just left here a few minutes ago," the butcher went on. "She'll be there soon. She's very rich. Give her the final dose and make sure that I get my twenty percent referral fee."

"I'll have no trouble remembering this time, Butch, and keep those victims coming. Okay, see ya," Peter concluded.

"Don't worry; we have plenty more victims to send you. Okay, Rypp, bye," Doctor Butchar also concluded.

Upon her arrival at Deprivayshun Psychiatric Hospital, Carmen was swiftly rushed to her room. By then, she had almost completely recovered from her sedation. She was doomed to spend the rest of her life there without any visitors, because the hospital decided that she had a contagious disease, and nobody from the outside should go near her – still no one from the outside knew her whereabouts anyway. Carmen was assigned to a room with three other patients – one was a towering man who she thought was about forty years old. Another one was a bedridden man who seemed to Carmen to be in a coma. The last one was a woman who Carmen realized was in a state of almost total confusion, because she referred to Carmen as her mother and made some other incomprehensible statements. They were all in similar situations as Carmen was, but she didn't know that then. Once in the room with the others, Carmen became acquainted with Sam Towhertz. Even though Martha Innaddayze didn't have all her faculties, she managed to say a few things that made sense, and Carmen was able to understand. Sam told Carmen about the comatose man. Of course, still no one knew that he was the real Doctor Ryppemuff.

Sam pointed towards a camera near the guard's cage and said, "Carmen, every time you talk, make sure that you whisper and face away from that camera. We're in Ward Two Seventeen – I heard a nurse mention the name a couple of days ago, and it seems like this is a prison ward, instead of a hospital ward. By the way, Carmen, why are you here?"

Carmen leaned back in her chair and replied, "I went to see someone named Doctor Sayahagain because I had a thorn in my left pinky. After doing nothing for me, Doctor Sayahagain referred me to a specialist named Doctor Byggliar for a second opinion. Doctor Byggliar didn't do anything for me either, and then he sent me to Doctor Sharlottan for a third opinion. Doctor Sharlottan ripped me off with a very high bill, and then he sent me to Doctor Butchar at Kuttemopen Hospital, where they performed several unnecessary operations on me. After they performed all that surgery, I was in terrible pain all over my entire body as a result of the operations. I was finally sent from Kuttemopen Hospital to Doctor Ryppemuff here at Deprivayshun Psychiatric Hospital. Between all the doctors involved, they have already taken about a million dollars from me, and all they have done is to cause me plenty of pain and misery. I'm still in terrible pain all over my entire body." Carmen then showed her finger to Sam and concluded, "And here I am, and look at my pinky – I still have the thorn under the skin, because they never removed it."

"Oh my God!" Sam exclaimed. "I'm here because I had a pain in my right foot, because one of my workers dropped a sledgehammer on my toe. I went through exactly the same steps as you did – I also started with Doctor Sayahagain, but I was sent to two different doctors before ending up at Kuttemopen Hospital. They also performed unnecessary surgery on me there, and I'm also in terrible pain all over my entire body. None of the doctors that I visited would even hear anything that I had to say. My toe still hurts terribly, because they never did anything about it. Between all the doctors involved in my case, they also took a lot of money from me, but my expenses have already been a lot more than two million dollars. They have also caused me plenty of pain and misery."

"This can't be real!" Carmen exclaimed. "We can't let them get away with what they have done to us. We have to do something about all this and retaliate."

"I totally agree with you, Carmen," Sam replied. "By the way, Martha has a very similar story. She doesn't remember much, except that she was at Kuttemopen Hospital, but she doesn't remember the rest of her ordeal, or how she got here. She's taking a daily dose of some medication that she says they prescribed to keep her from getting worse. The man in the bed next to her has been in that condition ever since I got here, over two weeks ago. Doctor Ryppemuff gives him a daily injection. At this point, I don't know what to believe around here."

"That's very interesting!" Carmen went on. "I wonder if there's anything in common between us. Maybe the comatose man is rich. I am a high-fashion model, and I own a cosmetics company. I am a very rich woman. Are you rich, Martha, and are you, Sam?"

"I guess I am," Martha interjected. "Oh, I don't know – I have no idea!"

"Yes," Sam answered, "as a matter of fact, I am very wealthy. I am a developer and I own a fortune in real estate. Doctor Ryppemuff told me that Martha has insurance to pay for her expenses here. Maybe you're right, and there's a connection here."

"They're probably ripping off some unsuspecting insurance company to pay for her imprisonment here," Carmen said. "I wonder if they do that, what they're doing to us, to other rich people to get money out of them!"

Sam thought for a few seconds and then replied, "That's an interesting thought, that's probably what it is. Anyway, it's getting late, and I see that Martha's getting sleepy. She's usually already fast asleep at this time. Let's go to sleep. Okay, good night."

"Good night, Sam and Martha," said Carmen.

"Good night," said Martha while staring at the ceiling.

The following morning, Peter Emppostar went into the ward and gave Carmen a big amount of the same rip-off information that he gave Sam when he was admitted. He had everything memorized, but he made slight alterations to make his speech fit different patients. "Is there anything that you don't understand, Miss Pynkeehertz?" he asked as he concluded.

Carmen was totally shocked and speechless, as Sam had been when Peter told him the same garbage. Peter assumed that she had no questions, so he left the room. As soon as Peter left, Carmen started another conversation with Sam and Martha, "Has either one of you tried calling someone outside to tell them what's going on here?"

"We're not allowed to communicate with anyone from the outside," Sam Replied. "I would like to escape, but it seems like it's impossible – the only door here is locked with five different locks. The walls are made of concrete blocks. The cups and plates are made of soft material. The utensils are also made of soft plastic, and must be accounted for after we use them, because they're collected and put back into use. There are security guards all over."

"I still think that there must be something that we can do, and we have to think of a plan to escape," Carmen insisted. They continued talking for a while, and Martha had joined in the conversation, but because of her condition, she wasn't able to contribute much to the idea of escaping. Before they realized it, it was late in the evening, and it was time to go to sleep, but they planned to continue talking the next day to try to figure something out.

Unhappy Patients

THE NEXT MORNING, AT 1234 Rich Lane, Doctor Sayahagain was getting ready to start his moneymaking day once again. A repeat patient named Sally Sonbernd walked in and introduced herself to the receptionist. Sally then told her why she was there. The receptionist, Betty Whilling, looked at Sally's records and noticed that she was only a coffee shop waitress. While Sally sat in the receptionist's enclosure, Betty went to the examining room and told the doctor that the next patient was poor. She then returned to her desk and told Sally to go see the doctor. Sally walked into the examining room and said, "Doctor Sayahagain, I don't feel any better after taking the medicine that you prescribed the other day for my sunburn."

Doctor Sayahagain looked at Sally's form just to see her name. "Well, now, Miss Sonbernd," he yell, "don't blame me if your system is intolerant to medicine! Double your dosage and take it for another week, and then we'll see!" The doctor then turned on his microphone so his receptionist could hear him and continued, "Your bill is $125, plus expenses plus other charges. Go see my receptionist and pay her. She'll give you another prescription for twice the amount of medicine. Good bye. Next!" Sally left the examining room without saying anything. She then walked out after paying her bill and taking the prescription.

After Doctor Sayahagain prescribed plenty of his "Ahs" and useless medicine to numerous easy victims, as he called them, another patient named John Suolenthom walked into the office. He stepped forward to see the receptionist. He moaned as he stood in front of her desk and told her that he was there because he was prescribed medicine the week before for a bee sting in his right thumb, and it didn't help him at all. "My thumb hurts a lot because it's swollen," he said. "I want to see the doctor right away."

Betty looked at John's records and noticed that he was a rich lock manufacturer. She then told him to have a seat in the enclosure where her desk was. She went to the examining room to tell the doctor about the rich victim. Doctor Sayahagain told her to skip all the other patients and send him in. Betty returned to her desk and told John to go see the doctor. The other patients were upset because John was called in as soon as he walked in. Betty told them that Mr. Suolenthom was having a severe heart attack and needed emergency treatment. The waiting patients accepted her explanation and continued to wait.

When John Suolenthom walked into Doctor Sayahagain's examining room, the doctor looked at his records simply to see his name and what he was complaining about – not to do something about it, but to make up a bogus name for his diagnosis of the patient. Doctor Sayahagain then started his "Ah" routine when John sat in the patient's chair, "Good morning, Mr. Suolenthom, please have a seat. Open your mouth and say, 'Ah' so we can get started."

"Didn't we go through this last week?" John asked as he shrugged. "I'm only here because my thumb is swollen. Can we skip the 'Ahs' this time?"

"Well, now, Mr. Suolenthom!" Doctor Sayahagain shouted. "If you can prove to me right now that you're a doctor, and you have already diagnosed yourself, then we can skip the 'Ahs.' Otherwise we have to go through several of them to make sure that we find your problem!"

John very reluctantly remained quiet and did as the doctor told him to do, and then he was put through a record number of "Ahs" in Doctor Sayahagain's medical career. The doctor then turned on the microphone and said, "Mr. Suolenthom, you're a tough patient. It took me a long time to find your problem, but I finally found it – based on what I saw in the back of your throat, you have an acute case of Stungosis. I'll send you for an emergency appointment with a highly recommended psychiatrist who specializes exclusively in the treatment of Stungosis. His name is Doctor Louzi. He's the best there is when it comes to Stungosis."

"Why a psychiatrist? Am I crazy or something?" asked John.

"Oh, no!" the doctor yelled. "Because of your condition, we have to prepare you for your physical treatment by sending you to a psychiatrist first. Your final bill, after a discount that I'm giving you for being such a good patient, is only $19,765. Please pay the receptionist, and she'll give you details for Doctor Louzi's appointment. Good bye."

John Suolenthom did as he was told because he actually believed that Doctor Sayahagain found something wrong with him caused by his allergic condition on his thumb. John was quite concerned because Doctor Sayahagain told him that he had to see a psychiatrist to prepare him for his physical treatment – he thought that the doctor found a very serious, if not fatal, condition. He walked out of the doctor's office very scared. After he left, Doctor Sayahagain personally phoned Doctor Louzi to remind him about his twenty percent referral fee and to give him the name of the bogus diagnosis.

In all, John Suolenthom saw Doctor Sayahagain, Doctor Louzi and Doctor Louziar. He eventually arrived at Kuttemopen Hospital where he was put through the same routine that Sam Towhertz and Carmen Pynkeehertz had been put through. The only difference was that his unnecessary surgery only had three phases – he was given a blood transfusion, a lung transplant and a triple bypass, simply because he had a swollen thumb due a bee sting, which was totally ignored by all the doctors.

John eventually ended up at Deprivayshun Psychiatric Hospital. He was assigned to the same room where Sam was with the other patients. He was in the same situation as everyone else in the room – being ripped off and suffering from total deprivation. Upon John's arrival, Sam introduced himself. He then introduced John to the others and told him everything that he had told Carmen when she arrived. Before long, they were telling each other all about their ordeals. Martha Innaddayze didn't say much, and the real Doctor Ryppemuff, of course, couldn't say anything at all.

Later on that day, Peter Emppostar went to Ward Two Seventeen to welcome John Suolenthom and brief him on hospital procedures. He told him the same thing that he had told Sam and Carmen, but he changed the speech somewhat to make it fit John's position. After Peter concluded, John was totally amazed, shocked and completely speechless after hearing all the ridiculous prices, as well as everything else that Peter told him. Peter assumed that John had no questions, so he said, "Good bye" and left. Right after Peter left, Carmen and Sam took the opportunity to speak with John about some kind of plan to do something about freeing themselves from that horrible place. They told John everything that they had talked about previously.

After hearing what they told him, John said, "I started my company manufacturing locks because I was always interested in locking mechanisms and how they worked. I invented a special lock, which is extremely difficult to pick, even by the most qualified locksmiths. However, up to this day, I have not yet found a lock that I myself couldn't pick. Therefore, I think it would be a simple task for me to open those locks on the doors so we can get out of this prison. The only problem I see is the heavy security they have around here." Right after that, they went on talking for several hours, and as the hours passed, it was time for them to go to sleep.

The next morning, at 1234 Rich Lane, Doctor Sayahagain was getting ready to start his day by severely ripping off his victims once again. His first patient walked in, and the doctor put him through his usually cruel "Ah" routine. During the next few hours the doctor ripped off numerous other patients.

Later on that day, almost at quitting time, a last-minute patient named Frank Icheethom walked into the doctor's office. He went straight to the receptionist's desk. As soon as he explained to her why he was there, he was given a form to fill out. He then told Betty Whilling, the receptionist, that he had already filled one out the week before. She then looked it up and pulled it out of a filing cabinet. Frank was then instructed to go to the examining room. He entered and sat next to the doctor. Doctor Sayahagain then started, "Open your mouth and say, 'Ah,' please." The patient did as the doctor told him, but it was getting late in the day, so the doctor was getting tired and decided to end his cruelty after taking only one "Ah" from Frank. Doctor Sayahagain then turned on the microphone and said, "That'll be $50 plus expenses plus other charges. Go see my receptionist. She'll give you the prescription for your medicine. Good bye."

"But, Doctor," Frank said as he wondered, "I'm here because I still have itchy rashes all over my left thumb, caused by some kind of allergic reaction. I was here last week, and the medicine that you prescribed for my itchy thumb didn't help me at all. Instead, it caused me to get a fever, headaches, blurry vision, rashes and a few other problems when I was in bed at night."

Doctor Sayahagain wanted to get rid of Frank as quickly as possible, so he finally looked at his application for the first time just to see his name. "Mr. Icheethom," he said, "if you were sick when you were home at night, why didn't you go to an emergency doctor?"

"Because I wanted to come here and tell you that the medicine caused all those problems," Frank answered. "I wanted to see if you can do something about it."

"How do you know that the medicine caused all that?" asked the doctor.

"Because every time I took the medicine, I got those symptoms, and the day I didn't take it, I was okay," John answered.

"Mr. Icheethom!" said the doctor as he started yelling. "You seem to be suffering from illusions and hallucinations! I have no other alternative but to send you to a psychiatrist for an immediate evaluation! Your bill is very high now because you made me work past my quitting hours! It is now $775, plus expenses plus other charges! Go see my receptionist! She'll tell you what the total is and give you instructions for your emergency appointment with the psychiatrist! His name is Doctor Louzi! Good bye! Next!"

Betty suddenly turned towards the doctor and spoke to him through the microphone, "He was the last patient, Doctor Sayahagain! There are no more patients to be called!"

"Oh, I'm sorry!" the doctor replied in a loud voice. "It's this patient's fault that I'm losing my mind." Frank was speechless, and after seeing and hearing the reaction by the doctor, he decided not to continue his pursuit of Doctor Sayahagain's unprofessional services. He walked out of the examining room and went over to the receptionist's desk. He appeared to have something on his mind, and put his head down as he walked.

As soon as Frank entered the receptionist's enclosure, she went through a series of numbers and gestures. "Mr. Icheethom," she said as she scolded Frank, "you wasted a lot the good doctor's time. You also put him through a lot of pressure and misery – you should be sent to jail for that. Your total fee for this visit is $1,865. Please pay your bill now, and I'll give you the information for you to go see Doctor Louzi."

"May I see the bill please?" asked Frank. "I'd like to see why it's so high." The receptionist handed it to him, but she didn't do it willingly. Instead, she did it with so much disgust, that it could be seen all over her face. Frank looked at the bill and started thinking again for a few seconds. "Hmm," he finally said, "this bill looks very interesting. I'm not even able to agree that it makes any sense." As soon as Frank said that, he tore up his bill and scattered the pieces all over the receptionist's desk. He didn't pay the ridiculously inflated bill, and walked out with a great deal of anger and disgust. He didn't take the information about the psychiatrist. The receptionist went running towards Doctor Sayahagain to tell him what happened, but the doctor decided to take the loss, because it was very late and he was tired.

As Frank was walking home, he decided never to go to any doctor again as long as he lived. He thought that he saved a little money by not paying the bill, but he had no idea what he really escaped from, and how much more he saved by not going to the next doctor! He saved a lot of money and a great deal of pain and misery. Maybe he even saved his own life – who knows?

The next day, when Doctor Sayahagain's office was full of patients, a man named Robert Berndhend walked in and went directly to the receptionist's desk. He explained to her that he was there because he was prescribed medicine the week before for a chemical burn on the palm of his left hand and it didn't help him at all. Betty looked at Robert's records and noticed that he was a rich scientist. She told him to have a seat right in the receptionist's enclosure, and then she walked to the examining room to tell the doctor about the rich victim – she couldn't use the microphone to talk to Doctor Sayahagain because Robert was in the enclosure. When Betty went to the examining room, Doctor Sayahagain told her to skip all the other patients and send Robert in. The receptionist returned to her desk and told Robert to go see the doctor. The other patients were upset because they saw that the patient who had just walked in was sent to see the doctor right away. Betty told them that Mr. Berndhend was having a severe brain hemorrhage and needed immediate medical attention. The other patients then felt that they had to accept what the receptionist had told them.

When Robert walked into the examining room, Doctor Sayahagain told him to have a seat next to him. The doctor immediately began the huge dose of his "Ah" routine, "Please open your mouth and say, 'Ah' for me."

"Oh my God!" Robert exclaimed. "More 'Ahs' again? I gave you twelve last week. Do I have to give you more 'Ahs' this time, Doctor Sayahagain? I'm only here because the medicine that you prescribed last week for the burn on the palm of my hand didn't work at all."

"Are you a doctor?" asked Doctor Sayahagain. "Did you diagnose yourself?"

"No, I'm not a doctor," Robert replied, "and I did not diagnose myself, but what does that have to do with the burn on the palm of my hand? For that matter, what does it have to do with the fact that the medicine didn't work?"

Doctor Sayahagain always had a convincing answer or argument. Of course, he didn't know why Robert was there to begin with, because he didn't bother to look at the paper, and he didn't pay attention to what Robert told him about the burn on the palm of his hand – he didn't care either. The doctor then said, "Your answers to my questions should let you see very clearly why I have to take more 'Ahs' from you. I am the doctor here, and I am the one who should diagnose you. Please let me do my job. I am an expert, and I know exactly what I'm doing. There's no one better than I am when it comes to what I do. We have to go through several 'Ahs' to make sure that we find the cause of whatever your problem is."

Robert reluctantly did as the doctor told him. He was then put through almost as many "Ahs" as John Suolenthom had been put through. After about half an hour of nonsense from Doctor Sayahagain, Robert was presented with a final dose of rigmarole. Doctor Sayahagain looked at Robert's form, for the first time during his rip-off scheme, simply to see what the patient's name was and to see what he was complaining about. He then turned on the microphone and said, "Mr. Berndhend, you're a good patient. It only took me about twenty two 'Ahs' to find your problem. You have an acute case of Bernosis, which is a very severe form of an extremely dangerous condition. I saw the problem when I looked in the back of your throat – right behind your tongue. I'll send you for an emergency appointment with a highly recommended psychiatrist who specializes exclusively in that field. His name is Doctor Louzi."

"Why do I have to go see a psychiatrist, when the problem is in my hand?" asked Robert.

"There are certain procedures that have to be followed in our profession, Mr. Berndhend," the doctor replied. "Don't worry, go see him, and you'll see that your problem will be resolved. Your final bill here, after a discount that I'm giving you for being such a good patient, is only $16,965. Please pay the receptionist, and she'll give you details for Doctor Louzi's appointment. Good bye. Next!"

"Wait a minute, Doctor Sayahagain, will Doctor Louzi finally look at and take care of the burn on the palm of my hand?" Robert asked. Betty didn't call the next patient because she heard Robert talking to the doctor.

The doctor, of course, answered Robert's question with another lie. All he wanted to do was to get rid of the patient and continue ripping off other patients. He then said, "He'll certainly take good care of your condition. He's the best there is when it comes to Bernosis – you'll see. Your bill is now much higher, because I had to answer your question. Go see my receptionist so she can tell you what the total is. Good bye. Next!" Following that, Robert did everything that he was told to do and left the doctor's office hoping that the next doctor would at least look at his burn. He was quite scared because he imagined that the doctor had found an infection in his throat, caused by the chemical burn.

From there, Robert Berndhend visited Doctor Louzi, Doctor Louziar and Kuttemopen Hospital. He was put through the same routine as John Suolenthom, Sam Towhertz and Carmen Pynkeehertz had been put through. He was lucky because they only performed two phases during his unnecessary operation at Kuttemopen Hospital because it was late at night and the doctors were getting tired – his prostate was removed and part of his colon was also removed, simply because he had a chemical burn on the palm of his hand, which, of course, was totally ignored.

No Hope for the Patients

ROBERT ALSO EVENTUALLY ENDED up at Deprivayshun Psychiatric Hospital. Peter Emppostar finally realized why it was that the hospital kept expanding endlessly – because the patients kept pouring in every day and never got out. That's why Doctor Ryppemuff once told Peter while they were eating breakfast at Gudphood Diner that the hospital will eventually have thousands of wards.

Robert was put through exactly the same initiation routine by Peter as the others had been put through. After Peter finished, he asked Robert if he had any questions. Of course, Robert was totally shocked, amazed and completely speechless as the others had been before him. Since he didn't respond, Peter said, "Good bye" and left.

After Peter left, Carmen, Sam and John approached Robert to get acquainted with him. Before long, they were talking about their ordeals once again. The others told Robert what they had discussed so far. After a while, they continued discussing the possibility of getting out of that infernal place. "I am a scientist, involved with chemicals," said Robert, "and I invented a very strong anesthetic which made me a fortune. I can put some ingredients together to create a drug that would knock the security guards out cold in less than a second. I can mix different ingredients to make a drug to make us immune to the anesthetic. I also know how to make a mixture of chemicals to turn hardened mortar into powder. We can use it on the mortar between the building blocks in the walls, and remove some blocks to make a hole so we can escape. It seems like we all have some special talent – let's see if we can put them altogether and come up with a plan."

"The only problem that I see, Robert," said John, "is that we don't have the chemicals necessary to make any drugs here."

"Well, leave it up to me," Robert went on. "You'll be surprised to know that simple things, such as makeup, plastic cups, rubber, urine, sweat, plastic floor tiles, paint, varnish, salt, ketchup, soap, bleach, sugar, gasoline, alcohol, ammonia and other things, have chemicals in them to make just about anything you want. I think that we can possibly get a hold of most of those things that I mentioned. The biggest problem is that we don't have any containers in which to mix and store the drug." Following that, they talked for a long time, but they hadn't yet finalized an escape plan.

As the days passed, the prisoners had managed to get away with keeping some plastic cups from their meals. They also started collecting and saving some of the ingredients that Robert Berndhend said that he could use as chemicals. By then, they had amassed a great amount. They put it all under Robert's bed, which was in a corner of the ward. Luckily, no one ever saw anything.

The prisoners also made several futile attempts to communicate with numerous hospital employees. They tried talking to janitors, food servants, linen changers, security guards, nurses, doctors, etc., but they found out that no one was willing to talk back to them, because the hospital employees were only allowed to tell them what the hospital administration had instructed them to say.

One morning, a food servant went into their room to take the breakfast orders from the patients. The servant was a woman who looked like she was in her forties. She was wearing a chef's hat, which covered her entire head, including all of her hair. Carmen Pynkeehertz noticed that the woman had been there several times before, but they never tried to communicate with her because someone else from the hospital staff had also been there at the same time. Carmen spoke to the woman to try once more to establish communication with someone who had contact with the outside world, "Good morning, lady."

The woman looked towards the direction of the security guard and noticed that he wasn't looking at them at that moment, so she replied in a whisper with her back turned towards the camera, "I'm sorry, but I'm not allowed to talk to the patients."

Carmen let out a big sigh of relief as she insisted on having some kind of feedback from the woman, "I understand, but at least tell us your name, please."

The woman looked towards the guard's cage, and when she saw that he wasn't looking at them, she said, "My name is Anna Lyphesayvar, but please don't talk to me. I have three children, and they depend on me for their full support. I can't afford to lose my job." Anna was the same woman who was turned down for a job at Kuttemopen Hospital at the same time Elizabeth Syckcolun met her there while Elizabeth was waiting for her husband, James, to be operated on. Anna was later hired by Deprivayshun Psychiatric Hospital.

"Thank you, Anna," said Carmen, "I understand, and we'll be careful from now on when we talk to you." Shortly after that, Anna left, and the foursome went into action. Carmen had established communication with Anna Lyphesayvar. She was someone who, they thought, could become an important link between them and the outside world.

"We're all rich," Sam Towhertz added, "or at least we were before we came here. Maybe we can offer Anna a great deal of money so she can help us communicate with our families. I hope Anna returns tomorrow to take our meal orders so we can make her an offer."

"I doubt it," said Carmen, "because I don't remember ever seeing the same servant two days in a row, but whenever she returns, we can talk to her." They continued talking, and after a while, they devised a plan that they thought they would execute whenever Anna returned.

The following morning, a servant went into the room to take their orders, but it wasn't Anna. Instead, it was a different woman. They were very disappointed, but Carmen approached the woman and said, "Good morning, lady, how are you?" The woman didn't answer.

"You're a very beautiful woman," said John.

"I'll give you $10,000 if you say something," said Robert as he moved closer to the woman."

"I'll give you a condominium for your family to live in if you just talk to us, as well as the $10,000 that Robert will give you," Said Sam.

"I'll make you look ten years younger," Carmen added, "in addition to what Robert and Sam will give you."

The woman still remained silent and maintained a face with a very cold look. She acted as though she were alone in the room. She never said a word to them. She walked out after taking the orders that the patients had filled out while they tried to communicate with her.

Several days passed, and every day a different servant went into the room to take their orders. They tried everything that they could think of to communicate with each servant, but not a single one would ever say anything. Finally, one morning, Anna Lyphesayvar returned to take their orders. The prisoners were relieved and ecstatic to see her there. As soon as Anna got close to them, Carmen approached her and said, "Good morning, Anna, we're very happy to see you here. How are you?" Anna very inconspicuously looked to see if the guard was watching, and she noticed that he was, so she didn't reply. The prisoners noticed and refrained from talking to her.

Anna continued occasionally looking at the guard very cautiously as she tended to her duties. After a while, she finally noticed that the guard wasn't watching anymore. "Good morning," she finally replied. "I'm sorry that I couldn't answer before, but the guard was watching."

"We understand, Anna," said Sam while letting out a sigh of relief, "thank you for risking your job by talking to us. If we ever get out of here, we'll help you, financially. We're not insane – they have us here simply to steal our money because we're all rich."

"How old are you, Anna?" asked Carmen.

"I'm thirty six, why?" Anna replied with a look of confusion on her face.

"Well, Anna, how old do you think I am?" Carmen asked.

"You look like you're about twenty seven," Anna answered.

"Anna," Carmen went on, "I'm delighted to hear that you underestimated my age. I'm actually thirty nine, and I can show you how you can look at lest ten years younger."

It seemed like Carmen hit the nail right on the head, because she had Anna's complete attention and cooperation. "Really?" Anna asked. "Wow! That would be great!"

Robert interjected and made Anna a fantastic offer, "Anna, as Sam told you, the four of us are very rich, and we can give you enough money so you can live very comfortably with your children for the rest of your life. All you have to do is deliver messages to our families."

"My goodness!' Anna exclaimed. "That sounds very appealing, but if they find out that I'm trying to help you, they'll put me in a room, just like they put you here, for the rest of my life. I don't have the means to pay for the room, but they would find the way to get insurance to pay for it plus all the other ridiculous expenses here. I can't accept your offers because I don't know what would happen to my three children if I'm locked up in this jail cell. You see, my husband left me for another woman when Bobby, my youngest child, was born. I applied for a divorce shortly after he left, and I got it right away. I went through very rough times before I started working here because my ex never helped me with their support. Now that I have a job to support them and myself, I really wouldn't want to lose it."

The prisoners understood Anna's position and decided not to pressure her anymore. A few minutes later, after they talked a little longer, Anna had to finish taking their orders and get ready to leave.

When their orders were completed, she left. Although the prisoners had noticed that the same servants didn't take their meal orders every day, after talking to Anna, they learned that the hospital purposely alternated the servants to keep them from getting too acquainted with the hospital patients. They then realized that Anna wasn't due back at least for the next two weeks. They had made tremendous progress with her, so they decided not to attempt to communicate with any of the other servants and wait until she returned.

The next morning, as expected, another servant walked into their room to take their breakfast orders. They didn't make any attempt to communicate with her at all. On the same day, late in the evening, a woman janitor walked into their room through the guard's cage to do whatever janitors did. Janitors did not alternate, and the same ones did the cleaning every day and every night at the same places. The prisoners were surprised to see her there, because they noticed that they had never seen her before. The woman had long and beautiful hair, almost down to her thighs. Her hair was done in such a way that it covered most of her face. Everyone noticed her hair, especially Carmen. The prisoners decided not to say anything to the janitor because they thought that they would be wasting their time with anyone other than Anna Lyphesayvar. They continued doing whatever they were doing while the janitor was tending to her chores. After a while, the woman was very close to the prisoners, and all of a sudden, they heard a very low voice – it was almost a whisper, "Good evening, Carmen, Sam, John, Robert and Martha." They quickly turned around in total amazement.

Carmen's face suddenly brightened up. She let out a huge sigh of relief and inadvertently said in an extremely loud voice, "Oh my God!" Security at night was much laxer – the number of guards outside was half that of the number during the day, and the guard in the cage was much more lenient, so he was napping and didn't hear Carmen when she spoke so loudly. Carmen then spoke in a much lower voice, "It's you, Anna. We couldn't recognize you with that long and healthy hair you have."

"It's me, in the flesh!" Anna replied.

"Wow!" Carmen exclaimed with a very low voice. "Without the servant's uniform that you used to wear, you're now showing your entire figure. You're very attractive, and that hair of yours makes you look great!"

"Thank you, Carmen, that's a real nice compliment," Anna replied with a big smile on her face.

"Imagine how good you're going to look if I could only help you look younger. By the way, we didn't expect you for another two weeks – why are you here now, and why are you working as a janitor?" asked Carmen.

"Well," Anna answered, "at first, I didn't want to get involved with your problems, but then I started thinking about two things. First, the future of my children, and secondly your future as prisoners here, so I changed my mind and decided to help you. After I made that decision, I wanted to help all of you so badly, that I didn't want to wait for another two weeks to be here only for a few minutes.

"I went to the administrative office of the hospital yesterday morning after I took your breakfast orders, and I told them that I needed more money to support my children and myself. I asked them for overtime hours with the hope that I would be able to come here somehow to help you, but they told me that there are too many servants as it is, and they're thinking of letting some go. I was then able to understand why it is that they have the servants do other chores and errands after we finish the business about the patients' meals — because they have too many of us, and it doesn't occupy our entire day. They also told me that there are openings for janitors at night, and the pay is higher because of a nighttime differential. When they told me that the night janitor who cleaned Ward Two Seventeen and the other two wards next to it was retiring this morning, I practically begged them for the job. Then they offered me a transfer from daytime servant, with the possibility of being let go, to nighttime janitor, with a higher salary and more job security – of course, I was delighted to accept the transfer. Even though this is an evil hospital, I still want job security because this is all I have, and I can't afford to be unemployed.

"My shift begins at six in the evening, but I had to take care of another ward before coming here. Now we can spend more time together, and with fewer security guards around. Well, here I am, ready to begin helping you."

"You're very brilliant, Anna!" Sam added. "You have already started to be rewarded for your good deed – by making more money and having more job security as a result of trying to help us. If we ever get out of this place, you'll be rewarded even further and very generously for what you have done – that is my personal guarantee, and I'm sure that the others will do the same."

After Anna told them the story, and Sam Towhertz guaranteed her that he would help her, John Suolenthom, Robert Berndhend and Carmen Pynkeehertz assured her that they would also help her very generously. Immediately after that, they went to work on their plan to escape. They knew that they had a fighting chance because they finally found a link between them and the outside world. "Anna, we need to communicate with our families," said Sam. "Can you give us paper and a pen so we can write the names, addresses and phone numbers of all the members of our families?"

"No way!" Anna answered. "It would be impossible to get any written messages out of here, because all the maintenance employees are thoroughly searched before entering and leaving the hospital. I can only bring memorized messages. It's a good thing that they don't go as far as using lie detectors when we come in and out."

The prisoners then realized that there was absolutely no way to have Anna memorize the names, phone numbers and addresses of all the members of their families. They decided that they would give her the name and address of Carmen's father, Mike Pynkeehertz. His address was 1321 Rich Lane. That information would be easy for Anna to memorize. They told her to tell him all about their situation – that was the only thing that they decided to do that night. They also told Anna that once Mike learned what was going on, he'd immediately go to a lawyer so he could demand Carmen's release. After securing her freedom, they'd go to work on the release of the rest of the prisoners.

After finishing her duties and memorizing the name and address of Carmen's father, Anna left for the evening. She'd visit Mike Pynkeehertz the next day before going back to work. The prisoners let out a sigh of relief, knowing that they'd be free soon.

Early the next morning, after not getting much sleep, Anna left her home and went to Mike Pynkeehertz's house. When she arrived, she rang the doorbell, but there was no one home. She left Mike a note saying that it was extremely urgent for him to call her regarding his daughter, Carmen. Anna then went shopping after she left Mike's house. She went home afterwards. When she got home, Mike had not called her yet. Later on that day, late in the afternoon, after managing to get a little more sleep, she went back to work.

The prisoners spent the day at Deprivayshun Psychiatric Hospital anxiously waiting for Anna's return. Eventually, she finally arrived, and they were nervously waiting to hear if she had given the message to Mike. As soon as Anna had a chance, she said, "I'm sorry, I went to see Mr. Pynkeehertz this morning, but he wasn't home. I left a note in his mail box for him to urgently call me regarding Carmen. After that, I went shopping, and when I got home, he hadn't called me yet, and I had to come back to work shortly after I got home." Anna went on about her duties as she continued talking to them as she worked. After she finished her shift, she left with the understanding that she would try again the next day. They were all very disappointed as the evening passed, but they hoped that the next day would be better.

When Anna got home, late at night, she was surprised to see that her children were still awake, but then she remembered that they had just finished school that day, and their summer vacation had started. Christine, her oldest daughter, who was sixteen years old, told her that a man named Mike Pynkeehertz had called thirteen times, asking for her. "Did he leave a callback number?" Anna asked very anxiously.

Bobby, the youngest of Anna's three children, replied before Christine was able to answer her mother's question, "I don't know."

"Yes, he did," Christine finally answered, "it's on the table, next to the phone."

Anna knew that it was late at night, but she felt sure that Mike wouldn't mind being waken up for such an emergency. She picked up the piece of paper with Mike's phone number written on it and went to her bedroom to call him. She dialed the number as soon as she sat in her bed. "Hello," Mike answered.

"Mr. Pynkeehertz, I am Anna Lyphesayvar," she started very nervously, "the one who left you a note in your mailbox yesterday in the morning. I'm sorry for calling you at this time and waking you up, but your daughter is being held captive in an evil hospital along with many other people."

Mike knew that Anna wasn't a crank caller, because she wouldn't have given him her telephone number, which was the same number that just showed up on his Caller-ID. He then let out a huge scream and turned towards his wife, Joan, "Honey! Listen to this! I have Anna Lyphesayvar on the line! She says that Carmen is being held captive in an evil hospital!" Joan suddenly rose, sat up in her bed, picked up an extension and listened in. Mike then told Anna that it was quite all right that she woke him up, and that he was glad that she called. Anna was very tired and needed to go to sleep, so she told Mike and Joan that she'd meet them at their house the next morning before going back to work so she could tell them all about it. Mike and Joan Pynkeehertz agreed to meet Anna in the morning. After they finished their conversation, they couldn't go back to sleep at all that night in anticipation of Anna's visit the next day.

The next morning, before breakfast, Anna appeared at Mike's and Joan's house. They both stayed home from work that day, and had been desperately waiting for Anna. They invited her in and offered her breakfast, which she happily accepted. While eating, Anna told them the entire story. Joan couldn't help herself and started crying as loud as she could. After Joan settled down, Anna told them what the prisoners wanted Mike to do, "Mr. Pynkeehertz, Carmen said that you should go see a lawyer so he can go to work on getting her released from the hospital."

"I'm not going to wait for any lawyer!" Mike shouted. "I'm going there myself! When you're ready to go to work, Miss Lyphesayvar, I'll go with you to get my daughter."

"No, please," Anna begged, "they'll fire me instantly, or take me prisoner, if they find out that I'm involved."

"Okay," Mike agreed, "in that case, give me the name and address of the hospital, so I can go there myself to get Carmen. We'll always remember what you have done for us, Miss Lyphesayvar." Following their conversation, Anna gave Mike the name and address of the hospital. She left immediately after that.

Mike left his home to go straight to the hospital as soon as Anna left. When he arrived at Deprivayshun Psychiatric Hospital, he went through several minutes of an extremely difficult security check while trying to get past the guard. After several minutes, he was finally allowed to enter the hospital, so he went to the information desk and started yelling, "I'm here to pick up my daughter!"

"There must be some mistake, Sir" said the receptionist. "No one ever gets released from this hospital unless they die. Is she dead?"

"She'd better not be! I want my daughter right now!" Mike yelled again.

"What is your daughter's name, Sir?" asked the receptionist.

"Carmen Pynkeehertz!" Mike answered.

The receptionist looked at the computer monitor, and after pressing a few keys, she saw Carmen's name and said, "Oh, I see. She's not allowed to have any visitors."

"Why not?" asked Mike in a very loud voice.

"According to what I see here, Sir," the receptionist replied, "she has a highly contagious disease. She shouldn't have any contact with anyone from the outside world."

"I want to see the manager! This is all I can stand!" Mike shouted again.

The receptionist left her desk in fear of being harmed by Mike Pynkeehertz. He then grabbed the phone from the desk and slammed it on the floor. In a minute or two, the security guards overpowered and handcuffed Mike. Then they took him inside to another part of the hospital. He ended up locked up in a windowless room where he waited for more than an hour while he was in a rage. Finally, a doctor walked in, accompanied by four huge orderlies. "Sir, my name is Doctor Ryppemuff," said Peter Emppostar. "I understand that you're suffering from hallucinations."

"I'm not suffering from anything!" Mike replied, while still in a rage. "I came here to get my daughter, Carmen Pynkeehertz!"

When Peter heard the name, he knew that he couldn't let Mike see the outside world ever again. "Mr. Pynkeehertz," he said, "no one ever gets out of this wonderful hospital alive. There must be some mistake."

"I want my daughter now!" Mike demanded. "And she better be alive and well!"

"Your daughter has a contagious disease, and shouldn't have any contact with anyone from the outside, Mr. Pynkeehertz," Peter replied.

"No! I will not accept that! Just let me take her home now!" Mike insisted.

"How did you find out that she's here?" asked Peter.

"Don't worry about how I found out!" Mike yelled. "Let me have her now!"

"I can see now that it's true that you're suffering from hallucinations," Peter went on. "We have to hospitalize you immediately to give you the best of care. There is no better place than Deprivayshun Psychiatric Hospital for people like you. You'll be in excellent hands here." Before Mike was able to say or do anything, he was instantly overpowered and sedated. He was then taken out of the room.

In a few minutes, Mike was brought to another room where he was doomed to spend the rest of his life. Peter purposely told the orderlies to place Mike in a bed in Ward Two Seventeen where his daughter, Carmen, was with the other prisoners. Mike was still under the influence of the sedation when he was put in a bed next to the real Doctor Ryppemuff. He was covered with a sheet, and the other prisoners didn't pay much attention, except that they wondered what the poor victim looked like. They also wondered how many unnecessary operations they performed on him before he was brought there – they didn't know that he was actually the fortunate one because he did not get any operations before he was thrown to the lions. About twenty minutes after he was brought into the room, Mike finally moved and groaned. Sam went to his bedside to try to comfort him, "My name is Sam Towhertz. How do you feel?"

"I'm a little groggy," Mike answered with difficulty. "I came here to get my daughter, but they injected something into me, and that's the last thing I remember."

"What is your name?" Sam asked.

"Mike Pynkeehertz," he answered.

When the others heard the name, everyone instantly went to Mike's bedside. Carmen started crying right away and shouted, "Oh my God! It's my father!" Mike saw Carmen and slowly rose to a sitting position. They hugged and cried for a long time. After a short while, when Mike and Carmen were fully recovered from such an emotional shock, Mike was introduced to everyone else. By then, he was fully recovered from the sedation. They quickly briefed him about the entire situation, and told him not to cause any disturbances that might hinder their escape plan. Mike thought that the whole thing was completely absurd, but he believed it all based on what had happened to him so far. He then became part of the plan to try to get out of there, but they had to wait for Anna to return that evening before doing anything else.

Shortly after Mike was fully briefed by the others about the horrible things in the hospital and their plans to escape, Peter Emppostar walked into the room to brief Mike about the ridiculous prices of everything on the menu – he told Mike the same story that he told everyone else before him. After Peter finished his rigmarole, Mike was devastatingly speechless. Therefore, Peter had a perfect record, because no one else before Mike was able to reply – they were all in a state of shock after hearing the ridiculous prices and everything else that Peter told them. Mike was no exception.

After Peter left, the prisoners had a long discussion. While they waited for Anna to return, they continued telling Mike what they had done and discussed so far. He then became part of the escape team. Mike also had knowledge of chemicals because he was a research specialist with a laboratory that specialized in new drugs. He agreed with the possibility of making the knockout drug, "Robert's idea about making a drug to knock out the guards might turn out to be a good way to escape."

"Yes, that's very true," Sam replied, "but we decided that we should try to communicate with our families, with Anna's help before doing anything else. You were our first attempt to contact someone, but as you can see, it didn't work out. We have to send another message to another family member. As soon as Anna returns, we'll give her another name and address."

That same evening, Joan Pynkeehertz called the police to tell them that her husband, Mike, was missing, but they told her that they couldn't do anything because he wasn't missing twenty four hours yet. They told her to go to Police Headquarters to report him as missing when the twenty four hours were up.

Shortly after that, Anna finally walked into Ward Two Seventeen. She was surprised to see Mike there as a prisoner. They told her what happened, and she was very concerned that the hospital administration, namely, Peter Emppostar, who she thought was Doctor Ryppemuff, would try to find out how Mike knew that Carmen was in the hospital. Because of that, they all realized that they had to work extremely fast.

After all the problems that the prisoners went through so far, at least Anna had a little bit of good news for them, "The other day, Robert told us about the things that he can use to make the knockout drug and the antidote. I took a big risk and hid some king-size plastic cups inside of the janitorial equipment when I came upstairs. I'll fill some of them with some of the cleaning solutions. I'll leave them hidden in the room under Robert's bed in case all else fails. I'll also leave a lot of empty ones under the bed so you can use them to mix the stuff – I thought that this would help."

"That's fantastic!" Robert exclaimed. "Thank you, Anna, you're a genius. I'll go to work on the drug and the antidote as soon as possible."

As the whispering continued, they decided that they would give Anna the name and address of another member of one family. They chose Sam's brother, Raymond Towhertz. They had Anna memorize his name and address. After a while, Anna finished her work. When she was getting ready to leave, she said, "I'm leaving some powder soap, as well as everything else that I used tonight. Altogether, I left a whole lot of stuff, and I'll try to bring some more tomorrow."

As soon as Anna left, the prisoners started examining, very carefully, what she had left behind. They had to use extreme caution not to arouse any suspicion from the guard. Robert, Carmen and Mike had knowledge of chemicals, but it was Robert who had the most knowledge and experience. He determined that with all the ingredients that Anna had left behind, plus everything that they had accumulated, all he needed was salt to make the antidote. Robert also concluded that he needed something strong, such as gasoline or something similar, to make the drug to knock out the guards.

Salt was not part of Anna's cleaning solutions, so the prisoners didn't know if she would be able to bring salt from the outside. They had to try to get salt somehow. Otherwise they wouldn't be able to make the antidote. Without taking the antidote, they wouldn't be able to use the knockout drug without passing out themselves, because the overpowering effects of the drug were going to be airborne.

"We have to find a way to get salt," said Sam. "There must be something we can do."

"I've got an idea!" Carmen exclaimed. "I just thought of something!"

"Good, let's hear it," Robert added before Carmen had a chance to continue.

"I have noticed that salted pretzels are on the menu," Carmen went on. "Let's order as many pretzels as we can, so we can use the salt that's on them by scraping it off."

"That sounds great," John replied, "but the only problem is that they might get suspicious if all of a sudden we order too many pretzels, when we have never ordered any before."

"That's true," Carmen replied, "but maybe there's some way to get some pretzels anyway."

"Well," Sam interjected, "let's order two pretzels each, and order some extra salt as well. After all, there's an extra charge for salt, so I think that they'll be happy to give us what we order. Besides, even if we order a lot of pretzels, people have the right to change their eating habits once in a while, but let's not order any more than two pretzels each anyway." Following Sam's suggestion, they all agreed that that would be the plan – to order two pretzels each, and some extra salt.

The next morning, when the servant took their orders, they did as they had planned, and there was no suspicion at all from the food server. Later on that morning, the servant went back to their room with everything that they had ordered. After the servant left, they scraped off the salt from the pretzels, and combined it with the extra salt that they ordered. Robert determined that they had enough salt, and it wouldn't be necessary to order anymore. Immediately after that, they started planning the process of mixing the ingredients together to make the antidote before making the knockout drug – which they couldn't mix yet because they still needed something that had a strong and overpowering smell, accompanied by fumes. They had the plan ready, but they decided to wait for Anna with news about Sam's brother, Raymond – they figured that it would be better and easier to get released from the hospital through legal means, rather than escaping.

Later on in the evening, Anna finally walked in. She noticed that the guard was looking at her, so she decided to wait before approaching the prisoners. As the minutes passed, little by little, she went closer and closer to the group, pretending that she was only tending to her chores as a janitor. After a little while, they all noticed that the guard wasn't looking towards them anymore – in fact, it appeared to them that he was leaning back in his chair, and seemed to have been napping. Sam then turned towards Anna and asked, "How did it go with my brother, Anna?"

"I'm sorry," she replied, "but I went to his house, and a neighbor told me that he was away on vacation for two weeks. He had just left this morning."

"Oh my God!" Carmen exclaimed. "One problem after another!"

After a few minutes, while discussing the situation, they decided to select another contact name. John felt that he had the perfect choice, "I should have thought of this earlier, I'm sorry, I didn't think of it – my brother, Eric, is a lawyer, and he's always available. No matter where he goes, his secretary is always able to contact him. I think that he should be able to get us out of this mess. Anna, his name is Eric Suolenthom, and you'll find him at 234 Salvayshun Street."

Anna memorized Eric's name and address and then said, "Okay, I got it – Eric Suolenthom at 234 Salvayshun Street. Anyway, I left more stuff under the bed. I even left a bottle of ammonia and another bottle half full of alcohol." Shortly after that, she left. Robert then examined what Anna had left behind. He was satisfied that he had what he needed to make the drug to knock out the guards. However, he wasn't sure how effective it would be, because what he had was alcohol and ammonia, instead of something stronger, such as gasoline – he knew that it would work, but he just wasn't sure how long the guards would be knocked out. After that, the prisoners continued their daily activities, and they had nothing else to do, except to wait. The night seemed like a century, and the next day seemed even longer.

Finally, the following night, it was time for Anna to return, but to their disappointment, another woman went into the room to do the janitorial work. They approached the woman, and Carmen asked her where Anna was. The woman looked at the guard. She noticed that he wasn't looking towards them, so she reluctantly answered Carmen's question, "Please, don't talk to me anymore. If they see me talking to you, they'll fire me. They told me that Anna went on vacation." That was a big obstacle to their plan, and the prisoners then knew that they were in big trouble. They had to act very fast, but they waited for the janitor to leave before doing anything else. However, they continued talking, but not about the plan. It was a lucky break for a change that the janitor didn't clean under Robert's bed, because if she had, she would have seen all the drug ingredients that they had under it – for that matter, she didn't clean under any other bed.

After the janitor left, Sam Towhertz assessed the situation and concluded that they should take action immediately, "We know very well that Anna didn't go on vacation. They probably found out that she was helping us and was probably fired or harmed, or both. Robert, I think that you should begin putting the ingredients together to make the antidote and the knockout drug as soon as possible."

"I know," Robert replied, "and I think that I should also make the mixture that turns mortar into powder in case we have to use it on the building blocks in the walls. We can escape through a hole in the wall by removing some blocks after the mortar between them is turned to dust. We can then bring the knockout drug with us to use it on anyone who may try to stop us." Robert Berndhend immediately started working on the mortar-powdering mixture. After a few minutes, he had mixed some ingredients together, and it was ready. He started working on the antidote next. After a little while, he had mixed all the necessary ingredients, and the antidote was also ready to be put to use, but it was late by then, and they went to sleep.

The next morning, shortly after getting up, they started working with the ingredients to make the knockout drug. They had several interruptions along the way, such as the servant taking their breakfast orders, eating breakfast and a few other minor problems. After they finished eating, and the servant took everything away, Robert continued working on the drug. It was a painstaking venture because the guard looked towards their direction several times, as Robert worked.

As the hours passed, it was already late in the afternoon, and the drug was almost ready. They decided to take the antidote before adding the final ingredient to the knockout drug, because when completed, it would give off overpowering fumes. After everyone, except Martha Innaddayze and the real Doctor Ryppemuff, drank the antidote, Robert Berndhend was about ready to add the final ingredient to the anesthetic. To make matters worse, the night janitor walked in just as Robert was getting ready to reach under the bed to take out the last thing that he needed to finish the drug. When he saw the janitor, he put everything back under his bed and waited for an opportunity to get back under it and finish the drug. He would have to do it with a great deal of difficulty due to the janitor's presence.

After a long while, Robert had been unable to get under the bed because the janitor was still in the room. All of a sudden, a big commotion was heard coming from the guard's cage. Everyone looked towards the guard. They saw a group of people in white coveralls bringing five more patients into the room. The patients were under heavy sedation and being rolled into the room in gurneys. The first patient brought inside was a woman. Following her, three children were wheeled in. Finally, the fifth patient was brought in, and it was also a woman. Mike Pynkeehertz saw the last patient who was placed into the room. He screamed in horror, "Oh my God! That's my wife, Joan!" Carmen and Mike immediately went to Joan's side and started crying.

Sam Towhertz then saw and recognized another patient, "Oh my God! That other woman is Anna! Those must be her three kids." At that very moment, the prisoners knew that they were doomed, unless they acted very quickly. With so many people around, they couldn't do anything with the knockout drug until the hospital staff left, so they waited until all the people in white coveralls were gone. After several minutes, they left the room, but the guard was looking at the prisoners, so they couldn't do anything at all. A few minutes later, the sedated patients were beginning to come to. It was then that Mike, Carmen and Joan cried as they hugged very tightly. Anna's children also started crying as soon as they came to. The guard kept watching them incessantly, but after several minutes, the prisoners finally saw him looking the other way. Then they decided to go into action because the janitor was at a good distance away from them at that moment. Robert was doing his best to attempt to give the new arrivals the antidote, but every time he tried, there was someone watching – either the guard or the janitor.

After a while, Robert finally noticed that no one was looking at him, so he thought that he had a chance at that moment. He attempted to reach under the bed to get the antidote, but just as he was about to grab it, the guard opened the door on the opposite side of the cage. When the door was fully open, the prisoners saw a doctor walking into the cage. It was Peter Emppostar. The guard closed the door and opened the door into the room to let him in.

As Peter entered the room, he walked towards the prisoners to talk to them. When he stopped in front of Sam's bed, he began talking with a look of great accomplishment and satisfaction on his face, "This is to show all of you that you can't play games with me. Ever since the day that Mike Pynkeehertz came to the hospital looking for his daughter, Carmen, I knew that there was an inside leak here. I have connections with the phone company, and we started checking phone records immediately. It didn't take me long to find out who the culprit was – when we checked Anna Lyphesayvar's records, we noticed that she had called Mr. Pynkeehertz's house. We only got that information back two nights ago while Anna was still in the hospital – probably right here in this room. We couldn't take any chances, so we had to detain her as she attempted to leave last night.

"Later, we went to her house and told her children that their mommy had been in an automobile accident, and she wanted to see them. Then, they were brought here. Finally, we went to Mike Pynkeehertz's house to get his wife, Joan. We used the same trick on her as we used on Anna's children, and we brought her here to the hospital, too – it was a good thing that we arrived in time, because she told us that she was about to go to Police Headquarters to report her husband as missing. She also told me that her husband had come here to Deprivayshun Psychiatric Hospital because someone named Anna Lyphesayvar told them that their missing daughter was here. Of course, I'm a genius, so I told her that I was from Kuttemopen Hospital, and I also told her that her husband was there.

"Once Joan and Anna's children were all here, it was easy to control them. We sedated them all as soon as they were brought to the hospital

– just to make sure that they were completely under our control. We had them in another room until we sedated them again to bring them here." Peter paused momentarily to think about what he was going to say next. At that moment, the group knew that Anna didn't deliver the message to John's brother, Eric, so they felt that they were doomed unless a miracle happened.

"We have to be very careful with mentally disturbed people such as all of you," Peter continued after a moment. "Mental illness is a very debilitating problem. Every one of you here is a menace to society, and we have to make sure that this doesn't happen ever again. I believe that we have detained everyone in the outside that knew that you were here in the hospital.

"This is a very elite and reputable medical facility, so I don't understand why you're behaving this way, because I am the best there is. I have been recognized as the top authority in the psychiatric society. My credentials have been written in every medical journal throughout the world. I have been on many talk shows as the most knowledgeable and respected psychiatrist alive. Newspaper, television and radio headlines have been so numerous, that I couldn't even begin to count them. I am the king, not to mention the fact that I am also a god, in this profession." Peter took another short break, and the prisoners were totally speechless. By then Anna's children had stopped crying.

A few minutes later, Peter went on, "The proof that I can offer you right here and now that I am the best, is your silence – you don't even know what to say to such a great man standing in front of you, because no one in the world compares to me. Anyway, to prevent any further problems here, I'm going to put all twelve of you in different rooms, and no two of you will ever see each other ever again as long as you live. Let me think for a moment to see how I'm going to handle this situation. I'll be right back." Peter then turned around, momentarily walked away from the prisoners and went towards the guard. Anna's children had already started crying very frantically again when Peter said that they would be completely separated from everyone else.

"Oh my God!" Robert desperately started thinking. "If we don't do something right now, we'll be doomed. If they separate us, we'll never escape." By then, it was already very late at night. Luckily, Peter and the janitor were far away from Robert's bed, and the guard was looking the other way. Robert managed to get under the bed to finish working on the knockout drug. He was extremely lucky because no one noticed when he went under the bed.

After a moment, Peter finally turned around and walked back towards the group. He then continued his cruelty, "If you think that you had a hard time here so far, just wait to see what you'll get in the near future – if you can survive. You should all be grateful to me for everything that I have done for you here. Instead, you have tried to do some stupid things – that's another sign of your severe mental illnesses. I think I'm going to write a long book about your cases. Such a book will educate the entire psychiatric world. They will be able to provide services that will almost rival my abilities. They will never be able to compare themselves to me, but at least, after reading my book, they may come close. I have already written many books, but this one will top them all. Okay, enough is enough. I'm going to get some orderlies right now to take all of you to separate rooms." By that time, the five sedated patients were fully recovered. They were either standing up or sitting in their beds. The prisoners were totally scared, devastated, worried and still speechless, except Anna's children, who were still crying very hysterically while holding onto their mother.

The Escape

PETER EMPPOSTAR LOOKED TOWARDS the guard's cage and was getting ready to walk away to get some orderlies. The janitor finally went to do her work around the prisoners before her shift was over. At that very moment, Robert Berndhend was coming out from under his bed with a large plastic cup in his left hand. Martha Innaddayze was standing right next to Robert. She immediately felt sleepy due to the fumes coming out of the cup in Robert's hand. She stumbled as she sat in her bed. Peter then took one last look at the prisoners before leaving. He saw Robert immerging from under his bed and spoke to him while bending down to look under it, "What were you doing under that bed? And what's all that stuff underneath? I think it's making me sleepy – what is it?"

There was no time to have the five newcomers to drink the antidote, so Robert suddenly shook the cup that he still had in his left hand. Using his right hand, he sprinkled a generous amount of the drug on Peter's face. Robert couldn't take any chances with the janitor, so he also sprinkled some of the drug on her face. Luckily, the guard wasn't watching. Robert then hid the cup, with whatever drug was left in it, behind his back while he was still holding it in his left hand. The invisible fumes from the drug overpowered everyone in the room, except those who had taken the antidote. Peter fell unconscious instantly. The janitor, Martha and the five patients who were brought in together also fell unconscious instantly.

Another lucky break was that the effects of the antidote were still in their systems, and the prisoners who drank it didn't pass out. The conscious prisoners had to act very quickly. Sam noticed that Robert still had the cup with the drug behind his back. He made a gesture for the rest of them to wait as he ran over to the guard's cage. When Sam arrived, he banged on the gate to attract the guard's attention. "Help!" he shouted. "There's something wrong with the doctor and some of the patients. Please come in and see what the problem is."

The guard looked towards Sam and the rest of the prisoners. He saw several people all over the floor, including Peter and the janitor. He then turned around to open the door on the opposite side of the cage. While the guard was facing away from the room, Sam took a good look inside of the cage. He saw something that looked like a slide, which was on the floor, and seemed to be going downwards.

The guard then called the rest of the guards who were outside, and in a few seconds, they rushed into the cage. The guard then closed the gate and opened the door into the room. As soon as all the guards entered the room, they stumbled from the effects of the invisible fumes, but it wasn't enough to knock them out. As they rushed over to the group, they saw the doctor, the janitor and four patients unconscious on the floor. They also saw Martha unconscious in her bed. When they got closer to the prisoners, Robert sprinkled another generous amount of the drug all over their faces. The guards instantly became unconscious and dropped on the floor. Luckily, all the guards passed out, because Robert didn't have much of the drug left.

The prisoners had to act very quickly again, because they didn't know the potency of the drug, and they didn't have much left. They also didn't know how long the effect of the drug was, so they didn't know how long the guards would be out cold. They had the plan all thought out. Everything else had failed so far, but they hoped that their plan would work for a change. They knew that there were monitors in the main lobby, because Anna Lyphesayvar had told them when she started helping them. They hoped that the monitors would be turned off, or that no one was watching them.

"I think we have a fighting chance now," said Mike. "We should try to run out through the cage and take some knockout drug with us to use it on anyone who tries to stop us."

"That's a good idea," John replied. "Now we don't have to use the mixture that turns mortar into powder, because we can get the keys from the guard to open the doors."

"That's right," Carmen added. "If we see any guards in the hallways, we can give them a dose of the good stuff that'll knock them out."

"Wait a minute!" Robert interjected. "We can't leave without the patients that are knocked out, and I just realized that there may be too many guards on all the other floors. We may not be able to knock them all out, because there isn't much of the drug left."

"I think I got the answer to our immediate problem," Sam interjected. "I just realized that when I walked over to tell the guard that the doctor was in trouble, I noticed something on the floor in the guard's cage that looks like a slide going downwards – it must be a laundry chute. I think we can use it to slide down, because we're only on the second floor. Even if we drop, it wouldn't be much of a problem. If it is a laundry chute, there may be some dirty laundry at the bottom to cushion our fall." Everyone agreed with Sam and decided to use his plan.

There were twelve prisoners in the room, but only ten were going to leave – five were knocked out by the drug, because they were the ones who were brought in after the other five took the antidote. The other two, Martha Innaddayze and the real Doctor Ryppemuff, were in no condition to leave – they were to be left behind for the time being.

After removing the keys from the guard's belt and opening the gate to the cage, Mike Pynkeehertz picked up his unconscious wife, Joan. Sam Towhertz picked up Anna Lyphesayvar. Robert Berndhend picked up Anna's oldest daughter, Christine. John Suolenthom picked up Anna's second daughter, Susan. Carmen Pynkeehertz picked up Anna's youngest child, Bobby. They all rushed as fast as they could towards the cage.

"I'll slide down first to make sure that it's safe," said Sam as he arrived in front of the others and placed Anna in the guard's chair. "I'm the biggest one here, so, if I can slide all the way down, then everyone else should be able to make it. Once I get to the bottom, I'll tap on the metallic chute three times very rapidly as a signal that everything is fine. Then you can slide the unconscious people down, one at a time. Wait each time until I tap three times again. After the unconscious people are all down, then the rest of you can slide down, one at a time, after hearing three taps."

They then proceeded as planned. Sam slid down the chute first, and Lo and Behold, everything went perfectly well. To his own pleasant surprise, he landed right into a laundry truck, which was just about full. He tapped on the chute three times. Almost instantly, he saw one of the children sliding down. After placing the child in a safe place, he tapped three times again, and the process continued until everyone was in the laundry truck. They decided to stay in the truck and wait for it to leave – even if it meant waiting what was left of the night. They covered themselves completely with bed sheets to prevent anyone from seeing them, because it was an open truck. To their amazement, the truck driver arrived about five minutes later – the timing couldn't have been any better. The driver got into the cabin and drove away to bring the laundry to a commercial wash a few miles away.

As the truck was disappearing into the darkness, the unconscious people were beginning to wake up. A few minutes later, a little before dawn, the truck driver decided to stop at a local diner to get some coffee. By that time, everyone was fully recovered. While the driver was in the diner, the prisoners decided to get out of the truck and run for it, in case the truck was followed – because they knew that the guards and Peter, who they thought was Doctor Ryppemuff, would also be recovered by then. They were having a streak of good luck for a change, and hoped that it would continue. Luckily, across the street from the diner, there was a car and limousine company. They went there and hired two limousines. They were then driven to John's house.

After about five minutes, they arrived. John got out, went towards his house and rang the doorbell. Margaret, his wife, opened the door and saw him standing there, totally disheveled. She started crying immediately, and they embraced very tightly. "Oh my God!" said Margaret. "It's you, John. "Where have you been?"

"It's a long story, Dear," John replied as he cried.

"You have been missing for about three months," Margaret went on. "The police looked all over for you for a long time. They still stop by occasionally to see if you have returned, and to tell me if they have any leads."

"I'll tell you what happened soon," John replied.

"Come on in and tell me all about it," said Margaret.

"Not now," John went on, "I need some money to pay the limousines outside. I also have some people in the limousines waiting to come in. We're all in big trouble." Margaret didn't say anything else. She then went inside and got some money for John. When she returned, John went back towards the limousines to pay the drivers and to bring the other people into the house.

A minute or two later, everyone entered the house. Once inside, the group told Margaret their entire ordeal. It was then that the five people who didn't take the antidote learned about their ingenious escape. They were very grateful to the others for having rescued them, especially Anna because her children were all safe and sound. Margaret was speechless for a long time, but she eventually regained her ability to talk, "I really don't know what to say, except that they have to be punished for what they did."

After a while, everyone had a chance to bathe. Margaret managed to get clean clothes for everyone. Following that, they sat at the table to eat. "We have to notify the authorities," said John while the other prisoners ate. "I'll call them right now." When John was about to pick up the phone to call the police, someone knocked on the door. He walked away from the phone and went to see who it was. As soon as he opened the door, to his amazement, there was Peter Emppostar, the fake Doctor Ryppemuff. When John saw Peter standing there, he yelled very loudly, "Oh my God! Here we go again!" John then made a futile attempt to shut the door and leave Peter outside, but two huge orderlies who were standing next to Peter rushed in to stop John from closing it. The trio then rushed in, followed by numerous other orderlies. Some of the orderlies instantly overpowered everyone in the house, but due to Sam's size and strength, it took four very large orderlies to totally subdue him.

Peter then mocked the prisoners with a great deal of pleasure. "So you thought that you could escape, huh?" he said as he started laughing very loudly. In a few seconds, he went on after he stopped laughing, "Just wait and see what will happen to all of you in the days to come. It took me a while to come out of the effects of the drug that you sprinkled on my face. As soon as I came to, I noticed that you were all gone. I reviewed the security tapes and saw your entire escape. I have to admit that it was a good plan, but not good enough against a genius like me.

"I called the police and told them that ten dangerously insane people had escaped from the hospital. I also told them that you were extremely resourceful and possibly armed. They put out an all-points bulletin to look for you. I knew that you'd have to be in one of your homes, so I went to two other houses before I hit the jackpot here – well, here I am.

"I will inject every single one of you with a very powerful drug that will keep you knocked out for at least twenty four hours – it's bear tranquilizer. I will call the media before I bring you back to the hospital so I can become a hero when they broadcast my personal capture of the ten dangerous and insane people who had escaped from my wonderful and lovingly caring hospital. After that, I'll bring you back to the hospital where you belong, but this time I'll put all of you in different rooms from the beginning. Then I'll call the police to see if there's a reward for your capture.

"When I reviewed the security tapes, I saw that the guard in Ward Two Seventeen wasn't looking at us when you sprinkled the stuff on my face – I fired him on the spot. I also saw that the four guards that were supposed to be watching the monitors in the main lobby weren't doing their job either – two of them were sleeping, one had gone into a linen closet with a nurse about twenty minutes before that and the last one was doing something with the receptionist right on top of her desk – I also fired them all. I'll have to hire fifty more guards to make sure that my wonderful hospital is well-guard against evil people like all of you. I'll also raise the prices of everything in the hospital in order to cover their salaries.

"If you thought that the prices were high when you were there, wait until you get back – you're going to see what 'High' really means. The extra cost will come out of your own bank accounts now, for being so stupid. Okay, enough is enough. I will now get the syringe ready to inject you, one at a time, and with pleasure." Peter took a syringe and a large bottle of bear tranquilizer out of his medical bag. He started getting the syringe ready with the intention of filling it with the drug. At that moment, Anna's children started crying very frantically – neither Anna, nor anyone else was able to soothe them, because everyone was being overpowered by the orderlies – because of that, Anna started crying as well.

At that very moment, half a block away, there was a police car approaching the house – Officer Gudkopp was making a routine stop to tell Margaret Suolenthom that they had no leads on John's disappearance, and to see if she had any news. As soon as he arrived, he saw an unusually large number of cars parked very disorderly all around the house. One of the cars had MD license plates. Among the cars, there was also an ambulance. Officer Gudkopp immediately thought that the ten escapees had stolen the ambulance and several other cars to make their getaway. He assumed that they were in the house terrorizing Margaret, so he remained out of sight and quietly called Police Headquarters for backup. He then waited for their arrival.

Within a few minutes, several police cars arrived. Many high-ranking officers were present, including the top brass, Commissioner Gudboz. The commissioner took a bullhorn and got out of his car. He was very cautious, so he took a body shield and approached the house. Several officers, also using body shields and drawn weapons, accompanied him.

Meanwhile, back in the house, as soon as Peter was ready to inject the first victim, everyone heard a very loud voice coming from outside: "THIS IS COMMISSIONER GUDBOZ! WE KNOW YOU'RE IN THERE! COME OUT WITH YOUR HANDS UP!"

Peter hid the syringe and the bottle of bear tranquilizer in his robe pocket and went to the door. He opened it, put his hands up and said, "I am Doctor Ryppemuff, and I have single-handedly captured the ten escaped dangerously insane people. I have them overpowered. Come in and see for yourselves."

The commissioner and the officers cautiously and swiftly rushed into the house. They saw that the orderlies were overpowering the ten people. The commissioner was aware of their escape, so he sided with Peter, "I am Commissioner Gudboz, and we can take it from here. Thank you, Doctor Ryppemuff, for your assistance. You'll be highly commended for your actions."

"Thank you for coming, Commissioner Gudboz," Peter replied, "but we don't need you, because we have everything under control. You can go now, and we'll handle it all the way from here. We'll take the escapees back to the hospital where they belong."

"I can't do that, Doctor Ryppemuff," said the commissioner, "because we have certain rules and regulations that we must follow regarding such incidents. We have to take the prisoners to Police Headquarters. Because they were on the lam, they belong to us for now."

"Excuse me, Commissioner Gudboz," Robert Berndhend interjected, as Peter and the Commissioner were talking, "we're not the bad guys – they are. That doctor is insane and held us as prisoners against our own will just because we're rich, and he's stealing our money. We can prove to you that..."

The commissioner abruptly interrupted Robert, "Sure, sure, that's what they all say. Tell it to the judge."

"That's right," said Peter Emppostar in a rather loud voice, "that's what all insane patients say about their good doctors!"

John then made an attempt to reason with the commissioner, "Commissioner Gudboz, I am John Suolenthom, and I live in this house with my wife, Margaret. Robert is right, we're not the bad guys – they are. That doctor held us as prisoners in an evil hospital to steal our money. You know that I have been missing for a few months – ever since I was captured and placed there, with the rest of these people, against my own will."

"Yeah, okay," the commissioner responded to John's desperate attempt to reason with him, "now I see the whole thing very clearly – your reported disappearance was just a farce to make us believe that you were missing, when you were actually put in a psychiatric hospital because you have some kind of mental disorder."

"You're very bright, Commissioner Gudboz," Peter added. "You hit the nail right on the head, and that's exactly what happened. He's totally and dangerously insane. If you don't let me keep the patients, they will become a HUGE problem for you."

"That may be so, Doctor Ryppemuff," the commissioner went on, "but I can't let you have them, because we have rules that we have to follow. My final word is that these people will be taken to Police Headquarters. They will be put in a jail cell for proper processing. Insane or not, they'll have the right to an attorney when they're in my hands." Peter's plan was beginning to backfire right in his own face. He decided that he shouldn't argue with the commissioner, and wait for the process to take place. He felt that the entire matter would be resolved in a day or two, and that the prisoners would eventually be released to him.

Shortly after that, while the orderlies were still holding the prisoners, the commissioner read them their rights. They were handcuffed and taken to Police Headquarters for processing. On their way there, some of the prisoners attempted several times to talk to some of the officers and tell them the truth, but the officers thought that they were insane and making it all up.

The Imprisoned Patients

UPON ARRIVING AT POLICE Headquarters, the prisoners were all placed in a very large cell. The Public Defender and the District Attorney were immediately notified, so they could assign counselors to the case for a speedy trial. Shortly after that, a man was let into the cell – he was a very young man, very neatly dressed in a suit and tie. He was carrying a briefcase. He was a man of average weight, height and looks. The only distinguishable characteristic was that he had a very small mole on his forehead. He nervously approached the prisoners, "Good afternoon, my name is Gene Lissenzwel, but you can call me Gene. I am a lawyer, and I am with the Public Defender's Office. I am here to defend you. I understand that you escaped from a mental institution. Everyone wants freedom, but they say that you're dangerous and shouldn't be free. You're all being charged with unlawful escape and an unprovoked assault on several hospital workers, including the Director himself. Please explain to me the circumstances under which you committed the alleged assault. Tell me the details during your escape as well." Gene Lissenzwel was the same young man who celebrated his last year of law school with his parents at Gudphood Diner while Doctor Ryppemuff and Peter Emppostar ate and talked there at the same diner. He was only twenty two years old, but he was already a lawyer because he attended summer school, and also because he took a heavy load during his college years.

Sam approached Gene, who was very concerned about that huge "insane" man who was about to stand next to him – Sam was well over six and a half feet tall and had a strong and robust physique. "My name is Sam Towhertz," he said as he stopped and stood next to Gene. "Please, Gene, hear what we have to say. We're not insane, Doctor Ryppemuff is."

"If that's the case, why were you in a mental institution, instead of Doctor Ryppemuff?" asked Gene.

"Thank you, Gene, for talking to us and especially for being willing to listen to us," Sam replied as he let out a sigh of relief. "We were in a mental institution because we're all wealthy, except for Miss Anna Lyphesayvar and her family. She was there for trying to help us escape, and her family was there because Doctor Ryppemuff took them as prisoners after he maliciously drugged her to lock her up with us."

Gene Lissenzwel was a good listener, so he listened well and spent a long time listening to what they had to say. After a while, they told him the whole story, and he thought that it was ridiculously unbelievable. Gene also felt that it was so crazy, that it had to be a figment of someone's imagination. However, he wasn't sure of that, because they were very well-spoken and used good manners – and especially because he didn't detect anything that indicated to him that they were insane. Gene then decided to test them out – he asked Sam to walk with him to an isolated corner where they could talk alone. When they got to the corner, Gene wasn't nervous anymore, in spite of Sam's towering size. Gene asked Sam a few questions and then asked him to go back to the group. When Sam joined the group, Gene called John Suolenthom to join him at the corner. When John was with him, Gene asked him the same questions that he had asked Sam – John's answers were identical to Sam's answers. Gene decided to try one more, so he called Carmen to the corner. He asked her the same questions, and again, her answers were identical to Sam's and John's answers.

After the results of that test, Gene was beginning to wonder if it was all true, so he decided to conduct a few more tests, which finally convinced him that they weren't lying. He then said, "I believe that you're all telling me the truth. I have to speak with my boss and tell him all about this, but in the meantime, we have to prepare for your arraignments, which will probably take place very soon."

Coincidentally, just as Gene Lissenzwel finished saying that to the prisoners, another young man, also dressed in a suit, was let into the jail cell. The man saw Gene, also well-dressed and holding a briefcase, and said, "Hello. I assume that you're the defense attorney."

"Yes, I am. My name is Gene Lissenzwel, and I assume that you're the prosecutor."

"Yes I am. My name is Thomas Nuattie, and I would like to talk to the prisoners." Because Gene was present, the prosecutor started talking to the prisoners. Gene still had some unfinished business with the prisoners – mostly, he had to talk to them about the arraignments, but he decided to hold off until Thomas concluded his visit. In another few minutes, Thomas finished with the prisoners and told Gene that the arraignments were going to take place in about an hour. The prosecutor left immediately after that. Gene then had to rush while preparing the prisoners and himself for the arraignments. Shortly after that, they were taken to the courthouse, where they spent a few hours.

After they finished in court, Gene said to the prisoners, "I'll return to your jail cell as soon as I have some information for you. Let's hope for the best, and see if we can get you out of jail and into your homes as soon as possible. We have less than four weeks for your court appearance, so I have to work very fast." Gene then left and went back to the Public Defender's Office, and the prisoners were brought back to the jail cell. After they were left alone, they started talking and realized that perhaps they had a fighting chance. They had finally met someone who seemed to believe them, so they were anxiously waiting for Gene's return.

After a while, Gene arrived at the Public Defender's Office and told his boss the whole story that the prisoners had told him, and that he believed them. "Come on now, Gene," said Benjamin Diphycolt, "don't you know that insane people have great talents? They know how to lie and sound real!"

"I don't believe they were lying, Sir," Gene replied.

"Gene," the difficult boss continued, "I remember the time when an insane prisoner had everyone convinced that he was an illegally ousted prime minister of a European nation. He sounded very real and had some people, just like you, totally convinced. They found out later that he had been a homeless man most of his life, and that he had also spent many years in mental institutions."

"Mr. Diphycolt," Gene insisted, "I know how you feel, but I put them through some testing of my own, and found out that they were telling the truth."

"Testing of your own?" Benjamin shouted. "Are you an expert in formulating tests? Are you an expert in interrogating witnesses?"

"No, Sir," Gene answered, "but believe me, because I know that they're telling the truth and they're not insane."

"You're a test and an interrogation expert," Benjamin went on, "and now, all of a sudden, you're also a psychiatrist, because you just concluded that they're not insane. What makes you so highly qualified, Gene?"

"Please, Sir," Gene begged, "let me help them, because I do believe them, and I'd like to defend them."

"Gene," the boss added, "you have been with us only four months, and you were fresh out of law school when you joined us. What qualifies you to make such statements?"

"Sir," Gene insisted, "if you'd only let me prove it to you, you'll see that I'm right."

"End of discussion, Gene," Benjamin demanded. "Just go back to them and put them through the system, so they can return to the hospital for treatment. If you keep this up, you may have a very difficult time trying to convince someone else to hire you."

"What did you mean when you said, 'Put them through the system,' Sir?" asked Gene.

"I meant that you should just be there to take their information and act as a clerk, not as a defense attorney," Benjamin replied, "and let the other side win the case. There's no sense in defending a bunch of low-lives. That'll make your life a lot easier – believe me because I've been doing it for years, and look where I am today!" Gene stopped arguing with his boss, but he knew that he had to do something about the prisoners. He walked out of Benjamin Diphycolt's office with a lot on his mind. Shortly after that, he left the Public Defender's Office and went home.

The following day, Gene went back to the jail cell and told the prisoners the bad news. He also told them that he wasn't giving up and that he was going to do his best to get them out of that mess. Following that, he started collecting as much information as he could from the prisoners so he could go back and approach his boss again. After Gene wrote down everything that the prisoners told him, he left the jail cell. After that, he had to do a lot of legwork to confirm everything that the prisoners had told him. After several phone calls and trips, he was definitely convinced that everything was true. He had enough evidence to bring the case to trial, but he decided that he was going back to his boss to tell him all about it. It was too late to go back to the office that day, so Gene decided to go home and approach his boss the next day. When he got home, he spent several hours putting all the material in order. He was all excited with the possibility that his boss would finally listen to him. He planned to show Benjamin Diphycolt all the hard evidence that he had.

The following day, first thing in the morning, Gene went back to work at the Public Defender's Office. When he arrived, his boss wasn't there yet, so he went to his own desk and continued going over his material. After a while, as soon as Benjamin Diphycolt walked in, Gene very reluctantly went into his private office to talk to him, "Sir, I have plenty of evidence to prove that the prisoners are telling the truth – I have it all here. When you see the evidence, you'll also be convinced that it's all true."

"That's enough, Gene!" said the difficult boss in an extremely loud voice. "Pack your bags and go look for another job! You spent four months assisting other lawyers, and I can't believe that you messed up on the first case that I assigned entirely to you! You'll never amount to anything in the legal profession! I'll have no recommendation for you, so, when you go out looking for employment, make believe that this job never existed! Good bye!"

Gene was totally devastated because he came from a poor family, and he needed the job to survive. He was in a state of near panic and decided to take one last shot, "I'm sorry, Sir, but I was hoping that you'd at least hear what I have to say."

"GET OUT!" the non-listener shouted. After collecting all his belongings, Gene walked out and decided to go home before telling the prisoners the bad news. Benjamin Diphycolt immediately assigned another attorney, who happened to be loafing around in the office at that moment, to put the prisoners through the system as quickly as possible. A few minutes later, the assigned lawyer left the Public Defender's Office and went to Police Headquarters to talk to the prisoners.

About an hour later, the newly assigned attorney entered the jail cell and approached the prisoners. He didn't have any unique physical characteristics, except that he spoke and moved around very fast. He started talking to the prisoners in a very rapid manner that sounded almost like a rattle, "My name is Jesse Louziloyar, but you may call me Mr. Louziloyar. I'm here to process you. Please let me have all your names so I can put you through the system very quickly. You'll see that with me here, you won't have to spend too much time in jail."

After a few minutes, Jesse had written down everyone's name. He also made a notation next to each prisoner's name in order for him to be able to distinguish between them. Otherwise he wouldn't be able to tell which name belonged to which prisoner. For instance, next to Carmen Pynkeehertz's name, he wrote: "The tall beautiful woman." Next to Sam Towhertz's name, he wrote: "The huge guy." Next to Anna Lyphesayvar's name, he wrote: "The woman with the long and beautiful hair." He also made unique and descriptive remarks for everyone else.

"Mr. Louziloyar," asked Sam Towhertz when he saw Jesse put all his papers in a briefcase, "what happened to our attorney, Gene Lissenzwel?"

"Mr. Lissenzwel is no longer with the Public Defender's Office," Jesse answered. "He was fired this morning for failing to process you properly."

"What did he do wrong, Mr. Louziloyar?" asked John Suolenthom.

"I don't know for sure," Jesse answered. "All I know is that he didn't want to obey my boss. Gene is a novice, just out of law school. You're better off with an experienced attorney like me. I have been with the Public Defender's Office over ten years, and I have never messed up yet – all my cases have been processed right through the system, very fast and without a single glitch."

"I'm glad to hear that, Mr. Louziloyar," Carmen Pynkeehertz interjected. "Does that mean that you'll get us out of here so we can go home?"

Jesse took out some papers from his briefcase and looked at them for a few seconds until he saw Carmen's description, and then he answered her question while putting the papers back in the briefcase, "You have to understand, Miss Pynkeehertz that it all depends on the judge. Okay, I have all the information I need. I'll be back sometime in the near future to tell you what you'll have to say when you appear in court. Good bye."

"Aren't you going to ask us any questions, Mr. Louziloyar?" asked Robert Berndhend, as Jesse started to walk away.

Jesse again took out the papers and looked at them momentarily until he saw Robert's description, and then he answered while putting the papers back, "Mr. Berndhend, there's no need for me to ask you any questions, because the judge won't believe anything that you tell him anyway. My advice to you is that you cooperate fully so you won't have to endure any more hardship. Okay, good bye"

"Listen to us for a minute, please, Mr. Louziloyar," Carmen begged. "We're not insane. We were held as prisoners in an evil mental institution just because we're all rich, and Doctor Ryppemuff wants to rip us off as much as he can. He doesn't want to lose the money that he's taking out of our bank accounts every month – that's the only reason why he wants us back."

For a change, Jesse didn't have to look at the papers to remember Carmen's name, and he said as he started laughing, "That was a good one, Miss Pynkeehertz. Okay, I really have to go now. I'll get back to you. Good bye." The lousy lawyer then walked out.

Sam let out a big moan and said, "Oh my God! That attorney is definitely not even going to try to defend us. He just wants to process us right through the system, as he said. With him on our side, we'll end up right back in that infernal place in no time."

Carmen agreed, "That's right, and now we're really doomed." Because of what Carmen said, the children started crying again very frantically, but that time they had all the prisoners there, who did their best to try to cheer them up, especially the women.

When Gene got home, after being fired from the Public Defender's Office, his mother was out visiting her sister, and his father was still at work. Gene didn't have a chance to tell them anything at that point. After he had something to eat, he went back to the jail cell and told the prisoners what happened at the Public Defender's Office. "I guess you don't know that they have already assigned another lawyer to represent us – do you, Gene?" asked Carmen.

"Wow!" Gene replied. "No, I didn't know that, but I'm shocked to hear that my ex-boss did it so quickly."

"Actually, Gene," said John, "the new attorney didn't even want to hear anything that we had to say. Robert asked him if he was going to ask us any questions, and he told him that there was no need for him to ask us anything, because the judge won't believe anything that we tell him anyway. Then he told all of us to cooperate fully so we won't have to endure any more hardship. At that point, Gene, we all knew that he wasn't on our side."

"What's his name?" asked Gene.

"Jesse Louziloyar," John answered.

"Oh, Jesse, no wonder!" said Gene. "You're right, John, he's not on your side at all. He's only on his own side – to make his job as simple as possible."

"Gene," Sam interjected, "we know very well that he will do his best to send us back to the hospital, because he didn't say that he was going to defend us, or even represent us. Instead, he said that he was going to process us and put us through the system very quickly."

"You're also right, Sam," Gene replied, "he's always sitting around in the office, doing nothing other than rattling his tongue very fast – he's good at that. Whenever he handles a case, he helps the other side win, and my ex-boss loves him for that – because he finishes every case very fast. And it's true that he doesn't defend anyone – he just processes all his clients right through the system to get rid of them as quickly as possible."

"Gene, do we have the right to hire you and fire Jesse Louziloyar?" asked Anna.

"Definitely," Gene answered, "but you'll have to fire him before you hire me, even without pay, so I can continue coming here to talk to you. I'll be your pro bono attorney if you decide to take me on.

I want to continue defending you because I believed that you were all telling the truth even before I checked all your stories. After I checked out everything that you told me, I found out that I was right in believing you. By the way, one of the things that I found out when I was checking out your stories was that Doctor Ryppemuff has taken control of all your bank accounts, including yours, Anna, which has the lowest balance."

"Oh my God!" Anna exclaimed. "He has also taken away the little money that I have in the bank! Okay, Gene, how do we fire Mr. Louziloyar if we're here, locked up in this jail cell?"

"It's very simple, Anna," Gene answered, "the next time he comes over, simply tell him that he's fired. He'll have no choice but to step aside." All the prisoners agreed to fire Jesse Louziloyar, and promised Gene that they would pay him very well after his successful attempt to defend them – after all, they had nothing to lose and plenty to gain. Gene then concluded his business in the jail cell and left.

Luckily, a little after Gene left, Jesse Louziloyar went back to the jail cell because he forgot to ask the prisoners their dates of birth. As soon as he walked in, all ten prisoners, one by one, instantly fired their useless attorney before he even had a chance to speak – Jesse's rattling tongue, as Gene had put it, seemed to have been inoperative at that moment, and he had no choice but to leave.

Later that day, Gene went back home and finally told his parents what happened at his job. He also told them the whole story about the prisoners. They were confident that Gene was right and they had faith in him, so they wanted to help him financially so he could continue representing the victims, but they didn't have much money in the bank after putting Gene through law school. Gene's father, Anthony, was a janitor, and his mother, Annette, was a housewife. They owned a small house, which they managed to buy many years before. The mortgage was almost paid off, and they decided to refinance the house and get as much money as they could so Gene could go on with his case.

Later on the same day, Gene went back to the jailhouse to tell the prisoners the good news – that his parents were getting an equity loan on their home to keep things going while he represented them pro bono – the prisoners were totally ecstatic to hear the news. They had grown fond of Gene. Most importantly, he believed them, and he was all they had. They told Gene that right after he left the jail cell, Jesse Louziloyar returned, and they never knew why he did, because they fired him instantly before he was able to talk. Gene was extremely glad to hear the good news, "I'm very happy that you fired him. I'm sure that he would have sent you right back to the hospital. Anyway, now that we can proceed with the case and bring it to trial, I will consult a psychiatrist named Doctor Gudsyke. He will come here alone and give you all a psychiatric evaluation so I can put him on the witness stand." After a few more minutes, Gene left, and the prisoners were totally hopeful at that point. Later on that day, Doctor Gudsyke went to the jail cell and gave the prisoners a complete mental evaluation.

The prisoners' court appearance finally came up. To everyone's amazement, Gene managed to convince the judge that he wanted to bring the case to a trial by jury. The judge then set up a date for the trial. By that time, Gene knew a great deal about all the doctors that the prisoners visited before they were imprisoned at Deprivayshun Psychiatric Hospital. When he got home that day, he asked his father if he could go to work a couple of hours late the next day, because he wanted to send him out to do an errand that he thought was extremely important to the case.

That same day, Gene asked the assigned prosecutor, Thomas Nuattie, to meet him at Judge Pharemynded's office later that day because he wanted to talk to the judge about the case. Gene told Thomas that he'd call him later to give him a time, and the prosecutor agreed to be there.

At about the same time, Jesse Louziloyar arrived back at the Public Defender's Office and told Benjamin Diphycolt that he had been fired by the prisoners. "Those people mean nothing but trouble," the difficult superior replied. "I'm glad that they fired you anyway, because I can use your great talents doing better things around here. They're all insane and belong back in the hospital. Without you there, they'll spend more time in jail, but they'll end up in the hospital anyway – you'll see. I'll keep a close look on the case as it progresses. Anyway, it's late and I want to go home. Good night, Jesse."

"Good night, Ben," said Jesse.

Shortly after that, Gene phoned the prosecutor and told him at what time he'd be in Judge Pharemynded's office the next day.

Early the following day, Gene's father left his house to do the errand that Gene had instructed him to do. When he finished, he went home and left something for Gene on the kitchen table. From there, he went to work. A little after his father left, Gene went home for a few minutes and saw what his father had left for him on the table. Gene then took it with him.

That same day, a little later, Peter Emppostar went to the courthouse to see Karl Ondetayke to try to pay him to forge a court order to get the prisoners released to him immediately, but when he arrived, he found out that the corrupt clerk had been fired for forging an affidavit. Peter then had no choice but to try to apply for a legal court order claiming that the prisoners were insane. Judge Pharemynded denied it because he didn't know anything about the case, and Peter didn't present a situation where the judge believed that Peter should have the prisoners back at that time.

Coincidentally, right after Peter left Judge Pharemynded's office, Gene entered and saw that Prosecutor Thomas Nuattie was already there. Gene showed the judge a great deal of evidence that proved that some of the prisoners had undergone very serious operations, and also that there were children involved. Gene told the judge that he had very powerful evidence that proved that the prisoners were not insane or guilty of any crime. He then made an unusual request – he asked the judge to make sure that all the prisoners, because of their condition, were kept together and as comfortable as possible while they were in jail. After carefully reviewing all the evidence, Judge Pharemynded showed Gene Lissenzwel that he was more than fair-minded. He prepared a court order in which he stipulated something that was extremely unusual – he ordered the police commissioner to put the prisoners in adjacent hotel rooms until the trial was over. However, he did order armed guards to be placed at the door of each room, and the windows to be safeguarded. The judge also ordered all the phones to be removed from their rooms, but he ordered the televisions to remain. The prisoners were to be treated as regular hotel guests and given three square meals daily – it was all at taxpayers' expense. Gene very humbly thanked the judge and left his office to go home to take a break for a while. He intended to go back to the jailhouse after his break, to talk to the prisoners again and give them the good news.

Before the prisoners were transferred to the hotel, Peter went back to the hospital to think about a plan to get the prisoners back. He thought of finding another way to forge a court order, but instead, he decided to go to the jailhouse and tell the captain in charge to release them pending the legal papers. When Peter arrived at Police Headquarters, he told the captain what he wanted, but the captain rejected Peter's request, "Without the actual court order, I cannot do it." Peter continued insisting that the captain should do as he requested, but because the captain didn't budge, Peter eventually gave up and went back to the hospital.

When Peter Emppostar arrived at the hospital, he started talking to people to see if anyone knew of any other way to get the prisoners back. A doctor suggested that he should go to court to get them back. Peter then had no choice but to listen to him. He went to court immediately to file a case against the prisoners. When Peter filed the case, one of the clerks handling it knew Gene Lissenzwel personally – they had met during one of the many visits that Gene made to the courthouse when he was assisting other lawyers while he was employed by the Public Defender. The clerk had already learned that Gene was the defense attorney, so he called his house to tell him about it. When Gene found out, he was very worried because then he knew that he would have to fight against the prosecutor and, most likely, an experienced attorney that Peter, who Gene thought was Doctor Ryppemuff, would be hiring to help him put the prisoners back in the hospital. Gene also knew at that point that there would be two separate trials, which meant that the prisoners would have to remain detained much longer – because preparing for both trials would delay the process. He had to think very hard to try to resolve that huge problem very fast.

Later that day, Gene finally thought of something that he wanted to try. He called Thomas Nuattie to ask him to meet him at Judge Pharemynded's office again, because he had something else to discuss with the judge. The prosecutor once again agreed to be there. Gene then went back to see Judge Pharemynded to make an even more unusual request than the one he had previously made. Shortly after Gene entered the judge's office, Thomas arrived, and Gene said, "Your Honor, I really don't know what else to do, but I have such a big problem that I would like to humbly ask you to do something that is extremely unusual."

"You were here earlier today," said the judge, "and I have already done something that is extremely unusual. Well, let's hear what you have to say this time."

"Thank you, Your Honor," Gene went on, "as I told you when I was here before, there are three young children involved in this case, as well as four adults who recently underwent various major operations. Now the defendants have to endure a criminal trial and a civil trial, because the doctor in charge of the hospital from which they escaped has filed charges against them to get them back. Your Honor, would it be too much to ask if I humbly beg you to combine the two trials into a single trial, and have the prosecutor and the doctor's attorney there simultaneously?"

The judge acted very confused and exclaimed, "Oh my God! That is something unheard of. Are you insane, Young Man?"

"Forgive me, Your Honor," Gene replied, "but I really think that the defendants wouldn't be able to endure two separate trials, because four of them are still in pain as we speak, and if the children remain as prisoners too long, I think that they will suffer severe psychological problems later on in life."

"Well," said Judge Pharemynded, "let me think for a moment to see what can be done here."

"Thank you, Your Honor," Gene responded with a great deal of respect.

After a few minutes, the judge finally said, "Okay, lets do it. I will call the Public Defender and the District Attorney and order them to combine the two trials. Congratulations, Young Man – you have already accomplished more than any other attorney that I know, because you have talked me into doing two things that I had never done before, and I have never heard of anyone else ever doing it either – these are two historical events."

"I have no words with which to show you my appreciation, Your Honor," said Gene. "I can only say that you are the most fair-minded judge that I have ever heard of in my entire life."

"Thank you, Mr. Lissenzwel," said the judge, "but I only did it because you shown me some evidence that revealed the condition of the defendants, and you told me the last time that you were here that you have very powerful evidence that proves that they're innocent and not insane, and I believed you. Well done, Young Man!" After they concluded, the judge went home because it was already very late in the day.

Gene went back to the jail cell and told the prisoners the bad news – that Peter had filed a case to get them back. He also gave them the good news – that there would be only one trial, instead of two. One trial would have been the prosecutor claiming that the prisoners caused malicious harm to Doctor Ryppemuff and other hospital employees. The other trial would have been Peter trying to get them back, because he claimed that they were insane and should be brought back to the hospital for treatment. Most importantly, Gene told the prisoners that they would be staying in a hotel very shortly until the trial was over. The prisoners couldn't find words that were adequate to show their appreciation. Gene left and went home.

That same day, early in the evening, several police officers walked into the jail cell and handcuffed the prisoners. The children started crying immediately, but one of the officers told them that they weren't there to do them any harm. Instead, they were there to take them to be much more comfortable in a hotel until the trial was over. The children then felt more at ease and stopped crying. The same officer also told them that he was sorry because the officers were obligated to handcuff them due to security regulations.

In a short while, they were placed in their rooms, and they had a chance to bathe and be comfortable, watching television and relaxing.

After several hours, Peter had already returned to the hospital. He was very tired, because it was already late in the evening, so he decided to go home. He was so busy and worried about the case that he forgot to go to Doctor Ryppemuff's room to give him his daily dosage of bear tranquilizer. Doctor Ryppemuff's receptionist, Mary Ohnowear, wondered why he didn't go upstairs to give his brother his daily injection – because of that, she became confused and deep in thought. Shortly after Peter left, she also went home.

The next morning, Mary arrived at the hospital an hour earlier than usual. She knew that Peter wouldn't be arriving for at least an hour. She arrived early because she wanted to go to Ward Two Seventeen to see who she thought was Doctor Ryppemuff's brother. The reason why she wanted to go see him was to see if she could find out why Peter, who she believed was Doctor Ryppemuff, didn't give him his injection the day before.

A few minutes after she arrived at the hospital, Mary went upstairs to Ward Two Seventeen and told the guard that Doctor Ryppemuff told her to check on his brother, because the doctor didn't give him his daily injection the day before. After a very rigorous security check, and after she lied to the guard, she was finally admitted to enter the room because the guard knew who she was. She then went to Doctor Ryppemuff's bedside. After about half an hour, Mary hurriedly left the ward and went back to the doctor's office before Peter arrived. It turned out that Peter didn't arrive at his usual time that morning because he left so late the night before, so Mary didn't have to rush to get out of Ward Two Seventeen in fear of being seen there by Peter – she was glad that it worked out that way.

A few days later, Gene Lissenzwel had looked through numerous documents and publications in anticipation of the trial. Due to the fact that he wasn't employed by a government agency or a law firm, Gene had to provide his own resources to get things done. The wealthy defendants weren't able to pay him at that point because Peter Emppostar had found the way to take control of their bank accounts – which was another task for Gene, if he was ever able to get them to go home and resume normal lives. Gene's means were very limited, and he had to work harder than most lawyers, but he was also very bright and precise, so he did his best.

Gene hired a private investigator whose name was Rebecca Fynedzowt to help him with the investigation. Rebecca seemed to have been born to be an investigator because she had eyes that constantly moved around – she seemed to be always looking at or for something. Her inquisitive attitude made her one of the best at what she did. She was very expensive, but Gene hired her because she was the best he knew. She was also very compassionate and did most of Gene's work on credit because she was a friend of Gene's aunt's, Annette's sister. She knew that she was taking a big chance, because there was no guarantee that Gene would ever be able to pay her for her services, but because she was a friend of the family, she was willing to do it even if she never collected a single penny from him.

After Peter Emppostar did everything that he had to do about his case against the prisoners, he obtained the representation of the most successful attorney in the country – his name was Ralph Byggshatt. After learning all the details of the case, Mr. Byggshatt felt that it would be a cinch winning a case against such a novice who had never tried a case before. Ralph also thought that he wouldn't have to do anything to prepare himself for the case.

Ralph Byggshatt found out that an inexperienced attorney from the District Attorney's Office was going to be on his side as a prosecutor during the trial. He didn't want to take any chances on losing the case, so he immediately called Prosecutor Thomas Nuattie and told him that he wouldn't have to do anything in court because Ralph himself would handle the entire trial. The young Prosecutor agreed because he thought that the experienced attorney would do a much better job, and he was sure that Ralph could win the case for both of them.

When Gene Lissenzwel found out that Ralph Byggshatt was the attorney that he'd be facing, he was even more devastated, but he had a great deal of courage and determination. He thought that he'd die fighting instead of giving up. Gene made numerous trips to the hotel to acquaint the prisoners with the court procedures. He wasn't very familiar himself, but he did his best. He briefed them on the trial and went over most of the material that he had. He also told them who he was faced against, and prepared them for the cross-examinations from the opposing attorneys. He made several trips to the courts to get as many ideas and as much information as he could by talking to lawyers that he knew. He also met others lawyers while he was there and watched some of them in action in actual courtroom cases. He was working extremely hard and many long hours every day.

Eventually, after many weeks of research and evidence-gathering efforts, Gene had everything ready to go to trial. When he filed the document certifying that he was ready for trial, it was the only thing so far that went on without any problems. Jury selection was to begin in two days, and the trial was going to take place shortly after that. Gene had never been through the process of selecting a jury before, so he had to read various publications related to that issue. Time was running out very fast, and Gene was getting totally exhausted.

After two days, finally, it was time to select a jury. To Gene's own amazement, the process only took one day, and it went on without any problems. The jury was selected, and the trial was to begin in a week. Ralph Byggshatt felt so confident that he even decided to take a week's vacation after the jury was selected and before the trial began.

Gene knew that he was going to fight a war with a bow and arrow against an enemy equipped with a tank. Because of that, he felt that if he ever worked hard before, nothing compared to the way he would have to work in the days that followed. As the date for the trial approached, Gene was both nervous and scared, but confident and hopeful. He was getting little or no sleep every day following the selection of the jury. The preparation for the trial was very stressful on him. He worked very hard, day and night, and had no idea what he was getting himself into.

The Trial

AFTER A WEEK, IT was finally Monday morning – the day of the trial. Gene was walking towards the courthouse. He was alone and loaded with a tremendous amount of paperwork. He had his own notes, which were hundreds of pages long. He also had several books, magazines, bank statements from various banks where the prisoners had their money, subpoenas and many other papers. Along the way, Gene Lissenzwel saw Peter Emppostar and Ralph Byggshatt, accompanied by an assistant. Peter was wearing a white robe over his clothes and a stethoscope partially protruding from his left robe pocket – he dressed that way to impress the jury and the judge. Peter and Ralph were very relaxed, and Ralph only had a small briefcase swinging in his left hand. They looked at Gene and started laughing very loudly while ridiculing him. Gene felt extremely insignificant, but he didn't show any emotions.

Upon entering the courthouse, Gene saw the prisoners sitting at the defense section, and he sat with them. Everyone was extremely nervous and worried, but Gene had to proceed no matter what the situation was. Gene had arranged his material in a certain order. He also had a list of his planned step-by-step sequence of events.

Shortly after that, Peter and Ralph walked in with their assistant and sat at the prosecution's and plaintiff's section. Prosecutor Thomas Nuattie was already there. As they had agreed, Thomas would let Ralph do all the talking and handle the entire matter from the beginning to the end. Ralph thought that he didn't have to review anything. Instead he started staring at Gene with a smirk on his face. He was a very tall and bulky man. He was good at intimidating people just by staring at them. He used his almost grotesque smirk that was his trademark during his career as a lawyer. Ralph was simply using his experience as a tactic to intimidate Gene to force him out of the race. Gene tried to ignore him, but found it very difficult.

A few minutes after Ralph started staring at Gene, Carmen Pynkeehertz noticed the situation and made a suggestion in a very low voice, "Hey, I have an idea, guys. I see that Mr. Byggshatt is staring at Gene – he wants to make him nervous before the trial begins. Let's turn the table on him and stare at his face incessantly." Everyone instantly turned towards Ralph simultaneously and started staring at him. Within minutes, Ralph stopped staring at Gene, but the prisoners kept staring at him. At that point, Mr. Byggshatt was the one who was feeling uncomfortable. The constant staring continued for several minutes, and Ralph had to stand up and step outside to get some fresh air – they had finally found his weak point by forcing him to take his own medicine.

Ten minutes later, Ralph went back into the courtroom, and the prisoners once again turned towards him and continued staring at him, but he was saved by the appearance of the judge. "All rise please!" said the court officer. "This court is now in session. The Honorable Judge Lykezdoks presiding!" The judge sat behind his bench, and the court officer said, "Please be seated."

Ralph laughed very lowly as he whispered into Peter's ear, "I know Judge Lykezdoks, and he will never rule against doctors."

"Case number 06-87536," said the court officer, "the People of the state of New York and Doctor Ryppemuff versus Anna Lyphesayvar, Bobby Lyphesayvar, Carmen Pynkeehertz, Christine Lyphesayvar, Joan Pynkeehertz, John Suolenthom, Mike Pynkeehertz, Robert Berndhend, Sam Towhertz and Susan Lyphesayvar."

Judge Lykezdoks, with a face full of wrinkles and a permanent mean look on his face, began presiding. He turned his face towards

Ralph Byggshatt and said, "Counselors, let me brief the jury before your opening statements." He then turned towards the jury and said, "Members of the jury, this is an extremely unusual trial – we have a criminal case, which involves an alleged assault perpetrated by the defendants against Doctor Ryppemuff and several other employees of Deprivayshun Psychiatric Hospital. We also have a civil case in our hands, where the doctor wants the defendants to go back to his hospital for proper treatment because he claims that they're insane. I don't like it, but another judge ordered the District Attorney and the Public Defender to combine the two trials into one, so let us proceed with it. It is up to you to decide whether or not the defendants assaulted Doctor Ryppemuff without provocation. You must also decide whether they should go back to the hospital for psychiatric treatment or go home as free citizens. However, before the trial begins, you have to remember that doctors are gods in this court – whatever they say is sacred, and whatever the opposition says has very little validity in my courtroom."

With such briefing by the judge, what kind of a chance did the defense have? It seemed as though all Gene's efforts would be for nothing, and he felt that he was being hanged without a trial.

Ralph looked at Peter and smiled. He then whispered in his ear again, "See? What did I tell you? There's no way that we can possibly lose this case." Ralph then turned towards Gene and tried to ridicule him with a smirk, but the prisoners noticed and turned towards him, and he instantly look down.

The judge then concluded as he turned towards the prosecutor, "Let's hear the opening statements now. Mr. Nuattie, you may begin."

Thomas stood up and said, "Your Honor, both, Mr. Byggshatt and I have agreed that he will handle the entire trial for both the prosecution and the plaintiff."

"Very well then," said the judge, "Mr. Byggshatt, proceed with your opening statement."

Ralph stood up and approached the jury. He began talking in a very loud and deep voice, "My name is Mr. Ralph Byggshatt! I am the best there is in the legal profession – just like my client is the best there is in the medical profession. I have won thousands of cases, and I am sure that you will see how easily I'll win this one. You heard what His Honor said – that doctors are gods – need I say anymore? I agree that doctors are gods, but I must respectfully add more to what His Honor told you – and that is that, as we all know, psychiatrists are even bigger gods. My client is a psychiatrist and he's the best there is. Therefore, he should be considered to be an 'Almighty God,' which is what he deserves.

"Those ten defendants maliciously attacked my client without any provocation whatsoever. After their vicious attack on our good doctor, or, I should say on our 'Almighty God,' they had the audacity to escape from where they were being cared for with love, tenderness, and consideration. After you hear the defense attorney's futile attempt to win this case, you must immediately render a verdict for the people – of course, you must also render a verdict for the plaintiff – he's a Psychiatrist, and he's the Director of Deprivayshun Psychiatric Hospital – the one with the biggest number of insane people, such as the ten defendants here."

After his opening statement, Ralph went back to his chair. He then made another attempt to intimidate Gene with his smirk, but the prisoners were ready and stared at him instantly – he had no choice but to look the other way.

"Young Man," said the judge as Ralph sat in his chair, "approach the jury and deliver your opening statement, if you know how."

It was Gene's turn to address the jury, but he felt as though he had been found guilty of a horrendous crime and was ready to be executed. He finally got up and walked towards the jury. His knees literally trembled as he walked, and it seemed like the longest walk that he had ever taken. After a few seconds, Gene finally stopped in front of the jury and began talking very nervously, "Ladies and gentlemen of the jury, my name is Gene Lissenzwel. I have never won a case before. In fact, I have never lost a case either because this is my first appearance in a courtroom as a defense attorney – as a matter of fact this is my first appearance as an attorney of any kind. My first job after law school was as a defense attorney with the Public Defender's Office. I was fired after four months on the job, simply because I believed that my clients were telling the truth and were not insane. I'm not even getting paid to represent them, because Doctor Ryppemuff has taken control of all their bank accounts, and they have no financial means to compensate me as long as they remain as prisoners – yes, as prisoners, because that's exactly what they are, and that's also what they were before they escaped from Deprivayshun Psychiatric Hospital. They may not be gods or 'Almighty Gods,' as Mr. Byggshatt claims that his client is, but they are innocent and definitely not insane – I intend to prove it during this trial. I may not have the experience and expertise that Mr. Byggshatt has, but I do have powerful evidence that I'm sure will show you that my clients are not guilty of any crime, and that they don't belong in a hospital because they are not insane. They are victims themselves – yes, victims of a crime that was being committed against them by the plaintiff when…"

Judge Lykezdoks abruptly interrupted Gene by banging on the presiding table very hard with his gavel. Gene then turned towards the judge. "Be very careful with what you say, Young Man!" the judge shouted very loudly. "You're walking on a very thin line! You're dealing with a highly respected professional here!"

"I'm very sorry, Your Honor," Gene responded, "but I do have the evidence that will prove that what I'm saying is true. Please allow me to continue, and I will eventually show this court all the evidence."

"I will allow you to continue, just as a matter of formality," the judge went on, "but be extremely careful, Young Man. Just don't make your opening statement too long, because we're all desperately waiting for you to lose this case so we can all go home."

Mr. Byggshatt, upon hearing the judge's remark, wanted to end the trial right there and then, "I object! Your Honor, I am hereby demanding that the jury should render an instant verdict for the plaintiff and the prosecution, so we can save this court the aggravation of going through a trial that I have already won. Such a verdict will also save us all a great deal of time and money, not to mention the fact that our good doctor will then be able to provide the best of care for the ten insane defendants as soon as possible – why prolong their agony?"

"Overruled!" Judge Lykezdoks replied. "While you're absolutely right, Mr. Byggshatt, let's give this novice a chance to speak. I know that the verdict is yours, but let's see if the case becomes interesting. Young Man, continue your opening statement."

If Gene ever felt devastated, nothing compared to the way he felt at that moment, but he maintained an overall serene appearance as he continued. "Thank you, Your Honor," he said as he faced the jury again and concluded his opening statement. "Ladies and gentlemen," he went on, "the plaintiff's counselor stated that these ten defendants maliciously attacked his client without any provocation whatsoever. Well, I intend to prove to this court that they acted in self defense. The counselor also stated that after their vicious attack on our good doctor, they had the audacity to escape from where they were being cared for with love, tenderness, and consideration. I also intend to prove that everything that he said is the complete opposite of the events that really took place at Deprivayshun Psychiatric Hospital. The defendants are being accused of malicious harm and unlawful escape because they're insane. They very ingeniously devised a way to defeat their captors with extremely limited resources – that alone should prove that they're not insane. Ladies and gentlemen, please, put any prejudice aside, and listen to all the evidence before rendering a verdict. Please, cast your votes based on what you see and hear during this trial, instead of casting them based on my lack of experience. Thank you for listening to me."

"Mr. Byggshatt, call your first witness," said the judge as Gene was walking back to his seat.

"We don't need any witnesses, Your Honor," Ralph replied, "because we had this case won long before we walked into this courtroom, and you confirmed that yourself a few minutes ago. However, Your Honor, as a matter of formality, I would like to call Doctor Ryppemuff to the stand."

Peter stood up and walked towards the witness stand. "Raise your right hand," said the clerk. Peter raised his hand, and the clerk said, "Do you solemnly swear to tell the truth, the whole truth and nothing but the truth so help you God?

"I do," Peter answered.

"State your name and occupation, please," the clerk went on.

"My name is Doctor Ryppemuff," Peter replied. "I am a psychiatrist and also the Director of Deprivayshun Psychiatric Hospital."

"Please be seated," the clerk concluded.

"Doctor Ryppemuff," said Ralph Byggshatt, "please tell the jury what the defendants did to you and numerous other hospital employees during the near-dawn hours of June 21, 2006, when the vicious assaults against you took place."

"Sure," said Peter, "they put some extremely dangerous drugs on our faces that nearly killed us – we felt the effects for days. In fact, I'm still dizzy as we speak as a result of that attack."

"No further questions," said Ralph; "your witness."

"I have no questions, Your Honor," said Gene, "but I would like to reserve my right to recall the witness at a later time."

"Very well," said the judge, "your right is reserved. Okay, Young Man, call your first witness – again, if you know how."

Gene didn't fail to give the judge his due respect, which at that point, the judge didn't deserve, "Thank you, Your Honor. The defense calls Miss Anna Lyphesayvar." Anna walked up to the witness stand and was sworn in. "Miss Lyphesayvar," Gene asked, "were you overpowered by the effects of the drug that made Doctor Ryppemuff and the guards pass out in the same ward where all the prisoners were at Deprivayshun Psychiatric Hospital when they escaped?"

"I object!" Ralph yelled.

"On what grounds?" asked the judge.

"On the grounds that the defense counselor is putting words in the witness' mouth," he answered. "The defendants were not prisoners in the wonderful hospital that my client runs – they were simply patients there."

"Excuse me, Mr. Byggshatt," Gene interjected, "they are prisoners, as we speak, because they are being held by the law – that makes them prisoners."

"Overruled!" said the judge as he looked at Gene with his eyes wide open. "Please, Miss Lyphesayvar, answer the question."

"I forgot the question, Your Honor," she replied.

"Clerk," said the judge, "read the last question asked by the defense."

The clerk read: "Miss Lyphesayvar, were you overpowered by the effects of the drug that made Doctor Ryppemuff and the guards pass out in the same ward where all the prisoners were at Deprivayshun Psychiatric Hospital when they escaped?"

"Yes I was," Anna answered.

"One last question, Miss Lyphesayvar," said Gene, "do you have any side effects as a result of the drug."

"No way!" Anna answered. "It only lasted for a little while. Even my three children, who are present here, have no side effects at all. They didn't feel any pain or discomfort even when they were overcome by the fumes, and my youngest child is only eight years old. The only thing that happened when we were exposed to the fumes was that we all felt like we were very sleepy. We were knocked out very fast."

"No further questions," said Gene, "but, Your Honor, I would like to recall this witness later."

"So noted," said the Judge. "Mr. Byggshatt, your witness."

"I have no questions at this time," Ralph replied. "I'll save my questions for the next time that the novice calls the witness."

"Very well," said the judge. "Call your next witness, Young Man."

"Thank you, Your Honor," Gene went on. "The defense calls Bobby Lyphesayvar."

Bobby walked to the witness stand, guided by the bailiff. As soon as Ralph Byggshatt saw Bobby, he stood up and yelled, "I object!"

"On what grounds?" asked the judge.

"What possible knowledge can that young brat have about anything?" Ralph asked.

"Overruled," said the judge.

Bobby was then sworn in. "Bobby," asked Gene, "how old are you?"

"EIGHT!" he answered in a very loud Voice.

"Come now, Little Fellow," the judge intervened, "there's no need to yell."

"How come you and that man yell all the time?" asked Bobby as he pointed at Ralph Byggshatt. Most people in the courtroom couldn't help it and started laughing, including the judge.

"Well!" Judge Lykezdoks exclaimed. "Ah, I really don't know the answer to that question, Young Fellow, but please don't yell anymore."

"Yes sir, Mr. Judge, I'm sorry," Bobby replied. "I thought that I had to speak loud, so everybody could here me."

"Okay, apology accepted," the judge continued as he turned towards Gene and said, "Please go on, Young Man."

"Bobby," said Gene, "Mr. Byggshatt said that you don't know anything, and he also called you a brat – do you know what all that means?"

"Sure, Mr. Lissenzwel!" Bobby exclaimed. "A brat is a child who doesn't behave and is very badly spoiled, but I'm not a brat, because my mommy and my big sisters taught me to be a good boy. Besides, I do know a whole lot of stuff, and I have already noticed that that man thinks he's a big shot," Bobby pointed at Ralph again and continued, "but I bet you that you will beat him right here in this courtroom – you'll see."

Some people laughed again, and Gene then continued, "Well, thank you for your confidence in me, Bobby. "Anyway, can you tell us what happened that night when everyone escaped from the hospital?"

"Sure! It was all very scary, and we started crying. That doctor wanted to separate all of us," said Bobby, as he pointed at Peter, "but all those people there sitting at your table were so smart that they put everyone to sleep, except five of them, and they got us out of there safe and sound," Bobby concluded as he was still pointing towards the prisoners.

"Bobby, did you also pass out when the prisoners made the doctor pass out?" asked Gene.

"Yeah, but I don't remember anything after that," Bobby answered. "I only know the whole story because I heard it later."

"Do you feel dizzy now, Bobby?" asked Gene.

"No, Sir, I never did, I feel fine," Bobby answered. "The only thing I felt was that I was very sleepy before I passed out."

"Thank you, Bobby," said Gene, "I can easily see that Mr. Byggshatt was totally wrong about you, because you do know a whole lot of stuff, as you said. No further questions. Your witness."

Ralph was so embarrassed by Bobby's verbal abilities that he had no questions. "I have nothing to ask," he said.

"Call your next witness, Young Man," said the judge.

"Thank you, Your Honor," said Gene. "The defense calls Doctor Sayahagain." The doctor approached the witness stand and was sworn in. "Doctor Sayahagain," Gene Lissenzwel asked, "were you subpoenaed to appear here as a witness?"

"Ah, yes, I was," the doctor answered, "and you know that, because it was you who issued the subpoena – I don't know why you're asking me that question."

Gene knew that he wasn't obligated to reply to the witness' remark, but he gave him an explanation anyway, "Doctor Sayahagain, the reason for the question is so the court records will show your answer. Now, Doctor Sayahagain, do you remember a patient by the name of Sam Towhertz?"

"No, but I have his records right here," the doctor answered.

"Doctor Sayahagain," Gene went on, "please bear in mind that I have a copy of your records here, which were also subpoenaed. Will you please tell the court the reason for Mr. Towhertz's visit to your office?"

"Ah, let me see," the doctor answered as he looked at the papers. "Well, it says here that I sent him to see a psychiatrist – I guess my receptionist wrote that in."

"That's fine, Doctor Sayahagain," Gene continued, "you sent him to see a psychiatrist, but why did he go to your office in the first place?"

Doctor Sayahagain started to get nervous and couldn't answer the question. He then turned towards the judge and asked, "Do I have to listen to this nonsense, Judge?"

"As much as I hate to say it," the judge replied, "but yes – you're under oath, and you're obligated to answer the question."

Doctor Sayahagain hesitated while shifting his body a few times in his chair. His leftwards lean became more pronounced when he was nervous. After a moment, he finally answered, "Ah, well, I can't remember that because it was a long time ago."

At that point, Gene was beginning to feel good about his performance because he had already caused the doctor to become nervous – he felt that he had accomplished something. He then continued his legal attack on the doctor, "Doctor Sayahagain, I can't believe that a supposedly highly respected professional, such as you, doesn't have the events that take place in his office written down on his records. Isn't it true, Doctor Sayahagain, that you don't even bother to ask your patients why they go to your office for your services, and instead, you tell them to open their mouths and say, 'Ah' right away regardless of why they're there?"

"That's absurd," the doctor answered while shifting his body a few times in his chair again. "I am very highly trained in my profession, and I always ask all my patients very extensively why they come to see me."

"Do you ask all your patients without exception why they go to your office, Doctor?" Gene asked.

"Not a single exception," Doctor Sayahagain answered. "There has never been a patient in my office that I didn't ask him why he was there."

"Doctor Sayahagain," Gene went on, "isn't it true that you send almost all your patients to see a psychiatrist as soon as you want to get rid of them for one reason or another, even if there's nothing mentally wrong with them?"

"That's totally ridiculous!" the doctor yelled. "I do send patients to see a psychiatrist, but very rarely, and only when I thoroughly examine them and find absolutely nothing physically wrong with them. Then I see that they're suffering from some kind of mental illness."

"Okay, Doctor Sayahagain," Gene continued, "according to what you said, there are rare occasions when you do send patients to see a psychiatrist. On those rare occasions, you tell them that they're suffering from particular mental illnesses. Then you tell them that the psychiatrist you're sending them to see specializes exclusively in the particular problems that you claim your patients are suffering from – of course, the mental illnesses that you claim they have are different for each patient. Am I correct so far Doctor Sayahagain?"

"Ah, yes, that is exactly right," the doctor answered.

Gene then made an attempt to trick the doctor into admitting what he really did, "Okay, Doctor Sayahagain, when you do send patients to see a psychiatrist, you always send them to the same psychiatrist, regardless of what you tell them that they're suffering from. You tell different patients that they're suffering from different mental illnesses, and you always tell them that that psychiatrist specializes exclusively in the particular problems that you claim your patients are suffering from…"

"Objection!" Ralph Byggshatt shouted. "Counsel is testifying."

"Sustained!" said the judge. "Young Man, is there a question coming anytime soon?"

"I'm sorry, Your Honor," Gene replied. "Okay, here's a question – am I correct again so far Doctor Sayahagain?"

Gene's attempt to trick the doctor didn't work, but he made him feel very nervous as the doctor shifted his body once again and answered with a very low voice, "Ah, that's absurd. "Ah, the very few times during my many years as a great physician that I was compelled to refer patients to psychiatrists, ah, I made absolutely sure that I sent them to different psychiatrists, ah, depending on what they were suffering from."

"Thank you, Doctor Sayahagain," said Gene. "No further questions. Your Honor, I'd like to reserve the right to recall this witness at a later time."

"So noted," said the judge, "and you may recall the witness at a later time – that is if the trial doesn't end soon when the jury renders a verdict for the plaintiff and the prosecution."

"Thank you, Your Honor," Gene concluded. "Your witness, Mr. Byggshatt."

"I have no questions for that witness," said the overconfident lawyer. "What's the sense? I have already won this case."

Judge Lykezdoks started treating Gene with some respect from that moment on – he didn't refer to him as "Young Man" anymore and said, "Call your next witness, Mr. Lissenzwel."

"The defense calls my father, Mr. Anthony Lissenzwel," said Gene.

Anthony stood up and started walking towards the witness stand, but Ralph also stood up and acted very menacing. Anthony saw him and stopped before he reached the witness stand. "I object!" Ralph shouted. "Is this a circus? Mr. Anthony Lissenzwel is a janitor at my favorite restaurant. I have seen him cleaning the floors many times while I was having dinner there – is this a courtroom or a dirty dining room? What can a janitor possibly say that will be relevant in this case?"

"Your Honor," Gene continued, "my father is a patient of Doctor Sayahagain's. What he has to say is totally relevant."

"Overruled!" said the judge. "Mr. Lissenzwel Senior, please come up to the witness stand."

Anthony stood next to the witness stand and was sworn in. Gene felt a little funny at first, asking his own father questions for which he already knew the answers. "Mr. Anthony Lissenzwel," Gene began, "before I ask you my first question, in response to the plaintiff's attorney's attempt to demean you for being a janitor, let me tell you that I am extremely proud to have you as a father, and…"

"I object!" Ralph Byggshatt shouted. What does Mr. Lissenzwel Junior's pride have to do with this case?"

"Let the man talk!" Judge Lykezdoks yelled. "There's nothing wrong with a little family pride."

Gene displayed a big smile on his face and said, "Thank you, Your Honor. I was about to say, Mr. Anthony Lissenzwel, that I am extremely proud to have you as a father, and I think that if there is a great man here, it is YOU. I am also extremely proud of your wife, my mother, who has never held a job in her life." Anthony became very emotional upon hearing Gene's statement. He was only in his late forties, but due to his nervousness and his life as a hard worker, he appeared to be much older at that very moment. He displayed several lines of wavy skin on his forehead. Gene's mother, who was in the audience, couldn't help it, and tears came out of her eyes when she heard her son talk that way.

"Mr. Lissenzwel," Gene then went on, "were you a patient of Doctor Sayahagain's?"

Anthony felt very funny as he answered his son's question, "Yes, Sir, I was."

"Mr. Lissenzwel," Gene continued, "please tell the court why you were his patient."

"Because you told me to go to him and pretend that I was a wealthy investor with an ingrown toe nail," Anthony answered.

"Okay, Mr. Lissenzwel," Gene went on, "please tell this court everything that took place in the doctor's office during your visit."

"When I told the doctor's receptionist that I was rich," Anthony began, "she told me to wait a minute while she went inside to talk to the doctor, but I wanted to hear what she told him, so I followed her. As I was walking into the examining room, I heard her whispering into his ears that I was a wealthy investor. As soon as I was inside, the first thing that Doctor Sayahagain said to me was to have a seat next to him. He didn't even ask me why I was there, and after I sat down, he told me to open my mouth and say, 'Ah.' He kept on repeating the same thing over and over again, but every time he said it, he used other words that were different each time. He made me open my mouth and say, 'Ah' nineteen times, and after the nineteenth time, he told me that my bill was $2,750, plus expenses plus other charges. He then told me to go see his receptionist and pay my bill, and that she would give me a prescription for my medicine. He then told his receptionist to call the next patient.

"At that point, I told him that the reason why I was there was because I had an ingrown toe nail. He then told me that he was the doctor and that he was the only one there capable of making a proper diagnosis, but he still didn't bother to look at my toe. He then told me that I was suffering from Inngrounosis, which was a very rare and dangerous form of a mental disorder. Even with my lack of education, and the fact that English is not my native language, I still knew that he had made up that name. He said that he was going to send me to see a psychiatrist named Doctor Louzi, who specialized exclusively in the treatment of Inngrounosis. He then told me that my bill was $3,950, plus expenses plus other charges. Again he told me to go see his receptionist to pay my bill and get the information about the appointment with the psychiatrist. I went to his receptionist, and she told me that the bill total was $4,775. I paid it, and she gave me the information for the psychiatrist. Then I walked out of his office."

"I object!" Ralph Byggshatt shouted. "This is totally outrageous. How can anyone believe such a ridiculous story? Mr. Lissenzwel Junior coached the witness, his own father, and told him exactly what to say. I guess counsel forgot to tell his father that there are laws against perjury, and I'm sure, Your Honor, that you will fine the witness for lying under oath. I am also sure that you will definitely hold his attorney in contempt for making up such an incredible story and attempting to present it here as evidence."

"Your Honor," Gene intervened, "if you please, bear with me a little longer, and I will soon show the court that the witness told the truth."

"Mr. Byggshatt," said the judge, "you're absolutely right. This is an incredible story – it is so incredible that I don't believe it ever happened. In all my years as a judge, I have never heard of a doctor practicing medicine in such a ridiculous way. However, it's up to the jury to either believe it or disbelieve it, but in view of the fact that this is an unusual trial, I'll make a ruling on this issue right now – overruled! Very well, Mr. Lissenzwel, I will allow you to continue, but if you don't have the proof in one hour, I will order the entire testimony given by Mr. Lissenzwel Senior to be stricken from the records. Furthermore, I will give you until the end of the trial, and if you can't prove it by then, your father will be fined for lying under oath, and you will be held in contempt of this court and very heavily fined as well. You may also be stripped of your right to practice law for the rest of your life. Bear in mind that if you can't prove it within the hour, after I order his testimony to be stricken, even if you can prove it afterwards, it will remain stricken – I'll show that judge who ordered this unusual trial that I can also do unusual things! You may continue now, Mr. Lissenzwel."

"Thank you, Your Honor," Gene replied, "and thank you, Mr. Lissenzwel. No further questions. Your witness, Mr. Byggshatt."

Ralph approached Anthony with a mean look on his face. He was definitely attempting to intimidate him. He said in a very loud voice, "Mr. Lissenzwel Senior, that is totally ridiculous! How can you sit there and say that the good doctor told you to open your mouth and say, 'Ah' nineteen times? Did you count the 'Ahs,' Sir?"

Anthony then remembered that Gene had told him what to expect from Mr. Byggshatt. He prepared himself mentally and answered very calmly, "Yes, Sir, I did."

Mr. Byggshatt stood a few inches away from Anthony's face and yelled at him while staring right into his eyes, "Mr. Lissenzwel, I don't believe a word of what you have said! You're lying, and I'm sure that Judge Lykezdoks will fine you later for lying under oath, as he said he would. Are you willing to take that chance, or are you going to change your testimony?"

Anthony maintained his calmness and then he remembered that the prisoners made Ralph nervous by staring at him before the trial began. He decided to turn the table on Ralph with a firm stare as he answered while still staring at him, "I am not lying, Sir, I am telling the truth."

Mr. Byggshatt gave up due to Anthony's deep stare, and then he walked away as he made his last statement, "I have no further questions for the biggest liar in town."

"You may step down, Mr. Lissenzwel Senior," said the judge. "Mr. Lissenzwel Junior, please call your next witness."

"Thank you, Your Honor," Gene replied. "The defense would like to recall Miss Anna Lyphesayvar."

"Very well," said the Judge. "Miss Lyphesayvar, you're still under oath. Please come up to the witness stand."

Anna walked towards the stand and sat down. "Miss Lyphesayvar, are you insane?" asked Gene.

"I object!' Ralph yelled again. "The witness is not a psychiatrist, and she can't tell anyone whether she's insane or not!"

"Sustained," said the judge as he looked towards Gene as if he were enjoying himself.

Gene then went on with a different question, "Miss Lyphesayvar, what is your occupation?"

"I am a janitor at Deprivayshun Psychiatric Hospital," Anna answered. "At least I was before I ended up in jail."

"I object!" Ralph yelled once more. "Is this a convention of janitors? That's the second janitor who was called by the defense counselor to testify in this trial. What do janitors know about the law?"

"I'm not going to ask my witness any questions regarding her knowledge of the law," Gene responded, "but even if I do, Mr. Byggshatt, I have every right to ask my witness any question that is relevant and permissible."

The judge looked at Gene with his eyes wide open again as he allowed him to interrogate the witness. "Overruled!" he said.

"Thank you, Your Honor," Gene went on. "Miss Lyphesayvar, why are you one of the prisoners, when you just told me that you worked in the hospital as a janitor?"

"Because I delivered a message to the parents of one of the prisoners in an attempt to help them escape from their prison cell," Anna answered, "but Doctor Ryppemuff captured me one night when I was going home and locked me up in a psychiatric ward."

"You attempted to help them escape from their prison cell in jail, at Police Headquarters?" asked Gene.

"No," Anna replied, "I tried to help them escape from their prison cell in the hospital."

"Miss Lyphesayvar," Gene continued, "do you mean to tell me that they were prisoners while they were in the hospital?"

"Yes, Sir, they were," she answered.

"Wouldn't you rather refer to them as patients?" asked Gene. "Please explain to the jury why you said that they were prisoners in the hospital."

"Yes, Mr. Lissenzwel," Anna went on, "they were prisoners in the hospital. They weren't patients. They were there against their own will, and they weren't allowed to have any visitors. They were only there because…"

Ralph Byggshatt suddenly interrupted Anna with a very loud voice, "I object! That is absolutely absurd! The patients were there because they're insane, and Doctor Ryppemuff was doing his best to cure them and send them home as soon as possible."

Judge Lykezdoks was becoming very interested in the story. He wanted to hear the end of it. Before Gene said anything, the judge said, "Overruled! Mr. Lissenzwel, please proceed."

"Thank you, Your Honor," Gene continued with another smile on his face. "Miss Lyphesayvar, please tell the court why the defendants were patients, or prisoners, as you prefer to call them, at Deprivayshun Psychiatric Hospital."

"Well," Anna replied, "Mr. Byggshatt just said that the prisoners were there because they're insane, and Doctor Ryppemuff was doing his best to cure them and send them home. The truth of the matter is that no one ever leaves Deprivayshun Psychiatric Hospital alive. What I was going to say before Mr. Byggshatt interrupted me was that the prisoners were only there because they're very rich. They were there without the possibility of ever seeing freedom again, and they were only there because the hospital was making tons of money from each one. The prices of all the things in the hospital are totally outrageous. I'll give you a few examples – the last price that I heard for coffee was $210, coffee stirrers $12 each, toothpicks $7 each. They even charge the prisoners for the use of the menu, the dinner table and the chairs they sit in while eating. The hospital also reuses the paper napkins and charges an outrageous price for them. The list goes on and on. Some of the prisoners there get monthly bills amounting to millions of dollars – that's the only reason why Doctor Ryppemuff wants the prisoners back – to continue stealing their money."

"Miss Lyphesayvar," asked Gene, "how do you know so much about what goes on with the prisoners, as you call the patients, at Deprivayshun Psychiatric Hospital?"

"First of all, I worked there," Anna answered. "Secondly, it was common knowledge shared by all the employees that all the prisoners there spend the rest of their lives without any visiting rights and without the possibility of ever being released again. They were totally barred from the outside world. I have seen many bodies being taken out of the wards, but I have never seen a live person leave the hospital, and no one else that I have ever spoken with has ever seen anyone get out alive. The defendants were totally deprived of everything by Doctor Ryppemuff while they were at Deprivayshun Psychiatric Hospital. They didn't even have any windows in their room so at least they could look outdoors. They couldn't read anything other than their dinner menus, because they didn't have any newspapers, books or magazines. They had no televisions, radios or telephones."

"How do you also know so much about the cost of the prisoners' hospital stay, Miss Lyphesayvar," asked Gene.

"Well," Anna went on, "before I became a janitor, I was a food servant, and I went all over the hospital doing other duties when I finished serving the prisoners' meals. Very often they had me help the clerks in the accounting department, and I saw the way that the prisoners were ripped off so badly that their bank accounts suffered catastrophic damages because of the huge monthly bills that they had to pay, which Doctor Ryppemuff himself took out of their bank accounts."

"Miss Lyphesayvar," said Gene, "please tell us some of the things that you have experienced as a result of being unlawfully imprisoned at Deprivayshun Psychiatric Hospital."

"I object!" Ralph yelled. "It has not been established that the prisoners, I mean the patients, were unlawfully imprisoned at Deprivayshun Psychiatric Hospital."

"Sustained," said the judge.

"I'll rephrase my question, Your Honor," said Gene. "Miss Lyphesayvar, were you admitted to Deprivayshun Psychiatric Hospital against your will?"

"Yes, I was," Anna answered.

"Miss Lyphesayvar," Gene continued, "please tell us some of the things that you have experienced as a result of being at Deprivayshun Psychiatric Hospital against your will."

"Well," Anna replied, "there have been many problems as a result of that, and I don't really know where to begin. My children have been getting nightmares almost every night now. My youngest child, Bobby, has to sleep in bed with me, so I can comfort him when he wakes up crying in the middle of the night. Even Mr. Towhertz, who happens to be a very big and strong man, gets nightmares very often – I know it because the commotion that he makes in the middle of the night in the hotel where we're staying can be felt right through the walls. I also know that many of the other prisoners are also experiencing similar problems."

When Anna finished her last sentence, there was a feeling of compassion among everyone for the prisoners. The only ones without any compassion were the plaintiff and his attorney. Even the prosecutor, Thomas Nuattie, had a sad face, which indicated that he totally disagreed with the patients' treatment in the hospital.

"Thank you, Miss Lyphesayvar," Gene concluded. "Your witness, Mr. Byggshatt."

Ralph stood up and remained standing where he was. His voice was so loud, that he could be heard at any distance, "Miss Lyphesayvar, of course you know that everything you said was a lie. Why did you make up such a crazy story, knowing very well that the jury won't believe a word of it?"

"I didn't make it up, Sir – it's all true," Anna replied.

"I don't want to waste my time talking to such liars anymore," said Ralph. "I'm sure that the jury is made up of intelligent people who will vote against all the crazy defendants anyway, and I'm also sure that you're not fooling our great judge either, Miss Lyphesayvar."

"I object," said Gene; "counsel is testifying."

"Sustained," said the judge. "Mr. Byggshatt do you have any further questions for the witness?"

"No further questions, Your Honor," Ralph replied.

"You may step down, Miss Lyphesayvar," said the judge. "Call your next witness, Mr. Lissenzwel."

"Thank you, Your Honor," Gene went on. "The defense calls Mr. Sam Towhertz to the stand." Sam stood up and walked towards the witness stand while limping, due to his swollen toe. He was then sworn in. "Mr. Towhertz, are you insane?" asked Gene.

"I object!" Mr. Byggshatt yelled. "I must repeat, the witness is not a psychiatrist, and he can't tell anyone whether he's insane or not!"

"Sustained," said the judge.

"Mr. Towhertz," Gene continued as he rephrased his question, "were you a patient in Doctor Sayahagain's office?"

"Yes, Sir, I was," Sam answered.

"Do you remember why you went to the doctor's office, Mr. Towhertz?" Gene asked.

"Yes, Sir, of course," Sam replied, "I had excruciating pain in my left foot, because one of my workers, Mr. August Hahmerdrawpper, dropped a sledgehammer on my toe. In fact, I still have pain in my foot, because none of the doctors I visited even looked at my foot – including Doctor Sayahagain."

"Did the doctor ask you why you were there?" asked Gene.

"No, he did not," Sam responded.

"Mr. Towhertz," Gene went on, "please tell the jury the events that took place when you entered Doctor Sayahagain's examining room."

"Well," Sam began, "the first thing he did was to tell me to open my mouth, and say, 'Ah.' When I did, Doctor Sayahagain told me to open my mouth and say, 'Ah' again. When I did it the second time, he kept on and on telling me to open by mouth and say, 'Ah' more than a dozen times. Each time that he told me to open my mouth and say, 'Ah,' he added different words or phrases to his demands to make me believe that he was looking for something. I actually fell for it while I was in his office, but later I realized that it was only a tactic to rip me off very severely, because later on, I learned from one of the nurses at Kuttemopen Hospital that Doctor Sayahagain charges $50 per 'Ah' plus a lot of other hidden charges. After he finished his 'Ah' nonsense, he said that my bill was $700, plus expenses plus other charges, and to go see his receptionist so I could pay my bill. At..."

"Did you pay your bill at that point, Mr. Towhertz?" Gene interrupted.

"Oh no," Sam answered, "at that point, I told him that I was there because my foot was in pain caused by one of my workers dropping a sledgehammer on my toe. Doctor Sayahagain didn't even hear anything that I told him, because he told me that whatever my problem was, it was all in my mind. He then told me that his receptionist would make an emergency appointment for me to go see a psychiatrist because I was probably suffering from Swelosis, and the psychiatrist specialized exclusively in Swelosis. Then he jacked up the bill to $900, plus expenses plus other charges, and then he wanted to get rid me. I told him that..."

"Did he tell you the name of the psychiatrist, Mr. Towhertz?" Gene interrupted again.

"Not at that point," Sam answered, "because, I told him that he was beginning to annoy me because my problem was not in my mind, but in my foot! Then he told me that he was spending too much time on my problem, and kept insisting that I should go see the psychiatrist because the more I waited, the worse my mental condition would get.

When he realized that he couldn't convince me to go see a psychiatrist, he said that maybe he missed whatever problem I had, so he told me to open my mouth and say, 'Ah' again to see if he could find the problem. When I did as he told me, he said that he found it in the back of my throat. Then ..."

"Did he treat you then, Mr. Towhertz?" Gene interrupted for the third time.

"No," Sam replied, "he changed his diagnosis and told me that I was suffering from Aikosis. He then told me that he was sending me to Doctor Louzi, who specialized exclusively in the treatment of Aikosis. Then he said that my bill was much higher because of all the delay. I was somewhat convinced that Doctor Sayahagain knew what he was talking about, and that he actually found some kind of infection due to my swollen toe, so I decided to go see Doctor Louzi. When I..."

"I object!" Ralph Byggshatt yelled. "What is this line of questioning all about? All that nonsense is irrelevant to this case. The witness will say anything to try to stay out of going back to the hospital where he belongs. Insane people know very well how to make up stories that sound real."

"Your Honor," said Gene Lissenzwel, "if you allow Mr. Towhertz to continue, I intend to prove that all this is extremely relevant. What's more important is that there's a direct connection between Doctor Sayahagain and Doctor Ryppemuff, and that four of the prisoners started with Doctor Sayahagain, where he made up names for their supposed mental disorders. Your Honor, I intend to prove all this later on during this trial."

"Overruled!" the judge shouted. "You may continue, Mr. Towhertz."

"Thank you, Your Honor," said Sam. "Anyway, what I was going to say was that I was such a fool because when I got to Doctor Louzi's office, I found out that he was a psychiatrist, and Doctor Sayahagain sent me there and told me that he was sending me to a medical doctor.

When I finally arrived at Doctor Louzi's office, he put me through a massive dose of stupidity, and then he sent me to another psychiatrist named Doctor Louziar. Then, after Doctor Louziar put me through a huge dose of nonsense, I ended up at Kuttemopen Hospital, where they totally ignored my original problem and cut me open to perform numerous unnecessary operations on me – I was almost butchered to death."

"Mr. Towhertz, why did you let them do that to you, when your only problem was a swollen toe?" asked Gene.

"Oh," Sam replied, "they did it by force, but it wasn't that easy because I tried to get off the operating table when I heard the surgeon read the list of procedures that they had planned for me. Because of my size and strength, it took several doctors and orderlies to overpower me, but they finally did, and immediately anesthetized me."

"Mr. Towhertz, what did you mean when you said that they cut you open to perform numerous unnecessary operations on you?" Gene asked.

"They did a triple bypass, stapled my stomach, removed my spleen, removed my prostate, removed half of my colon and drained fluid from my brain," Sam answered.

"All that because you had a swollen toe, Mr. Towhertz?" asked Gene.

"Yes sir," Sam answered.

"What was you condition after such operations?" asked Gene.

"After all that," Sam continued, "I was in terrible pain all over my body for over two months. When I told the doctors at Kuttemopen Hospital that I had pain all over my body and also in my foot because they never did anything about my swollen toe, Doctor Butchar told me that they had nothing to do with my foot. He then wanted to send me back to Doctor Sayahagain so he could treat my foot. When I told him that that's where I started, Doctor Butchar told me that it wasn't his fault that I didn't know what I was doing. He then told me that he was going to send me to Doctor Ryppemuff at Deprivayshun Psychiatric Hospital, where I would be well taken care of. Doctor Butchar then sent me to spend the rest of my life as a prisoner in that infernal place. The pain in my foot was still there, even when I ended up as a prisoner at Deprivayshun Psychiatric Hospital, because they never did anything about it. In fact, my foot still hurts right now. No one at Doctor Sayahagain's office, Doctor Louzi's office, Doctor Louziar's office, Kuttemopen Hospital or Deprivayshun Psychiatric Hospital ever even looked at my foot."

"Thank you, Mr. Towhertz," said Gene Lissenzwel. "No further questions. Your witness, Mr. Byggshatt."

Ralph stood up and yelled at the witness from his current position, "Mr. Towhertz, you're under oath! Why are you making up such a ridiculous story? Is there any other reason besides wanting to be free and go home? Why are you lying?"

Sam looked at him straight in the eyes and answered with a very firm voice, "I am not lying, Sir, I am telling the truth."

"Doctor Sayahagain told us another version of your story, Mr. Towhertz," Ralph continued. "How can you sit there and call him a liar? He's a doctor, and as you heard, Judge Lykezdoks said that doctors are gods – that alone is enough to know that you're lying. Now, I'm going to give you another chance to tell the truth. Why are you lying?"

"I am not lying, Sir," Sam repeated, "I am telling the truth."

"Well, Mr. Towhertz," Mr. Byggshatt concluded, "I'm going to answer the question for you with the truth, so the jury can hear it – you're lying because this is a pure conspiracy to harm the names and reputations of all good medical giants, such as Doctor Sayahagain and Doctor Ryppemuff. No further questions, Mr. Liar."

"Objection," said Gene. "Counsel is testifying."

"Sustained," the judge replied. "The jury will disregard Mr. Byggshatt's statements. Mr. Towhertz, you may step down. Call your next witness, Mr. Lissenzwel."

"Thank you, Your Honor," said Gene. "At this point, I would like to call Miss Carmen Pynkeehertz to the stand." Carmen was sworn in. "Miss Pynkeehertz," Gene went on, "please tell the court the names of all the doctors and hospitals that you visited before you ended up in jail as a prisoner."

"Yes, Sir," Carmen replied, "I started with Doctor Sayahagain. After that, I went to Doctor Byggliar and Doctor Sharlottan, and then I saw several doctors at Kuttemopen Hospital – namely, Doctor Butchar, Doctor Manypewlatar, Doctor Oargandeelar and some other doctors whose names I didn't know. After that, I ended up at Deprivayshun Psychiatric Hospital, where I met Doctor Ryppemuff and other doctors whose names I never knew either."

"Thank you, Miss Pynkeehertz," Gene continued. "Were you properly treated by any of the medical doctors or psychiatrists who you have been seen by during your entire ordeal?"

"I object! Lack of foundation," said Ralph.

"On what grounds?" asked the judge.

"On the grounds that the counselor is putting words in the witness' mouth" Ralph replied. "It has not been proven in this court that the witness has gone through any ordeal. On the contrary, she has been taken care of with love, tenderness and consideration."

"Sustained," said the judge.

"I'll rephrase my question, Your Honor," said Gene. "Miss Pynkeehertz, were you properly treated by any of the doctors or psychiatrists who you have been seen by during your entire path from Doctor Sayahagain until you became a patient at Deprivayshun Psychiatric Hospital?

"No way!" Carmen answered. "I was not properly treated by any of the doctors involved. I still have the problem for which I went to see Doctor Sayahagain in the first place – which was a thorn stuck in my left pinky, and that's why I went to his office. I still have the thorn in my pinky – here, take a look." Carmen then showed her finger to everyone in the courtroom.

Gene Lissenzwel asked Carmen Pynkeehertz to explain in detail her entire ordeal. After she testified, he called John Suolenthom, who testified about his own ordeal because of his swollen thumb due to a bee sting. Gene then called Robert Berndhend, who testified about his nightmare caused by a chemical burn on the palm of his hand. Following that, Gene called all the remaining prisoners, one by one, to the witness stand and asked them to testify about their ordeals.

Right after the last witness testified, there was an even greater feeling of compassion felt by everyone that could bee seen all over their faces. Of course, Peter Emppostar and Ralph Byggshatt were the only ones who showed no emotions of any kind.

Gene had no further questions and turned the witness over to Mr. Byggshatt. Ralph had no questions, but he finally had a valid objection, which he used as a diversionary tactic. "I object!" Ralph yelled. "More than one hour has passed, and the defense has failed to prove that what his father said was true."

"I agree," said Judge Lykezdoks. "Do you have the proof, Mr. Lissenzwel?"

Gene had originally thought that his father's testimony was crucial to the case, but at that point of the trial, he felt that he had much more powerful evidence, which he intended to use later on. He answered after a brief pause, "Not at this time, Your Honor. It will take me more time before I'm able to present the evidence that will prove that it was true."

The judge put his head down briefly, and after carefully evaluating Gene's answer, he lifted his head again and said, "Sustained! Strike Mr. Anthony Lissenzwel's entire testimony from the records!" He then turned towards the jury and said, "Ladies and gentlemen of the jury, you're hereby ordered to disregard Anthony Lissenzwel's entire testimony. Mr. Lissenzwel, please proceed. You may call your next witness."

"Thank you, Your Honor," Gene continued. "The defense calls Doctor Gudsyke."

"I object!" said Mr. Byggshatt. "Doctor Gudsyke is not involved in this case. He has nothing to do with the plaintiff or the defendants!"

"Overruled!" said the judge even before Gene had a chance to respond. "Doctor Gudsyke, please come up to the witness stand."

Doctor Gudsyke walked towards the witness stand and was sworn in by the clerk. "State your name and occupation, please," the clerk went on.

"I am Doctor Gudsyke," he replied, "and I am a psychiatrist."

"Please be seated," the clerk concluded.

"Doctor Gudsyke," asked Gene, "how long have you been a psychiatrist?"

"Twenty two years," Doctor Gudsyke answered."

"And what can you tell us about yourself, Doctor?" Gene asked.

"I have treated mental patients very extensively all during my twenty two years," the doctor replied, "and I have taught psychiatry at several medical schools throughout the country and in some foreign countries as well. I have written several training manuals and text books related to the field of psychiatry, many of which are in use today at several psychiatric and learning institutions. I also wrote a complete book on the subject. Copies of all my credentials are on His Honor's bench."

"Thank, Doctor Gudsyke," said Gene Lissenzwel. "Have you ever met these ten defendants, before?"

"Yes I have," the doctor answered.

"When and where did you meet them?" asked Gene.

"A few weeks ago in a jail cell at Police Headquarters," the doctor answered.

"Doctor Gudsyke," asked Gene, "can you please tell us why you met them in their jail cell?"

"Yes, of course," the doctor went on, "I was consulted by you to give them a complete psychiatric evaluation."

"And what were your findings, Doctor Gudsyke?" Gene asked.

"I found absolutely no signs of any mental disorder in any of the defendants," the psychiatrist replied. "I found them to be perfectly mentally normal."

"Thank you, Doctor Gudsyke," Gene concluded. "No further questions. Your witness, Mr. Byggshatt."

"Doctor Gudsyke," asked Ralph Byggshatt, "are you the Director of a psychiatric hospital?"

"No, Sir, I am not," the doctor answered.

"Well," Ralph continued, "Doctor Ryppemuff is. Therefore, he's far more qualified than you are. Wouldn't you say that, Doctor Gudsyke?"

"I do not know whether or not he's far more qualified than I am, Mr. Byggshatt," Doctor Gudsyke answered, "but I assure you that the mere fact that he's holding that title doesn't make him superior to me in the field."

"Now, Doctor Gudsyke," Ralph went on, "Doctor Ryppemuff says that the ten defendants are dangerously insane, and he has far more experience with them than you do – you only spent a short time on only one single visit with them in a jail cell. Our good doctor has spent several months with them. What makes you so highly qualified to say that they're not insane, when Doctor Ryppemuff says that they are?"

"Mr. Byggshatt," Doctor Gudsyke answered, "I have spent twenty two years dealing with mental disorders, and none of the defendants showed any signs of mental illness whatsoever. It doesn't take me several months to determine that – only a few minutes. Sometimes, I only need a few seconds to determine when someone is suffering from mental illness. Would you like me to tell you what I think about your own mental condition, Mr. Byggshatt?"

Ralph became very nervous at that very moment and said, "Ah, no further questions," and ran back to sit next to Peter Emppostar.

"Thank you, Doctor Gudsyke," said the judge. "You may step down."

Gene finally wanted to reintroduce his father's testimony, but he had to do it in a sneaky way, "Your Honor, at this time I would like to exercise my right to recall Doctor Sayahagain to the witness stand."

"Doctor Sayahagain," said Judge Lykezdoks, "you're still under oath. Please walk up to the witness stand."

The doctor walked over to the stand and sat down with a sense of worry that could be seen all over his face. His body was leaning leftwards more than ever, and he was staring downwards. "Thank you, Your Honor. Doctor Sayahagain, was my father's testimony true?" asked Gene.

"I object!" Ralph yelled. "Mr. Lissenzwel Senior's testimony was ordered to be stricken from the records!"

"I'm not asking for his testimony to be reintroduced," said Gene, "I'm only asking the witness if it was true."

"I object again!" Ralph yelled even louder. "Counsel should know that he cannot refer to his father's testimony during this trial, because it was stricken from the records."

"Sustained," said the judge. "I will not allow it. Doctor Sayahagain, please disregard Mr. Lissenzwel's question. Mr. Lissenzwel, please rephrase your question or move on to another question."

"Thank you Your Honor." Gene rephrased his question and went on, "Doctor Sayahagain, let me ask you a different question, was Mr. Anthony Lissenzwel your patient in your office at one time?"

"I object!" Ralph yelled once again. "How many times do I have to say that Mr. Lissenzwel Senior's testimony was ordered to be stricken from the records?"

"And how many times do I have to say, Mr. Byggshatt," asked Gene, "that I'm not asking for his testimony to be reintroduced? I'm only asking the witness if Mr. Anthony Lissenzwel was his patient in his office at one time."

"Overruled!" said Judge Lykezdoks. "Please answer the question, Doctor Sayahagain."

"Ah, well, yeah, he was my patient," the doctor answered."

"Doctor Sayahagain," Gene continued, "a man in your position, I'm sure, knows that there are penalties for lying under oath – it's called 'Perjury.' If I can show this court right now that when my father went to your office, he had a different experience than what you told this court, then you'd be guilty of perjury – are you willing to take that chance, Doctor Sayahagain?"

"Of course I am," the doctor answered, "I know he was lying, so, I have nothing to hide."

"Doctor Sayahagain," Gene continued his attack on the lying doctor, "I have in my possession an audio tape that clearly details my father's entire visit while he was in your office. I intend to introduce it as Defense Exhibit A. Are you willing to change your testimony, or should I proceed with the exhibit?"

"I object!" Ralph Byggshatt shouted. "I have to repeat – Mr. Lissenzwel's testimony was thrown out! Even if the defense has a tape containing his testimony, it's already stricken from the records!"

"This tape does not contain Mr. Lissenzwel Senior's testimony!" said Gene in an unusually loud voice. "It contains his visit to Doctor Sayahagain's office, which is not the testimony that he gave in this court, but simply his visit to the doctor's office."

"Overruled!" said the judge. "Please answer the question, Doctor Sayahagain!"

"I forgot the question, what is it?" asked the doctor.

"Clerk," the judge ordered, "read back what Mr. Lissenzwel asked the witness."

The clerk read: "Doctor Sayahagain, I have in my possession an audio tape that clearly details my father's entire visit while he was in your office. I intend to introduce it as Defense Exhibit A. Are you willing to change your testimony, or should I proceed with the exhibit?"

The doctor then looked at everyone in the courtroom. He looked towards Mr. Byggshatt several times – he seemed to be looking for help from the supposed big shot, but the doctor didn't get any assistance at all, not even a sign or a gesture. After a few moments, he finally answered, "That's a bunch of nonsense. I am a well-respected doctor, and nobody distrusts me. No one would dare bring a tape recorder into my office, and I didn't see your father carrying one when he was there. That was a nice try, Mr. Lissenzwel, because what you have is a blank tape. I am not changing my true testimony."

"Your Honor," Gene continued, "at this time, I would like to prove to this court how Doctor Sayahagain treated my father, which is the complete opposite of the testimony given by the doctor himself."

"I object!" Ralph Byggshatt yelled. "Doctor Sayahagain is a highly respectable professional and he doesn't lie. Are you calling him a liar, Counselor?"

"When I present the evidence that I have," Gene replied, "you come to your own conclusion, Mr. Byggshatt, and you decide whether he's a liar or not."

"Overruled!" said the judge. "I want to see the evidence, and I'm sure that the jury wants to see it also. Please continue, Mr. Lissenzwel."

"Thank you, Your Honor," Gene went on as he took a cassette out of his pocket. "I would like to introduce this tape as Defense Exhibit A."

"So entered," said the judge.

"Thank you, Your Honor" Gene continued. "I would like this court to hear the tape right now, so we can all hear how Doctor Sayahagain mistreated my father, in the same way that he mistreated the prisoners who eventually ended up imprisoned at Deprivayshun Psychiatric Hospital."

"I object!" Ralph shouted again. "It has not been established whether or not the defendants were imprisoned at Deprivayshun Psychiatric Hospital."

"Overruled!" said the judge. "At this point it seems that they were, but we'll find out sooner or later. Bailiff, insert the tape into the cassette player and play it immediately. I'm anxious to hear what the tape says." The bailiff did as the judge told him, and the tape started playing.

Receptionist, in a whisper: "He's a wealthy investor, hit him hard."

Doctor Sayahagain: "Have a seat next to me. Open your mouth and say, 'Ah.'"

Anthony: "Ah."

Doctor: "Open your mouth and say, 'Ah' again."

Anthony: "Ah."

Doctor: "I didn't hear you. Open your mouth and say, 'Ah' again."

Anthony: "Ah."

Doctor: "Let's try it again. Open your mouth and say, 'Ah' once more."

Anthony: "Ah."

Doctor: "Okay, now we might be getting somewhere. Open your mouth and say, 'Ah' again."

Anthony: "Ah."

Doctor: "That was much better. Do it again."

Anthony: "Ah."

Doctor: "Wow, you're a good patient, but I'm not sure yet. Open your mouth and say, 'Ah' again."

Anthony: "Ah."

Doctor: "That was a lot better. Let's do that one again."

Anthony: "Ah."

Doctor: "Try a little different this time. Open your mouth and say, 'Ah' again."

Anthony: "Ah."

Doctor: "That was too loud. Do it lower. Open your mouth and say, 'Ah' again."

Anthony: "Ah."

Doctor: "No, no, that was much too low. Open your mouth and say, 'Ah' again, so I can hear you."

Anthony: "Ah."

Doctor: "That was better, but still too low. Open your mouth and say, 'Ah' again."

Anthony: "Ah."

Doctor: "Much better, but do it a little louder. Try again."

Anthony: "Ah."

Doctor: "Almost right, a tiny bit louder. Try again."

Anthony: "Ah."

Doctor: "Okay, that was perfect. Do the same one again to make sure."

Anthony: "Ah."

Doctor: "Okay, let's proceed. Oh, wait a second! Open your mouth and say, 'Ah' again to make sure that I got the right 'Ah' this time."

Anthony: "Ah."

Doctor: "No, that wasn't the same one. Open your mouth and say, 'Ah' again."

Anthony: "Ah."

Doctor: "Try the one before that to make sure that we get it right."

Anthony: "Ah."

Doctor: "I told you that you're a good patient. You did perfectly well. Now, do it again so I can write it down."

Anthony: "Ah."

Doctor: "That was perfect. That'll be $2,750, plus expenses plus other charges. Go see my receptionist. She'll tell you what the total is and collect the money from you. She'll give you the prescription for your medicine as well. Good bye. Next!"

Anthony: "But, Doctor, I'm here because I have an ingrown toe nail in my left foot."

Doctor: "Mr. Lissenzwel, I am the doctor here and I am the only one capable of making a proper diagnosis. You're suffering from a very rare and dangerous form of a mental disorder called 'Inngrounosis.' I'll tell my receptionist to make an emergency appointment for you to go see a psychiatrist immediately. His name is Doctor Louzi, and he specializes exclusively in the treatment of Inngrounosis. That'll be $3,950, plus expenses plus other charges. Go see my receptionist. Good bye. Next!"

Receptionist: "Mr. Lissenzwel, you're a very lucky man, because the total for your bill is only $4,775. Thank you for your payment. Here's the name and address of your psychiatrist. Good bye."

After the tape stopped, Peter Emppostar put his head down and whispered into his attorney's ear, "We're dead. "What are we going to do now?"

"I don't know," Ralph replied in a low voice for a change.

"What am I paying you for?" asked Peter. Mr. Byggshatt was completely speechless, and there was a huge silence in the courtroom, which lasted for more than a minute.

Mr. Byggshatt then took the opportunity to attempt to void the entire recoding. "I object!" he shouted. "I move to dismiss that entire farce!"

"On what grounds, Mr. Byggshatt?" asked the judge. "I doubt if your objection has any validity, but I want to hear it anyway."

"On the grounds that it's too ridiculous," Ralph answered.

"I agree with you, Mr. Byggshatt," said the judge, "it is totally ridiculous – I can't believe that any doctor can practice medicine in such a ridiculous way. However, it is true because the tape speaks for itself, and it doesn't lie. Your objection is even more ridiculous – therefore, OVERRULED! Mr. Byggshatt, I don't want to hear any more of your ridiculous objections. From now on, you may only object when you have a valid objection! I want to hear the end of the trial. Please continue, Mr. Lissenzwel."

Gene then concluded, "Your Honor, I think that, as you said, the tape speaks for itself. I have no further questions for this witness. Your witness, Mr. Byggshatt."

"I have no questions for that witness," said the "Big Shot" lawyer.

"Doctor Sayahagain," said Judge Lykezdoks, "bear in mind that charges will be filed against you for perjury. You may step down. Mr. Lissenzwel, call your next witness."

"Thank you, Your Honor," said Gene as he smiled with a great sense of satisfaction. "At this point, I would like to recall Doctor Ryppemuff to the stand before I call my final witness."

"I object!" Ralph yelled.

"On what grounds?" asked the judge.

"On the grounds that he's the plaintiff," Ralph replied.

"Mr. Byggshatt!" the judge shouted. "I told you before that I didn't want to hear any more of your ridiculous objections, and I think that the one you just made is ridiculous. Be very careful from now on. Overruled! Doctor Ryppemuff, you're still under oath. Please walk up to the witness stand and have a seat."

Gene had something on his mind, but no one knew what it was at that point. He approached the witness and asked, "Sir, what is your name?"

"I object!" Ralph shouted. "We all know what the good doctor's name is!"

"Your Honor," said Gene, "it is very important to this case that the witness answers the question. I will make it very clear when I call my next and final witness."

"Overruled!" the judge also shouted. "Doctor Ryppemuff, please answer the question."

"My name is Doctor Ryppemuff!" Peter answered in a loud voice.

"Sir," Gene said, "I'm sure that a man in your position knows the consequences of lying under oath. There are laws against it. Perjury is a punishable offense. Now, would you like to change your answer?"

"No, no, no! I told the truth! My name is Doctor Ryppemuff!" Peter yelled again.

"Very well, Sir," said Gene; "no further questions. Your witness, Mr. Byggshatt."

There was a sound in the courtroom, as people wondered why Gene didn't ask the doctor anything other than what his name was, and Mr. Byggshatt had no reason to question his own client. However, he used one last tactic in an attempt to win the case, "I have no questions for that witness. Your Honor, how long are you planning to let this farce go? You even told this court a long time ago that the verdict was mine. What happened to you all of a sudden?"

"Mr. Byggshatt!" the judge shouted once more. "I am hereby holding you in contempt of this court! You're now walking on a very thin line! Be extremely careful from now on!" The judge then turned towards Gene and said, "The witness may step down. You may continue, Mr. Lissenzwel."

Gene was extremely happy to see that Judge Lykezdoks had completely turned the table, and Mr. Byggshatt had become the underdog in the judge's eyes. "Your Honor," said Gene, "at this time I would like to introduce as Defense Exhibit B, copies of various bank account records – the accounts belong to all the adult defendants present in this courtroom. The statements clearly show the enormous amounts of money that were withdrawn from them every month by Deprivayshun Psychiatric Hospital while the prisoners were in the hospital, whether they were patients or prisoners there, and without authorization."

"So entered," said the judge.

"Your Honor," Gene continued, "I would like this court to issue court orders to reimburse all my clients with everything that was taken out of their accounts, plus interest."

"I will review all the statements, Mr. Lissenzwel," the judge responded, "and I will make a ruling later, but at this point, I don't see how I can justify issuing such court orders. Let's see whether or not you can find a reason that will show me that I should do it."

Gene then proceeded with extreme confidence at that stage of the trial, "Thank you, Your Honor. Before this trial began, when I heard that Mr. Byggshatt was the attorney that I would be facing, I really wanted to throw in the towel, but I realized that the prisoners had faith in me, and I was all they had. I felt much smaller than David was, and I viewed Mr. Byggshatt as being much larger than Goliath was – that visualization actually gave me the strength to work very hard, day and night, while preparing for this trial. I didn't want to leave any stones unturned, so I went all over and did everything that I could think of. I even hired an extremely competent private investigator, who was able to produce wondrous results. Her name is Rebecca Fynedzowt, and she turned out to be a key figure during my search for evidence. She provided me with a witness that will give this court the strongest evidence that I have, which will certainly clear my clients of all charges against them. She's the final witness that I would like to call – she's Doctor Ryppemuff's receptionist. Her name is Mary Ohnowear."

"I'm very anxious to hear her testimony," said the judge. "Is she here, Mr. Lissenzwel?"

Gene was even more anxious, so he answered the judge's question while pointing at Mary, "Yes, Your Honor, there she is."

Ralph Byggshatt, of course, didn't want the court to hear her testimony – whatever it was, so he shouted as usual, "I object!"

The judge showed a face of disgust as he looked and yelled at Ralph, "ON WHAT GROUNDS?"

"On the ground that the witness has nothing to do with this case," Ralph answered, "and she might be prejudicial to Doctor Ryppemuff."

Gene did his best to have the judge allow Mary to testify. He knew that her testimony was extremely crucial, and without it, he didn't know if he could win the case. "Your Honor," he said, "this witness is directly connected to this case. She works in the same hospital as the plaintiff, and she has complete knowledge of most of the activities there."

Mr. Byggshatt also did his best to have the judge disallow Mary from testifying, "The hospital is not on trial here, the doctor is – I mean, the prisoners are. What possible connection could there be between them and Miss Ohnowear?"

"Your Honor," Gene insisted, "the witness is also directly connected with the plaintiff and the defendants. She has full knowledge of all the actions taken by Deprivayshun Psychiatric Hospital against all the prisoners. Therefore, she has a very strong connection to this case."

"Overruled!" said the judge. "Miss Ohnowear, please come up to the witness stand."

Mary walked towards the witness stand and was sworn in. "Thank you, Your Honor," said Gene Lissenzwel. "Miss Ohnowear, please tell us your name, occupation and place of business."

"My name is Mary Ohnowear," she replied, "and I am Doctor Ryppemuff's receptionist. I work at Deprivayshun Psychiatric Hospital."

"Miss Ohnowear," Gene continued, "please tell this court all the events that took place in the hospital about sixteen months ago on the evening that you told me that you had to work overtime."

"I object!" Ralph shouted. "The prisoners only escaped from the hospital a few weeks ago, and none of them was there sixteen months ago. What possible connection could there be between events that allegedly took place then and this trial?"

"OVERRULED! SHUT UP, BYGGSHATT," the judge ruled without the need for Gene to even open his mouth. "You may answer the question, Miss Ohnowear."

"Yes, Sir," Mary happily replied with great satisfaction. "That day, Doctor Ryppemuff left as he usual, after his day at work. About an hour later, he went back to the hospital. With the help of an orderly and a gurney, he brought his sick brother into his office. It sounded very strange to me because I had never heard Doctor Ryppemuff say that he had a brother. I thought that maybe he never mentioned his brother because he was ashamed of him because he was sick. I didn't think much about it at that time, but I did mention it to the doctor, and he told me that he'd rather not talk about it. After that, I…"

"Did he tell you why he didn't want to talk about it, Miss Ohnowear?" asked Gene as he interrupted her.

"No, he did not," Mary answered, "and I never mentioned anything to anyone. Anyway, after Doctor Ryppemuff had his brother in his office for a little while, he told the orderly to bring him to the nearest room that had an available bed. His brother was then placed in a bed in the same room where those prisoners were eventually placed, one by one, about a year later. After he placed his brother there, Doctor Ryppemuff went back to his office and told me that he was becoming forgetful and needed me to remind him of certain things that he was starting to forget. He even offered me overtime hours, and I think he did that in exchange for my silence about his memory loss. I'm now ashamed that I accepted the overtime, but I need the money because I have younger brothers and sisters that I'm helping my mother to support, because my father died two years ago. Anyway, the first thing that I had to tell him was where the bathroom was. It was a little strange, but I thought nothing more about it. He often asked me to refresh his memory about simple things, and I was beginning to wonder if he was becoming senile, but he gradually stopped asking me for any more help with his memory. It was as…"

Gene interjected again and asked, "Miss Ohnowear, please tell us if at anytime you felt that the doctor was lying to you about his memory."

"No, not at all," she answered, "at least not at that point, because I had no reason to believe that he was lying. All I thought was that he had recovered his memory completely, and I didn't think about it anymore after he stopped needing my help. As time passed, Doctor Ryppemuff told me that he was giving his brother a daily injection because he was in a coma, and as we speak, he's still in the same condition. A few weeks ago, right after the prisoners escaped, Doctor Ryppemuff was so busy during his attempts to get them back from jail and into the hospital, that he didn't give his brother his daily injection. I was very curious about his sick brother, so I wanted to see him and try to talk to him. The following…"

"Why did you try to talk to him, Miss Ohnowear," asked Gene as he interrupted her again, "when he was in a coma?"

"Well," Mary replied, "I didn't really know that he was in a coma – I only knew what the doctor told me, and even though I had no reason to doubt him, I was curious to see if I could possibly communicate with his brother."

"Thank you. Please continue," said Gene.

"Okay," she went on, "the following day, before Doctor Ryppemuff arrived, I went upstairs to his brother's room. When I finally entered Ward Two Seventeen, where Doctor Ryppemuff's brother was, I went to his bedside and noticed that he was coming to. After a few minutes, he was able to talk with tremendous difficulty, but he couldn't get up at all, and he couldn't move very well. He told me that he was the real Doctor Ryppemuff, and that there was a man who was identical in appearance to him whose name was Peter Emppostar. He…"

Mary was interrupted by a commotion caused by an attempt that Peter immediately made to leave the courtroom, but Judge Lykezdoks saw him and yelled, "Bailiff, stop Doctor Ryppemuff from leaving this courtroom, and put him back in his seat." The bailiff ran and caught up with the fake doctor just before he reached the exit door. He overpowered Peter and put him back where the judge wanted him. "Stay there with him, Bailiff, until the trial is over," the judge ordered. "Miss Ohnowear, please continue your testimony."

"Yes, Sir, Your Honor," said Mary with an even greater sense of satisfaction. "Okay, the man in a coma also told me that Mr. Emppostar injected him with a syringe one evening in his car on his way home, and after that, he didn't remember the rest. It took him almost half an hour to tell me all that, and he passed out again as soon as he told me everything. At that very moment, I realized why Mr. Emppostar had told me the farce about his memory lapses – it was simply because he was trying to adjust his life to impersonate Doctor Ryppemuff as an exact copy of him. He certainly did a good job because he had me totally fooled all that time, and I was unaware that he was a fake. Anyway, when Mr. Emppostar arrived that day, I had already returned to the doctor's office, and he went to Doctor Ryppemuff's room and gave him another injection.

"I didn't want to say anything at the time. I was going to wait a little bit, and think very thoroughly about what I had to do before going to the police, knowing very well that I was going to be without a job – in fact, I am now unemployed, because after this, there's no way that I'm going back there. Before I had a chance to think about what I was going to do, and when I was going to call the police, your private investigator, Rebecca Fynedzowt, was digging around looking for evidence, and she got to me first. She approached me in the hospital's parking lot when I was going home after work one evening. She was so good at getting information from people, that, even though I resisted, I finally told her everything. Then she took me to your office, Mr. Lissenzwel, where I repeated the whole story to you – well, here I am, and I have just repeated it again."

Following Mary Ohnowear's testimony, everyone was totally astonished to hear that Doctor Ryppemuff was an impostor. Even the defendants were completely surprised because they had no idea that he was a fake during all the time that they spent at Deprivayshun Psychiatric Hospital. Peter Emppostar, Gene Lissenzwel, Rebecca Fynedzowt and Mary Ohnowear were the only ones who knew the truth until Mary testified in court. Gene didn't want anyone else to know it before the trial, to make sure that the information didn't leak out.

Gene Lissenzwel let out a big sigh of relief. He felt good because Ralph Byggshatt didn't object at all during Mary's testimony – perhaps because Judge Lykezdoks had warned him about his ridiculous objections. Gene then concluded, "Thank you, Miss Ohnowear. No further questions. Your witness, Mr. Byggshatt."

Even Ralph was so shocked that he had no questions for the witness, "I have nothing to ask."

"Your Honor," said Gene, "in view of my last witness' testimony, I must ask for a dismissal of all charges against all my clients. I must humbly ask the court to declare them sane and to allow them to go home."

"I object!" Ralph yelled.

"ON WHAT GROUNDS?" asked the judge.

"On the grounds that, that, that, that, never mind," Ralph replied.

"Very well, then," said the judge. "Based on the testimony given by all the prisoners, I can see that there was a specific pattern in the way that they were taken to Deprivayshun Psychiatric Hospital – four of them went through the same path, as they testified, but two of them were there because they tried to help the others. The other four were there because they are related to those who tried to help the original four.

"I also believe that the testimony given by the four prisoners who were almost butchered to death at Kuttemopen Hospital should be enough proof that none of the doctors involved were capable of properly treating their patients, or at least, if they were capable, then they were unwilling to treat them properly.

"Doctor Sayahagain made Mr. Anthony Lissenzwel say, 'Ah' nineteen times. Following his 'Ah' routine, the doctor presented him with an astronomical bill. The doctor never asked him why he went to see him. When Mr. Lissenzwel told him why he was there, the doctor ignored him completely and sent him to a psychiatrist. He then told him that that psychiatrist specialized exclusively in the mental disorder that Doctor Sayahagain claimed the patient was suffering from. I believe that if Mr. Lissenzwel had gone to the psychiatrist, he would have followed the same path that four of the defendants followed before they ended up under the imprisonment of Doctor Ryppemuff, or Peter Emppostar, at Deprivayshun Psychiatric Hospital.

"I further believe that the defense attorney has already shown this court enough proof that Doctor Sayahagain makes up a name for a bogus diagnosis, which is different for every patient. He then tells all his patients that he's going to send them to the same psychiatrist – Doctor Louzi. Then he tells each patient that Doctor Louzi specializes exclusively in the treatment of that particular illness. Doctor Sayahagain told Mr. Sam Towhertz that he was suffering from Swelosis, and then later he changed his diagnosis to Aikosis, while he told Mr. Anthony Lissenzwel that he was suffering from Inngrounosis. He sent them both to Doctor Louzi, and Doctor Sayahagain told them both that Doctor Louzi specialized exclusively in all three phony mental disorders that he made up names for. He did exactly the same to all the prisoners who went through him before they ended up as prisoners at Deprivayshun Psychiatric Hospital under the abuses of Doctor Ryppemuff – or Peter Emppostar, whatever his name is.

"I believe that Mr. Lissenzwel Junior has also proven that the defendants are not insane at all, and they acted in self defense when they escaped. Therefore, this trial is over! Defendants, I hereby declare you not guilty and not insane. You're free to go home."

The entire courtroom erupted in an uproar. The judge continued after the noise settled down somewhat, "Thank you, ladies and gentlemen of the jury, you're dismissed." After a few minutes, when the noised settled down even further, the judge concluded, "Bailiff, arrest Doctor Ryppemuff, or Peter Emppostar, whoever he might be, pending an investigation. Mr. Lissenzwel, before you leave, come to my desk because you have shown this court plenty of good reasons why I should prepare court orders for you to go to all the banks and have all the defendants' accounts released to them immediately. I'll also have a court order ordering Deprivayshun Psychiatric Hospital to reimburse every cent that was taken out of their accounts, plus interest, while they were put through their horrible ordeals as prisoners there. I will also prepare court orders demanding that all the doctors involved, and Kuttemopen Hospital, reimburse every cent, plus interest, to all the defendants. Case…"

"I object!" Ralph Byggshatt suddenly shouted. "Your Honor, Doctor Ryppemuff, or Peter Emppostar I should say, has only given me a retainer fee of $500,000. He still owes me another $500,000 for representing him. Now that he's going to jail, and the defendants' bank accounts are being released to them, where am I going to get my money from?"

"SHUT UP EX-BIG SHOT!" said the judge. "You know very well that that's your problem, and it's another case. I'm not here to try that case, but the case of the poor ex-prisoners, which has already been resolved. Go home, LOSER, and DON'T bother me anymore! CASE CLOSED!"

The judge banged on his desk with his gavel while Peter Emppostar was being handcuffed and taken away. Gene's parents had been patiently sitting in the courtroom all throughout the trial. They were so proud of their son that Annette couldn't control her crying, and even Anthony had tears in his eyes.

A few minutes later, Gene went to the judge's bench and picked up several court orders ordering the banks to release several bank accounts back to their rightful owners. He also picked up from the judge the court order to force Deprivayshun Psychiatric Hospital to reimburse all the money that was taken out of the prisoners' accounts, plus interest, back to them. The judge also had the court orders to have all the doctors and Kuttemopen Hospital reimburse all the money that they took from the defendants, plus interest.

Following the trial, it was almost impossible for all the participants to get past the numerous members of the media. They had been watching the trial from the beginning, because Mr. Ralph Byggshatt alerted them so he could be immortalized as the winner – the plan certainly backfired right in his face.

As soon as the commotion settled down, Gene spoke with Sam regarding his swollen toe, Robert regarding his chemical burn on the palm of his hand, John regarding his bee sting on his right thumb and Carmen regarding her thorn in her left pinky. "My parents have been very fortunate," he said. "They never had a bad experience with a doctor before, because a very good doctor was recommended to them by my mother's sister. The doctor's name is Doctor Honnastt. My entire family and all my relatives are her patients. I'll give all of you her phone number so she can take care of your problems, if you're interested."

All the ex-prisoners showed their appreciation to Gene and agreed to go to Doctor Honnastt from then on. At that moment, Carmen mentioned that they had to do something to help Martha Innaddayze, because she was still locked up in the hospital. Gene told them that he'd talk to District Attorney Jonathan Gudgovaygint about it, and they all promised that they would do whatever they could do to help her.

Just Compensation for Everyone

THE DAY AFTER THE trial was over, Ralph Byggshatt's name was plastered all over the radio, television, newspapers, magazines etc. as having lost a big case against a lawyer who had just finished law school and had never tried a case before.

The same day, Judge Lykezdoks told Jonathan Gudgovaygint to order an investigation regarding the truth about the man who was heavily sedated at Deprivayshun Psychiatric Hospital. He also told him to pursue the matter against Doctor Sayahagain for lying under oath. Gene had already told The DA about Martha Innaddayze. The District Attorney went to work on the three cases right away.

After their freedom, all the ex-prisoners returned to their homes to try to resume normal lives. The four wealthy ex-prisoners, Carmen Pynkeehertz, John Suolenthom, Robert Berndhend and Sam Towhertz, knew that Gene Lissenzwel's parents had to refinance their home in order to support Gene during the trial. Without wasting any time, as soon as their money was available to them again, they financially compensated Gene extremely well for his courageous and victorious efforts in defending them.

Gene did not charge Anna a fee for defending her and her children. He did it pro bono because she was barely making ends meet when she was captured and turned into a prisoner. Besides, when Gene was paid, he himself was very financially well-off. She told him that he should accept at least some financial compensation from her because she had some savings, which had already been released back to her.

Gene insisted that he didn't want to take it because she had been such a great participant during the entire process. The fact is that Gene did not charge a fee to anyone – the generous compensation that he received was given to him voluntarily by the wealthy defendants.

A few days later, after things settled down somewhat, Gene had more than enough money to take care of a few things. He paid Rebecca Fynedzowt everything that he owed her for her investigative work, plus a very generous bonus for her patience and great performance. Gene also repaid his parents by paying off the loan that they had taken against their home, plus the balance of the old loan that they still had on it. He also bought them their first automobile ever, so they wouldn't have to take their long walks to the supermarket and return home loaded with bags full of groceries – of course, they each had to learn how to drive and get a driver's license. His parents felt that their long sacrifices while Gene was going to school finally paid off, but they were happier about their son's great success rather than their own personal gain

Sometime later, when District Attorney Gudgovaygint checked Doctor Ryppemuff's records at Deprivayshun Psychiatric Hospital, he found out that the fingerprints that were on file were those of the man under sedation. After a few more pieces of evidence, the DA concluded that every word was true about Peter Emppostar, and the real Doctor Ryppemuff was the man under sedation.

Peter Emppostar, after all, did not get away with that almost perfect case of identity theft. It all happened because he failed to replace the fingerprints that were on file with his own fingerprints. It was hard to believe that after he ingeniously did so many things to impersonate Doctor Ryppemuff, he would overlook such a minor detail.

The real Doctor Ryppemuff was taken to Gud Hospital and rehabilitated by Doctor Honnastt. After his release, he went back as Director and Head Psychiatrist of Deprivayshun Psychiatric Hospital, and he still practices there today.

Jonathan Gudgovaygint was informed by Gene that Martha Innaddayze was also a prisoner at Deprivayshun Psychiatric Hospital. He discovered during his investigation of Doctor Ryppemuff that she wasn't allowed to have any visitors. He found that to be very strange, because after speaking with her, he thought that she was of sound mind, but somewhat forgetful. He took the matter to Judge Pharemynded and obtained visiting rights for her. The only problem was that no one knew of any relatives that she may have had. The District Attorney contacted Gene Lissenzwel to ask him to recommend a good private investigator. Gene gave his name and telephone number to Rebecca Fynedzowt, and after she called the District Attorney, he hired her immediately to try to locate living relatives of Martha Innaddayze. Because of Rebecca's fantastic abilities, after only two hours on the job, she was able to locate Martha's parents, Mark and Julie Innaddayze. They had moved out of the state shortly after Martha disappeared. They returned when they heard the good news. Gene worked out a power of attorney agreement so Martha's father could manage her affairs while they worked on getting her out of Deprivayshun Psychiatric Hospital. When Martha's parents finally exercised the court order that District Attorney Gudgovaygint had obtained to allow them to visit her, they were totally delighted to see their daughter again, but they were also completely devastated to see that Martha didn't even know who they were.

The fake Doctor Ryppemuff, also known as Peter Emppostar, was brought to trial. He was found guilty of all charges brought against him, and also declared to be terminally insane and a danger to society. He was sent to Deprivayshun Psychiatric Hospital to spend the rest of his life there without ever having any visitors. He was confined to a private room with no contact with anyone from the outside. Ironically, he was sent to spend the rest of his days in the same hospital where he impersonated Doctor Ryppemuff.

District Attorney Gudgovaygint eventually filed charges against Doctor Sayahagain for perjury. The judge gave the doctor the option of pleading guilty and paying a fine, but the doctor didn't want to risk the possibility of losing his medical license by having a bad mark on his record. He chose to go to trial and take his chances in court. He asked Gene Lissenzwel to defend him, but Gene turned him down, and the doctor hired another lawyer. Luckily for Doctor Sayahagain, the incriminating testimony that he gave in court was inadvertently distorted and rendered useless. Therefore, there was no proof that he ever lied under oath, and the charges were dropped. He didn't have to pay a fine or serve a prison term and was allowed to continue practicing as usual.

After partially recovering from their ordeals, one by one, Sam Towhertz, Robert Berndhend, John Suolenthom and Carmen Pynkeehertz, as well as all the other freed defendants and their families, eventually contacted Doctor Honnastt, and she became their regular doctor. Sam's swollen toe had already become totally disfigured due to the time that it went untreated. Robert's chemical burn on the palm of his hand caused a severe tissue abnormality also due to the same reason. John's bee sting in his right thumb caused the finger to be almost useless due to a buildup of puss that turned into a hard lump. Carmen's thorn inside of her left pinky also caused a lump that became hard and yellowish. They were all cured by Doctor Honnastt with just one visit to her office. Doctor Honnastt also successfully treated the defendants who had been victims of Kuttemopen Hospital's malicious practices. It took some of the ex-prisoners a very long time to resume normal lives, but with Doctor Honnastt's help, eventually they were all back to normal. Doctor Honnastt did such a great job that she was making an astronomically good living. She treated all her patients honestly and caringly – that's real proof that doctors can, and many do, make a good living while maintaining their honesty.

Sam Towhertz, right after recovering from his ordeal, donated a condominium to Gene's parents in the same building where his penthouse was. They occupied it as soon as they could and still live in it today. They didn't want to sell their original house because it had too much sentimental value – it was because of it that they were able to obtain money to support Gene during the trial. They let Annette's sister move into it free of charge because she had recently lost her husband, and her income was just barely enough to get by.

Anna Lyphesayvar was helped by Carmen Pynkeehertz to improve her looks. She looked at least ten years younger after Carmen finished with her. She was also rewarded by everyone involved. Sam Towhertz also donated a condominium to her in the same building where his penthouse was. She moved into it with her three children at once. The others donated plenty of money, as they had promised her, for helping them. She was very well-off, financially and otherwise, as a result of her willingness to help the prisoners. If she had looked the other way when the prisoners reached out for her help, she'd be most likely without a job, because the hospital dismissed several food servants shortly after she became a janitor, and she only became a janitor because she wanted to help them. Following the wealthy ex-prisoners' generous donations, Anna had so much money, that she decided to stay unemployed and devote her full attention to her three children until they no longer needed it.

Christine, Susan and Bobby Lyphesayvar, Anna's three children, became huge celebrities when they returned to school after their summer vacation was over. It happened because of their ordeals in the hospital, during the escape, in the jail cell, in the hotel and in the courtroom. They didn't get any more nightmares about their suffering during their imprisonment.

Following his great victory, Gene Lissenzwel's case against Ralph Byggshatt was documented in many law journals throughout the country. He started receiving offers to join several very prestigious law firms. He kept all the offers in mind, but he decided to try to make it on his own.

Kuttemopen Hospital, Doctor Louzi, Doctor Byggliar, Doctor Sharlottan, Doctor Butchar, Doctor Manypewlatar, Doctor

Oargandeelar, Doctor Sayahagain, Doctor Louziar and Deprivayshun Psychiatric Hospital were acquitted of numerous crimes that they were charged with during a new trial that was brought against them by District Attorney Gudgovaygint. In spite of all the evidence against the defendants, the DA was unable to strip them of theirs licenses – they were never found guilty of the major crimes that they committed. Most of the evidence that District Attorney Gudgovaygint had was deemed inadmissible and thrown out. The defendants' victory was also achieved by having numerous doctors testify on their behalf and say that everything that the DA was able to prove that they did was totally justified in the medical profession, and no one could dispute otherwise. They were heavily fined for their participation in numerous minor crimes that they were found guilty of, but were allowed to continue doing business as usual. Some of those crimes included: lying to the patients, sending them to other doctors for no reason, failing to treat them properly, and various other minor violations.

Doctor Ryppemuff was not a defendant at the trial because he was sedated during the events that led to all the harm that was done to the victims, but District Attorney Gudgovaygint planned to pursue the matter against him because he felt that the doctor was guilty of other crimes – such as the possibility that Martha Innaddayze was also being illegally held as a prisoner at Deprivayshun Psychiatric Hospital.

Eventually, the DA was finally unwilling to file charges against Doctor Ryppemuff because he felt that he didn't have enough evidence against him, and also because he had been unable to punish the other doctors involved even though he had found plenty of evidence against them. The DA then felt that if Doctor Ryppemuff had committed crimes – which he was sure of – then the doctor got away with everything that he had done.

Benjamin Diphycolt was fired as Head of the Public Defender's Office. Rumors were that he had been seen pumping gas at a local gas station. Gene Lissenzwel was offered the job as Public Defender, but he happily declined it. Someone else was hired shortly after Gene turned the position down.

Jesse Louziloyar was also fired from the Public Defender's Office and was unable to find employment elsewhere. Because he never saved any money, he borrowed his parents' life savings to open his own law firm. He was unable to gain the confidence of any prospective client due to his deceptive and rattling way of communicating with people. Prospective clients also noticed his unwillingness to make a good effort to defend anyone, which was reason enough for everyone to decline his services as a lawyer. Only a few months after Jesse opened his law firm, he lost his lease due to non-payment of his rent, and he had to close his law practice. After being unable to find employment anywhere, even doing other things, he ultimately went to the gas station where his ex-boss, Benjamin Diphycolt, worked and begged the owner for a job. Jesse was hired as a floor sweeper, but only because Benjamin talked the owner of the gas station into hiring him. The only reason why Jesse had been hired as a lawyer at the Public Defender's Office, and stayed there for over ten years, was because Benjamin Diphycolt was very similar to him in many ways, except that he didn't have a rattling tongue as Jesse did.

Ralph Byggshatt continues practicing law, but he is now working as an assistant to a new lawyer who recently graduated from law school and works for the Public Defender's Office.

Judge Lykezdoks continues presiding as usual, but with much more compassion for everyone, rich or poor. He now gives everyone in his courtroom an equal opportunity right from the onset of every trial.

Mary Ohnowear, as soon as she testified during the trial, had to leave her employment at Deprivayshun Psychiatric Hospital in fear of any retaliatory actions against her by the hospital's administration. Sam Towhertz hired her to work as an administrative assistant with twice her previous salary. Her life completely turned around for the better.

As time passed, because Benjamin Diphycolt and Jesse Louziloyar once worked for the Public Defender's Office, they eventually met Ralph Byggshatt, who started working there shortly after they left. They became friends and got together on a regular basis. One day, they decided to try to extort money from the government. They started planning a fraudulent scheme against the Public Defender's Office. They planned to charge the new Public Defender with age discrimination because Ralph was already near his retirement age. Ralph also claimed that he had to endure severe mental cruelty due to sex discrimination, because a woman was the boss after Benjamin was fired from the Public Defender's Office. Benjamin and Jesse also charged the Public Defender with sex discrimination because they claimed that she refused to rehire them, but the truth was that they had never applied to be rehired anyway. In addition, they claimed that when they went there to apply for a job, they were physically assaulted by other lawyers, because such lawyers were afraid of being replaced by superior attorneys, as Benjamin and Jesse considered themselves to be. Ralph also claimed that he was a victim of physical assault by other employees. The reason was that he claimed that the Public Defender wanted to get rid of him because he posed a threat to her, and because he truly believed that he was a good lawyer. They had a list of charges that was very long, but none of the charges ever amounted to anything.

They spent several months planning their scheme. Because Gene Lissenzwel had been so victorious before, when they had everything ready to execute their plan, they decided to contact him to represent them. When they presented the case to Gene and tried to fool him, he immediately realized that they were lying, and everything was fraudulent. Gene turned them down, and they hired another lawyer, Sebastian Nosenathyn, to represent them.

When the case finally went to trial, the three attorneys and their counselor were so inefficient, that their plan backfired right in their faces as soon as the trial started – the judge noticed too many irregularities and realized that there was a fraudulent conspiracy meant to steal taxpayers' money. The judge learned during the trial that their counselor was also involved in the conspiracy, because another bright young attorney who had recently joined the Public Defender's Office was able to produce wondrous evidence against the co-conspirator. All four attorneys were arrested before they left the courtroom.

Once in jail, they contacted Gene Lissenzwel again to ask him to represent them, but Gene turned them down because he knew that they were guilty. The Public Defender then assigned an experienced attorney with over twenty years of service in the office to represent the four jailed attorneys. The assigned attorney fed Benjamin Diphycolt and Jesse Louziloyar their own medicine – they were put right through the system very fast, together with Ralph Byggshatt and Sebastian Nosenathyn during the attempted extortion. They all ended up in jail, where they're still serving a long sentence.

The Lawsuit

FOLLOWING HIS VICTORIOUS TRIAL, Gene Lissenzwel immediately started preparing for a lawsuit against all the doctors and hospitals involved. He had plans to include all the ex-prisoners and Martha Innaddayze in the lawsuit. He had constant communication and meetings with all the ex-prisoners and Martha's parents, Mark and Julie Innaddayze, because Martha was still in the hospital and Mark had power of attorney to act on her behalf. Gene collected plenty of information from the malicious doctors by sending seven fake patients to Doctor Sayahagain's office with voice-activated cassette recorders. Of course, Gene made up occupations and financial status for all seven, in order to make his case against Doctor Sayahagain even stronger. There was absolutely nothing wrong with any of the patients, but they were instructed by Gene to tell the doctor that they each had a different problem – one had a scratch on his finger, which he covered with a home-made dressing, one had a small mark on his arm and was afraid that it might have been malignant, one had a splinter in his elbow, one had an ingrown toe nail, one had an earache, one had a stomachache and the last one had back pains – of course, all their ailments were faked.

All the fake patients visited the doctor the same day, but a few minutes apart. When the patients visited Doctor Sayahagain, he never asked any of them what their reasons for their visits were. He did look at all their applications to see their financial status, so he could determine how much he was going to rip them off. Every patient had the tape cassette recording every word that was spoken by both the doctor and the patient. After putting them through his usual "Ah" deception for several minutes, Doctor Sayahagain told them the amount of their bills and said, "Go see my receptionist and pay the bill. Good bye! Next!" As soon as the doctor said, "Next," the patients told him what their problems were, but he didn't even bother to examine any of them. He told six out of the seven patients that they were suffering from bogus names that he made up for their supposed mental illnesses.

He then told them that he was going to send them to see a psychiatrist for immediate emergency appointments. The psychiatrist was always the same – Doctor Louzi. Doctor Sayahagain told the six patients that Doctor Louzi specialized exclusively in whatever mental disorders he told them that they were suffering from, which were different for all six patients. One patient wasn't sent to the psychiatrist because he didn't have any substantial money or medical insurance to pay for the psychiatrist's ridiculous bill. The doctor didn't examine him either. Instead he told him to go home and rest for a while. Of course, he ripped him off with an inflated bill and gave him a prescription for useless medicine.

Right after the six patients left Doctor Sayahagain's office, they visited Doctor Louzi. As soon as they walked into his office, he put them through several minutes of very expensive rigmarole. Again, all the patients had the tape cassettes recording every word that was spoken by the doctor and the patients. After Doctor Louzi ran out of nonsense to tell them, he told them that their mental conditions were so grave that they needed to see a highly respected specialist named Doctor Louziar. He then told them that Doctor Louziar specialized exclusively in their particular problems, which, of course, were different for all the patients. From there, all six patients went to see Doctor Louziar.

Upon visiting Doctor Louziar, the patients experienced a routine that was almost identical to that of Doctor Louzi's routine, but much more expensive. As with the first two doctors, everything was recorded. After putting the patients through a massive amount of nonsense, the doctor referred them to Kuttemopen Hospital for immediate evaluations. Gene had instructed the patients not to go to the hospital because they would undergo various unnecessary operations against their will, and by force.

Gene also sent his fake patients to visit Doctor Byggliar, who put them through the same routine as Doctor Sayahagain had done, except that he didn't use the "Ah" method of ripping off his victims. After ripping them off, Doctor Byggliar sent them to Doctor Sharlottan, who also ripped them off. Everything was recorded again during their visits to both doctors. After Doctor Sharlottan stole their money, he sent them to Kuttemopen Hospital, but Gene had again instructed the patients not to go to the hospital because of the dangers that they would face there.

Counting all the seven patients' visits to all the doctors, Gene had already spent $335,680 to cover their various inflated rip-off fees that the five doctors they visited had charged them. It was a good thing that Gene was literarily a rich man when he was paid by the wealthy prisoners after he successfully defended them – of course, Gene kept track of all his expenses, for which he expected to get reimbursed by the plaintiffs after the lawsuit was won, as he hoped and expected. At that point, Gene had enough evidence against Doctor Sayahagain, Doctor Louzi, Doctor Louziar, Doctor Byggliar and Doctor Sharlottan. He still had to get evidence against Doctor Butchar, Doctor Manypewlatar, Doctor Oargandeelar, Doctor Ryppemuff, Kuttemopen Hospital and Deprivayshun Psychiatric Hospital. He didn't have any idea how he was going to get that crucial evidence that he needed from each one without exposing the patients to malicious harm.

One day, Gene started going over his notes with the help of the ex-prisoners. Anna had been a food servant and later a janitor at Deprivayshun Psychiatric Hospital. She provided Gene with the names of many of the servants, janitors and other hospital employees. Gene organized a spy team made up of some of the ex-prisoners to surveil the facility. It was a task that had to be handled extremely carefully, because the hospital had heightened security after the trial.

With Anna's help in being able to identify those hospital employees who she had mentioned, they started the difficult task of trying to learn more about their schedules and habits. During the many days of surveillance, Anna was able to recognize some of the servants, janitors and other employees as they went in and out of the hospital. It took several days to conclude the surveillance. By then, Gene and the others had to think of a way to try to communicate with those who Anna had recognized. They had to be extremely careful not to upset any of the observed employees, which would cause them to alert the hospital.

A few days later, Gene Lissenzwel asked all the others to meet him at Sam Towhertz's office, which was very spacious, and Sam had told him to use it anytime he wanted. They met the following day, and Gene asked if anyone had thought of something that would help. "I think I have a good idea," said Anna Lyphesayvar as she raised her hand, "Maria Jannytarboz might be willing to help us. She's the supervisor of the janitors, and she was one of the employees that I recognized during the surveillance. She has a lot of freedom to move around within the hospital, and she even has the keys to lots of places – at least, she did when I was there. Right after we completed surveilling the people coming in and out of the hospital, I realized that she's the first person that we should approach. I know her personally, and she's very unhappy with her job. She's actually very smart and knowledgeable – I know that, because we were very close friends. She hasn't left her job because she's a little afraid of making a change."

"That's a great idea!" Gene exclaimed. "I imagine that she would be reluctant to talk to us, in fear of losing her job, but I think that we can make her silence go away by offering her plenty of financial compensation – if that's what's bothering her at the job. If the problem is due to working conditions, then I'm sure that some of us can hire her with a higher salary and better working conditions. After winning the trial, I have become a little more financially independent, and I am now ready to hire a good secretary and assistant. Considering that Maria is a supervisor, and based on what you just told us about her, Anna, I'm sure that she has good qualifications. I'm willing to hire her and put her through some formal legal training, so she can work for me."

"I can also hire her if you don't need her, Gene," said Sam.

"I'm also willing to hire her," Robert interjected.

"Ditto," Carmen added.

"Me, too," said John.

Gene then proceeded with the discussions and said, "You're all great! Thank you, all. Let's go to work on Maria then. Maybe we don't have to contact anyone else. Let's think of a way to approach her without frightening her. Do you think she'll be afraid to talk to you, Anna, now that everyone knows what happened during the trial?"

"Well, I think I can surprise her at the right time and place and talk to her," Anna answered.

"Okay then," Gene went on, "I'll hire my private investigator again, Rebecca Fynedzowt, to get as much information about Maria as she can." After several more minutes of discussions, Gene ended the meeting, and everyone else went home. He then hired Rebecca to go to work on the case as soon as possible. After that, he went to work on other cases. After several hours, he called it a day and went home.

Several days later, Rebecca had watched Maria Jannytarboz many times as she went in and out of her home and the hospital. She saw Maria get out of her house a few minutes after she got home from work, almost every night, to go to Gudphood Diner to have her dinner alone.

Rebecca gave Gene a complete log of Maria's activities. She also told him that when Maria went to the diner, she sat at a table a few times near Rebecca. Gene had already figured out what he was going to do – he had originally planned to send Rebecca with Anna to the diner every night until they met Maria, but because Rebecca told him that Maria sat at a table near her, he changed the plan, because Maria may have seen Rebecca there and recognize her is she saw her again. He then decided to send Carmen with Anna instead.

The next day, Anna and Carmen went to the diner to have dinner and wait for Maria, but she never showed up. They went four nights in a row without any success. On the fifth night, they were sitting at their usual table, and, Bingo! There was Maria, who had just walked into the diner. Maria was about to pass by their side to go to her favorite seat at the rear of the dining area. Carmen and Maria looked at her, but she didn't see them, so Anna suddenly stood up in front of Maria and said, "Oh my God! It's you, Maria!"

"Wow! Is that you, Anna?" asked Maria.

"Yup, it's me!" Anna answered. "How are you, Maria?"

"I'm Okay," Maria replied. "You look great! And how are you?"

"I'm fine," said Anna. "Maria, this is my friend, Carmen."

"Glad to meet you, Carmen," said Maria.

"Glad to meet you, too, Maria," said Carmen.

"I'm not sure that it's safe for me to be talking to you, after what happened," Maria went on. "If I get caught, I'll lose my job for sure, and who knows what else would happen to me."

"No, don't worry, Maria," Anna responded. "Please listen for a minute. We have a lot to talk to you about."

"Please," Maria insisted, "you shouldn't talk to me because I'm afraid that there might be someone here from the hospital. They might say something and get me in trouble."

Carmen was the mastermind during their conversation. "Don't worry, Maria," she added, "we guarantee you that everything will be okay. Sit here with us, and we'll explain everything to you. We'll treat you to dinner. This won't take long, I promise." Maria reluctantly and fearfully sat at their table because she was still afraid of being caught there with them. Carmen and Anna made sure that she was facing away from everyone else, but Anna then suggested that they should go to one of the diner's private booths to continue their conversation. They walked to a private booth, and as soon as they had their privacy, the waitress went over to take their orders, and they took a few minutes to make their selections.

While they were waiting for their dinner, Carmen took the opportunity to tell Maria why they were there, "Maria, we're not going to discuss anything in detail at this time, but let me tell you something very important – we didn't just happen to run into you here – we actually came here five nights in a row, hoping that you would show up. We didn't want to meet you at your home because we thought that that would be an invasion of your privacy. Besides, we didn't want to scare you by knocking on your door. Now, Maria, please don't be alarmed by what I'm going to tell you next – we did it in order to meet you somewhere other than at your home. Okay, we actually had you under surveillance a while ago, and we learned that you come here almost every night, so we decided to meet you here. Anyway, Anna told us that you're not happy with your job. We can tell you that we can change all that for you, and we can offer you a wonderful change in your life if..."

"Yes, Maria," Anna interjected, "Carmen is right, I know what I'm talking about. I am very happy with a group of people that I have met since I left the hospital. They have done wonders for me. You even said that I look great – well, I owe it all to Carmen. I am now rich, compared to the way I was before I left the hospital. I even live in a very nice building now, in my own condominium. I am now devoting all my time to my children, because I don't even have to work anymore, at least until my kids stop needing my help. I owe it all to the people that I just mentioned, including Carmen."

"All we want you to do, Maria," Carmen continued, "is to come pay us a visit in one of our colleagues' office, so our attorney, Gene Lissenzwel, can explain it all to you – Gene was the attorney who successfully defended us during the trial. I can't tell you too much right now because the story is too long, but if you're ready, we can offer you a job, where you will be earning double what you make now, and working conditions are much better. Please say you'll go. We need your help in a big way."

"Well," Maria replied, "it's true that I hate my job, and my pay stinks, so, okay, I'll go and listen to what your attorney has to say. When should I go?"

Anna stood up and went to where Maria was sitting before Carmen had a chance to answer Maria's question. She gave her a big hug and said, "Thank you, Maria."

At that very moment, their dinner was brought to their table, and after the waitress left, Carmen said, "We want you to do it as soon as possible, Maria, for everyone's sake. Tell us when you can go, and I'll see to it that we put top priority on that meeting."

"I can go anytime, really," Maria replied.

"Maria," said Anna, "let's make sure that we can communicate with you after we finish our meeting here. Please give us your phone number so we call you." Maria gave them her phone number, and Carmen and Anna gave her their phone numbers as well.

After a while, they finished their dinner, and Carmen made the final decision, "Maria, now that we can call you, and you can call us, let's go home, and Anna and I will speak with Gene so he can set up the meeting." After they agreed on everything, they finished their dinner. Carmen then paid for their dinner, and they left the diner.

Later on, that same evening, Carmen called Gene from her home and told him all about their great accomplishment. He told her to call Maria and ask her if she could meet him first thing the next morning, but Carmen suggested that they should talk to Maria right there and then, "Let's put her on a three-way call, Gene."

"That's a great idea!" Gene replied. "What's her number?" Carmen gave Gene Maria's phone number, and he dialed it as she said each digit.

"Hello," Maria answered.

"Hi, Maria, this is Carmen. I have Mr. Lissenzwel with us on the line."

"Hello, Mr. Lissenzwel," said Maria. "I'm glad to speak to you."

"Hello, Maria, I'm very glad to speak to you, too, but please call me Gene," he said.

"Okay, Gene" Maria replied, "Carmen and Anna told me that you need me. What can I do for you?"

"Maria," Gene went on, "first of all, I would like to tell you how grateful we all are to you for talking to us. Secondly, the story is too long to go into detail now. All I can tell you right now, based on what Anna told us about you, is that you can benefit a great deal if you decide to join us. Please make every effort possible to come to a meeting with us tomorrow morning, so we can tell you all about it. You can call in sick tomorrow, and I will personally go to your house to bring you here if you want. We can compensate you very generously for any losses that you might incur."

"Well," Maria replied, "if you're associated with Anna, defended her and won, then I'll do it."

"Okay, Maria," said Gene, "I'll pick…"

"I'm sorry, Gene, for interrupting you," Carmen interjected, "but I think that you're much too busy to go get Maria. Anna is Maria's friend, so I'll call her after we finish here and ask her to go with me to pick up Maria first thing in the morning." After that, they all agreed to meet in the morning and concluded their conversation. Carmen then called Anna right away, and Anna agreed to accompany her to pick up Maria in the morning. Gene called all the other parties to the lawsuit, as well as Rebecca Fynedzowt, to have them present at the meeting, and everyone agreed to be there.

The following day, early in the morning, everyone arrived at the meeting. Gene assigned seats for everyone at a very large round table at Sam Towhertz's office. Gene opened the discussions as soon as everyone was present, "Most of us in this room have recently been victims of some unfair treatment by someone else. I am also included, and we have someone to thank for being where we are today. The only one in this office who doesn't know why we're here is Miss Maria Jannytarboz. Maria, everyone here is my client, except you and Rebecca Fynedzowt. This is what we're doing here – we're working on a lawsuit against several doctors and two hospitals, because all my clients have been, as I said before, victims of some unfair treatment by someone else. We will be demanding a very large sum of money for every one of my clients. Let me tell you the story, Maria…" Gene told her as much as she needed to be told, and after a few hours of questions and answers, Maria was totally briefed, and she knew most of the story.

They had been talking well into the afternoon and thought that it was time to get something to eat. They chose to order takeout, so they could continue their discussions while eating their lunch right at the conference table. They called Gudphood Diner, and lunch was delivered to them in minutes. "Maria," Gene continued while they were eating, "we're willing to make you part of our group. I understand that you're not happy with your job. Let's put my offer to the test – is there anyone here who's willing to hire Maria with double her present salary and better working conditions?"

All those who were financially able to hire Maria, and needed someone to work for them, raised their hands, including Gene. He then continued by making an instant offer to her, "I'll tell you what, Maria, if you're willing to work for me right now, I can put you on my payroll starting this morning, with a salary twice as high as your present pay.

You can be my first employee as a combination of my secretary and my assistant. You don't have to quit your job at the hospital until we finish the lawsuit or until anyone here detects that you're in danger by staying under the employment of Deprivayshun Psychiatric Hospital. While we conduct our evidence-gathering venture there, I'll put you through a formal training program that will prepare you to work for me. You can attend a seminar at night at a local college that will provide you with the necessary training – I'll cover the expenses. How does that sound, Maria?"

"That sounds so overwhelming," Maria replied, "that I think it's God-sent. How can I refuse such an offer?"

"Okay, that settles it!" Gene continued. "You're hired! Okay, I'll start giving you a weekly paycheck effective this morning, and you will continue getting your pay from Deprivayshun Psychiatric Hospital, which is all yours to keep. You will be earning three times your old salary as long as you stay in the hospital, but I'm sorry to tell you that after you quit the hospital, you'll only be getting twice your old salary. Is that a problem, Maria?"

"No!" Maria answered. "How can it be a problem when you're making me such a great offer, and you're overwhelming me with generosity? I want to leave that dreadful place as soon as possible! After the way that I have been treated at the hospital for years, I was beginning to wonder if there weren't any more kind and generous people in this world. I'm so glad that I agreed to listen to what Anna and Carmen had to talk to me about when I met them in the diner last night. Wow! I now feel like I hit the jackpot! Thank you, Anna, Carmen, Gene and everyone here."

Most of the people in the office made pleasant remarks in response to Maria's statements, and she felt extremely comfortable to be there. "You're very welcome, Maria," Gene went on. "Anyway, we need to plant surveillance equipment all throughout the hospital. I would like to cover as many areas as possible. Anna told us that you had the keys to several doors in the hospital – is that still the case?"

"Yes," Maria answered. "As a matter of fact, they gave me the keys to two other places a couple of days ago."

"Great!" said Gene as he continued. "Okay, Maria, there are so many cameras, microphones and other bugging devices that are so small, that they can be placed almost anywhere. You can carry a very small camera that looks like a shirt or blouse button, and no one will ever suspect anything. As you already know, Rebecca Fynedzowt is our private investigator, and she's the best there is. She's the one who will be handling the bugging equipment and collecting data with her computers." After that, Gene spent another couple of hours conducting the meeting, but some people had to leave early, so he decided to conclude the conference with the intention of returning the following morning to discuss in detail how the plan was going to be executed. Before Maria left, Gene gave her his home telephone number, and she gave him hers. Gene then continued working on other cases before he went home.

Later on that evening, Maria phoned Gene from her home and said, "Gene, I was called from the hospital just after I got home, and they told me that if I don't go to work tomorrow, I'll be fired."

"Okay, Maria," Gene replied, "we can't take any chances – we don't want you to get fired, because it is very crucial for you to continue your presence in the hospital. Rebecca is the expert with the bugging equipment, so, go to work tomorrow, and I'll personally go to your house with her after the meeting to explain to you what you'll have to do."

"Okay, Gene," said Maria, "I'll see you tomorrow night then, and thank you."

"No, Maria, don't thank me, I should be the one thanking you. Okay, see you tomorrow," Gene concluded.

The following morning, the meeting was conducted without Maria. When it was over, all the details had been worked out.

When they concluded, Gene and Rebecca went to Gudphood Diner to get something to eat before going to Maria's house. When they arrived at the diner, they hoped that Maria would show up to have her dinner, but since they had agreed to meet her at her home, they didn't expect her. Rebecca then realized that they should have arranged to meet Maria at the diner, instead of meeting her at her home.

About an hour later, as they expected, Maria never showed up, so they left the diner after they ate. Shortly after they left, they met Maria at her home. They spent about two hours talking about how the plan was going to be executed. After everything was explained to Maria, and she understood, Rebecca gave her several miniature bugging devices, all of which had cameras built into them. Gene and Rebecca then left and went to their homes. After they left, before going their separate ways, Rebecca told Gene that all the devices that she gave to Maria were self-destructing, and they would only last about a month.

The next day, Maria went back to work. She had a tiny camera on a decorative pin on her lapel. As soon as she had a chance, she started planting the bugging devices all over the hospital. There was absolutely no suspicion from anyone, and everything went as planned. Before the end of her shift, Maria had done everything that Gene and Rebecca had instructed her to do, except that she still had to plant as many devices in Ward Two Seventeen as she could – that was the most difficult part of the plan, because she very rarely went to that ward. After she finished her work, she went straight home.

When Maria Jannytarboz got home that night, she phoned Gene and told him what she had accomplished and what she still had to do. Gene complimented her and told her that he was sure that she'd find the way to finish the job. With the help of Rebecca Fynedzowt, Gene Lissenzwel started collecting a huge amount of information from within the hospital as soon as Maria planted some bugging devices there. He still needed Martha Innaddayze's room monitored before he felt satisfied that he would be able to get all the evidence that he needed against Deprivayshun Psychiatric Hospital.

The following day, Maria went back to work. She already had a plan in mind to get into Martha's room to plant the devices. As soon as she arrived, she went directly to Ward Two Seventeen and spoke to the guard at the cage, "I'm here to inspect the room, because I received a complaint from one of the night nurses that the night janitor is not doing a good job in this ward." The guard had no reason to distrust the janitors' supervisor, and because he knew who she was, he let her in. Maria went around the room making believe that she was inspecting every single inch of it – it was a perfect plan, because the guard didn't even bother to look at her during her entire visit, and she was able to plant several devices at various locations. After she finished, she approached the cage, and the guard let her out without saying or suspecting anything at all. Maria then went about her duties in the hospital, and after her shift was over, she went home. When she got home, she called Gene and gave him the good news. Gene complimented her very highly again, and they called it a night.

In a matter of a few days, because of all the data that was collected, Gene thought that he had enough evidence to use against Deprivayshun Psychiatric Hospital and Doctor Ryppemuff. The only reason why he needed evidence against Doctor Ryppemuff was because Martha Innaddayze was included in the lawsuit, and she was admitted before Peter Emppostar took over – the other victims who had been at Deprivayshun Psychiatric Hospital had all been handled by Peter. The cooperation of Maria Jannytarboz made it unnecessary to try to approach any other hospital employee. She had played a major roll in Gene's plan to unmask the culprits – namely, Doctor Ryppemuff and Deprivayshun Psychiatric Hospital.

At that point, Gene believed that he had enough evidence against Deprivayshun Psychiatric Hospital and many of the doctors – namely, Doctor Byggliar, Doctor Louzi, Doctor Louziar, Doctor Ryppemuff,

Doctor Sayahagain and Doctor Sharlottan, but he still needed evidence against Kuttemopen Hospital, Doctor Butchar, Doctor Manypewlatar and Doctor Oargandeelar. He knew that the last pieces of evidence that he needed would be very crucial. He also knew that they would be the most difficult to obtain. He couldn't risk sending any fake patients there for fear of what would happen to them. Moreover, neither Gene nor anyone else in the group knew anyone in the hospital. They had a huge dilemma in front of them, and Gene didn't know how to handle it just then. He had to think about a new plan.

As time passed, while having meeting after meeting and getting nowhere, Gene felt that he had to include Kuttemopen Hospital, Doctor Butchar, Doctor Manypewlatar and Doctor Oargandeelar. He didn't want to exclude any of them from the lawsuit. He discussed it with Rebecca Fynedzowt to see if she could come up with something. Ever since Gene hired Rebecca the first time, to get evidence during the initial trial, she had been Gene's almost full-time employee, and it was decided that she would do some investigative work in or around the hospital.

One day, Rebecca finally contacted Gene early one evening with something that might have been of interest to him, and they agreed to meet at Gudphood Diner for breakfast in the morning. The following day, they arrived at the diner, and as always, they chose to use one of the diner's private booths. As they sat at the table, a waiter took their orders. While waiting for their food, they started their discussion. "Gene," Rebecca began, "this is what I have accomplished – I was never able to get into the hospital because security there is very high. I couldn't get inside, pretending to be someone visiting a patient, because I was unable to get anyone's name. I made several futile attempts to communicate with hospital employees when they were going in and out of the hospital, but even some visitors that I was able to contact outside of the hospital were reluctant to talk to me. Anyway, the...."

"In a way," Gene interjected, "you're not surprising me, Rebecca, because I didn't think that it would be an easy task. I'm sorry, go ahead"

"Okay," Rebecca went on, "the only thing that I was able to find out after numerous trips to the hospital was that they need help in the janitorial department. That was the only thing that I got out of a young fellow who works there as a linen washer."

"I think that information can be very useful to us," Gene added. "Let's see what we can do with it." At that moment, the waiter served their breakfast, and they went on with their discussion between mouthfuls.

"Gene," Rebecca continued, "I agree about this information being important, because I remember how useful a janitor turned out to be at Deprivayshun Psychiatric Hospital – it was Anna, and she turned out to be the key figure in the entire matter during our surveillance mission there, because she was the only one who was able to point out to us who we should contact. Don't forget, she played a major role during the prisoners' heroic escape by bringing some of the most important ingredients that they needed to make the drugs that they used to escape. And now, as we speak, we have a janitors' supervisor still planted at Deprivayshun Psychiatric Hospital, and she has done a great job so far. I think janitors, all of a sudden, are very important. I'm sure that you want to plant someone to work at Kuttemopen Hospital as a janitor, huh, Gene?"

"Absolutely," Gene answered, "and that was my plan when you told me that they need a janitor there. Now we have to find someone to apply for that position."

"It has to be someone trustworthy and smart enough not to get caught," Rebecca pointed out.

As the minutes passed, Gene and Rebecca were trying to put a plan together, and Gene said, "Maria Jannytarboz would be an excellent contender to apply for the janitorial job at Kuttemopen Hospital, but she has two strikes against her – first, she should remain at Deprivayshun Psychiatric Hospital in case she's needed for anything else before the lawsuit begins. Secondly, it would be very risky for her to attempt to transfer between the two hospitals, knowing that they're in cahoots with each other regarding their malicious practices."

"I agree, Gene," Rebecca replied, "and I also thought of her before I came to see you. Another person that I thought about was Anna Lyphesayvar, but, as you put it before, I think that she has two strikes against her as well – first, she has been through too much already during her ordeal as a prisoner. Secondly, it would be very risky for her as well because she used to work at Deprivayshun Psychiatric Hospital, and someone may recognize her at Kuttemopen Hospital, and then she definitely would be in danger." After they finished their breakfast, they decided to call it a day and continue their discussion the next day at Sam Towhertz's office.

The following day, after Gene and Rebecca took care of some personal errands that they had pending, they met again at Sam Towhertz's spacious office. While they were there, they continued working out the plan. "Rebecca," Gene began, "someone popped into my mind last night while I was going over some of my notes. Someone who shouldn't have any strikes against her – well, maybe a little one, but it I think it can easily be corrected."

"And who may that be, Gene?" asked Rebecca.

"You!" he answered.

"Me?" she asked while totally surprised.

"Yes, you," Gene replied, "and I think that you're excellent for the job, unless you don't want to get your hands dirty, washing floors."

"Ha! I don't mind getting my hands dirty!" Rebecca exclaimed. "I wasn't always as financially comfortable as I am now, and I have gotten my hands dirty plenty of times before. Okay, so, what was that little strike against me that you mentioned before, Gene?"

"Well," Gene explained, "you're much too well-spoken and well-mannered to be a janitor, but I think that maybe you can fake a different personality."

"I'm beginning to get all excited about the possibility," said Rebecca with her eyes wide open. "I think that it could be very challenging for me to be there. Okay, I'll do it!"

"Okay, that settles it!" Gene exclaimed. "We have to move very fast before the janitorial job at the hospital is filled by someone else. I certainly believe that you would do an excellent job as a spy – because you're such a great private investigator. With your expertise, I don't see how this plan could fail now. With you there, your job in deciphering the information that the bugging devices will gather will be much easier for you."

"Okay, then," said Rebecca, "let's not waste any more time. I'll go to the hospital and apply for the job first thing in the morning."

"I agree," said Gene; "this is very urgent."

"Gene," Rebecca added, "I'm leaving. I have to go shopping. I'll see you tomorrow after I apply for the job."

"Okay, Rebecca," Gene replied as he concluded, "I still have to put some facts together for another case that I'm working on, and then I'll call it a day also. Good luck with your interview tomorrow. Good night."

"Good night, Gene."

The next day, Rebecca went directly to Kuttemopen Hospital to apply for the janitorial job. She entered the hospital and was stopped by a very large security guard, who seemed very strong and displayed a muscular physique. He talked to her very rudely and with a stone-cold look on his face, "What is your business here, Miss?"

Rebecca was surprised because she didn't expect such rudeness from the security guard. "I came here to apply for the janitorial job," she replied.

"I didn't know that they had an opening here for such a position. Who told you that they need a janitor here?" asked the guard.

"One of the janitors told me yesterday," Rebecca answered.

"You know the name of whoever told that?" he asked

"I don't know," Rebecca responded. "I didn't ask him his name because I didn't think that it would be necessary for me to know that. I met him when he was leaving the hospital, and he told me that they're looking for someone to be a janitor here."

After several questions from the guard, Rebecca was beginning to lose hope, but she didn't give up. She then became very aggressive and started giving the guard reasons to feel mentally inferior. After several questions and answers, she said in a firm tone of voice, "Well, if you don't know anything about it, that doesn't mean they don't have a position available. Why don't you just call someone and find out?"

"Yes, I was just about to do that," Curtis Hewgegaard replied as he made a gesture to another guard to approach him. When the other guard went to his side, Curtis told him to escort Rebecca to the personnel department and to stay with her all throughout her visit.

A few minutes later, Rebecca found herself in the personnel department, surrounded by several hospital employees. She felt a sense of distrust coming from everyone, and to make matters worse, the guard had his eyes on her all the while. Almost as soon as she entered, a very stern woman approached her and spoke to her with a firm voice, "How can I help you?"

"I came here to apply for the janitorial position," Rebecca answered.

"What janitorial position?" the woman asked.

"Someone told me yesterday that there's a position available in the janitorial department in this hospital," Rebecca explained, "and I came here to apply for it."

"Well, you're much too late," said the woman with an unfriendly look on her face. "We did have two openings, but that was several weeks ago. You must have been misinformed."

Rebecca was totally devastated, and she paused for a few seconds before saying anything. When she finally thought of something to say, she went on, "Oh, wow, maybe he didn't know! Do you have any other openings?"

"Yes we do, are you a doctor?" the woman asked with a smirk on her face in an attempt to ridicule Rebecca.

Rebecca noticed that the woman wasn't serious about such a question, so she decided to play her own game, "No, why? Do they need a doctor here? Should I be a doctor?"

The woman didn't expect such a reply from Rebecca, and she was speechless for a few seconds, but then she said, "Well! Okay! One of our doctors, Doctor Telsdetrooth, contracted terminal cancer not too long ago, and he quit the hospital as soon as he found out, and the position hasn't been filled yet. If there's nothing else, Miss, then, good bye!" Rebecca walked out without saying a word, and the guard escorted her directly to the exit door. All throughout her visit to the hospital, no one even bothered to ask her what her name was. She felt defeated and was afraid of going back to Gene with such terrible news, but she knew that she had to tell him, sooner or later. From there, she went to some stores to take care of some personal errands.

Gene Lissenzwel had been so busy, that he still had not been able to open his own office. Sam Towhertz didn't spend much time in his office because he conducted most of his business from his penthouse. He only used his huge office when he had a business affair that he couldn't conduct in his penthouse. He told Gene on several occasions that he was more than welcome to use his office.

Later that afternoon, Rebecca went directly to Sam's office, where Gene had told her that he would be that day. A little later, as soon as she arrived at the office, Gene saw her face and immediately knew that something had gone wrong. "I goofed and I didn't get the job," she said.

"Don't worry; it's not the end of the world. What happened?" asked Gene.

"The job had been filled several weeks ago," Rebecca replied.

"Wow! We're back at the starting line again," Gene added in a sad tone of voice.

"Aha!" Rebecca exclaimed. "That's exactly what I thought as soon as I didn't get the job. I really don't know what to do next, but I'm not giving up. We'll find the way to get in there."

"That's the spirit," said Gene, "I feel the same way, but it's getting late, so let's continue first thing tomorrow morning. Good night, Rebecca."

"Okay, Gene," said Rebecca, "we don't belong here. Let's scram. Good night." Rebecca went home very disappointed. She had accomplished absolutely nothing that day, and she felt that she had failed somehow. After she got home, as she was getting ready to go out to have dinner, her phone rang. When she answered it, she was sure that it was Gene, so she said, "Hello, Gene."

"Hi, Reb, this is Vivian, how're you doing? And who's Gene?" she asked.

"Oh, hi, Viv," Rebecca replied, "I'm sorry, I thought you were someone else – he's my boss, Gene Lissenzwel. I'm okay, and how're you doing?"

"Well!" Vivian replied. "For a minute there, I thought that you had gotten yourself a boyfriend. I'm great, and how's your investigative company doing?"

"My business is doing great," Rebecca answered, "but I'm having a little bit of a problem as we speak. I've been trying to get into a medical facility for over a week, and today I failed to get in, after a lot of effort. I have to think of a new way to get in there. It's very crucial that I get in for a case that involves a lawsuit that Gene is putting together. I really don't know what to do next. And how's your advertising company doing, Viv?"

"Fantastic!" Vivian Halpfall answered. "I'm so busy that I'm still at work at this hour, and I'm dead tired."

"Hey, Viv, I got an idea!" Rebecca exclaimed. "I'm also exhausted, and I was just getting ready to go out to get something to eat as my phone rang. Why don't I wait for you, and we can both go out to dinner together, if you don't have any other plans?"

"Wow! That's great!" Vivian responded. "I was just about to go out to eat also, but I thought I'd give you a call before leaving, because something just came up that I thought you might be interested in. I'll tell you what – I won't say anything about it until we get together for dinner, how's that?"

"Great!" said Rebecca. "Let's meet at the usual place – Gudphood. Okay, I'll see you there in about half an hour or so, Viv."

"Okay, Reb, see you there."

About forty minutes later, Rebecca and Vivian met at Gudphood Diner, and went to their favorite private booth at the rear of the dining area. The waitress took their dinner orders after they sat down, and while they waited for their food, they started chatting. "Wow!" Vivian exclaimed. "I'm glad I called you! It's been more than a month since we got together for dinner."

"Yeah, you're right!" Rebecca agreed. "I'm glad you called me, too! We used to get together right here in this booth at least once a week in the past. I guess after we both became successful, we don't have much free time anymore."

"You're right," Vivian continued, "sometimes success tears people apart. Anyway, Rebecca, the reason for my call pertains to investigative work. I know that you're busy, but another job couldn't hurt you, at least I don't think it would."

"Hmm!" Rebecca wondered. "Don't tell me that you want someone tailed, Viv!"

At that very moment, their dinner was served. After the waitress left, they started eating and continued talking between mouthfuls.

"Anyway, no, I don't need anyone tailed," Vivian finally replied. "The reason why I mentioned investigative work was because when I was getting ready to leave my office, a call came in, asking me to place an ad for an investigative position. I copied down the information before I left my office in case you're interested."

"Oh, sure," Rebecca replied, "I'm definitely interested, and I don't think that another job will hurt me in any way. Thanks for thinking of me."

"It's the least I can do for you after you have given me so much work," Vivian went on, "which has increased my business tremendously. When I got the call, I figured that you could jump on it before it hits the newspapers. Here's the information."

Vivian gave Rebecca a slip of paper with the information written on it. Rebecca looked at it and almost screamed. "Oh my God!" she said as she got up, went around the table and hugged Vivian.

"Well!" Vivian exclaimed while displaying a big smile. "I'm glad you like it! What's the excitement all about?"

"You have no idea, my dear friend, how much I like it," Rebecca replied. "Do you know anything about a recent case where some people were wrongly held as prisoners in a mental institution?"

"Sure," Vivian answered, "I read all about it in the newspapers. I read that the young attorney who got them out was fantastic."

"Okay," Rebecca went on, "I was directly involved in that case, and yes, that young attorney, Gene Lissenzwel, was fantastic and still is. In his…"

"Oh," Vivian interjected, "that's who you meant when you mentioned Gene before."

"Yes, it was him that I was talking about," Rebecca replied.

"At that moment," said Vivian, "I didn't know who you were talking about, Reb. You also said that he's your boss – now I can understand why you're so busy. Because of the publicity he got after he won that trial, you must be getting a lot of work from him."

"Yes," Rebecca continued, "you have no idea how busy he is, and how much work he's giving me! He's very busy working on many cases at the same time, and he still finds time to leave his office early many times. Anyway, what I was about to say was that in his short time as an attorney, I have already made a fortune with his cases alone. Up until now, I was doing investigative work for him that he needs for a huge lawsuit that he's preparing against all those doctors and hospitals involved in that famous case that he won. There are only three more doctors and one hospital that we have to collect evidence against. I have been trying so hard to get into the hospital to spy on them. I even applied for a job to be a janitor there, but they didn't have any positions available for a janitor. With this ad that you gave me, I hope to change my life somewhat. If I get this job, I won't have to be a janitor anywhere. It sounds very promising after all the disappointments that I got while trying to get into that seemingly horrible place."

"Well," said Vivian, "now you don't have to get your hands dirty by being a janitor, because this will be right up your alley – doing investigative work. You should feel much more comfortable spying on people than washing floors."

"You're absolutely right, Viv," said Rebecca.

"It seems like this ad was God-sent then," said Vivian, "and it couldn't have been sent to a better person than you."

"Thank you, Vivian," Rebecca replied with a smile on her face. "I won't forget what you have done for me. Let's get together more often from now on – that'll give me a chance to keep you informed about this job, if I get it."

"Great! I'll be looking forward to it," Vivian added. Following that, they continued chatting for a while. Rebecca then told Vivian the entire story about the prisoners and the trial, and Vivian was shocked after hearing the horrible things that Rebecca told her. They then finished their dinner and left the diner.

When Rebecca got home, she immediately picked up the phone to call Gene, but then she put it down as quickly as she had picked it up. She decided not to tell him anything yet for two reasons. First, in case it was a wild-goose chase. Secondly, if she got the job that she was hoping to get, then she would rather tell him in person because she knew that he would be very disappointed to hear that she would be working for someone else. Rebecca went to bed that night with great expectations.

The next morning, shortly after Rebecca got up, she was about to pick up the phone to call Gene to tell him that she wouldn't be able to meet him that morning, but her phone rang before she had a chance to call him. "Hello," she answered.

"Hi, Rebecca, it's Gene. I'm calling to see if you want to meet me at Gudphood for breakfast, instead of meeting me in the office, so we can continue talking about our plan to try to infiltrate Kuttemopen Hospital. What do you think?" he asked.

"I'm sorry, Gene," Rebecca answered, "I was about to call you to tell you that something extremely urgent came up last night, but you beat me to the phone. I'm afraid that I can't meet you this morning. I'll do my best to meet you later on in the afternoon if I can. I'll tell you all about what came up then. Is that okay?"

"Yes, of course, Rebecca," Gene answered. "I hope everything works out well. Good luck with whatever you have to do, and let me know if you need any help. Thank you for letting me know that you won't be here, and I hope to see you sometime later. Okay, see you."

"Thank you, Gene. See you later, I hope," she concluded. After her conversation with Gene, Rebecca had her breakfast and left her home to take care of some errands before going to apply for the job. She made a stop at a nearby beauty parlor, and then she went to a discount store to buy a few personal items. From there, she went straight to apply for that much-needed job, as she deemed it.

Later that day, late in the afternoon, Rebecca was out in the street after she applied for the job. The first thing that she did was to call Gene. She had some news to give him, but she didn't know how he was going to react, so she wanted to meet him in person. She dialed his number, and he answered. It was very late, almost evening, so Rebecca was glad that he was still there. "Hi, Gene, it's me, Rebecca. I just finished what I had to do. I'd like to come in to talk to you now. Is that okay?"

Gene didn't notice anything unusual about Rebecca's voice, so he wasn't sure whether she had good or bad news to tell him. "Yes, of course, Rebecca" he replied, "it's still early, and I'll be here. Is everything okay?"

"Ah, yes, everything is fine," she answered. "I'll be there shortly, Gene. See you in a few."

"Okay Rebecca, I'll be waiting," he said. A little while later Gene was in the office doing some work while waiting for Rebecca, and a woman with bright-orange hair and sunglasses walked in. Her face was slightly turned away from him. Gene was curious to see the woman there and asked, "Can I help you, Miss?"

"Yes, you can," said the woman as she turned her face towards Gene.

"Oh my God!" Gene exclaimed when he saw her clearly. "Is that you, Rebecca?"

"In the flesh!" she replied.

"What is this all about?" he asked.

"I'm actually starving," said Rebecca, "because I haven't eaten since I had my breakfast very early this morning. Let's go to Gudphood and have something to eat. I actually have some news for you, Gene, and I don't know how you'll react to it! I'll tell you all about it while we're in the diner." They didn't say much more after that and immediately left the office to go to the diner.

As soon as they arrived, as they were about to enter into a private booth, the waitress saw them and said, "Good afternoon. Oh my God! Is that you Rebecca?"

"Yes, it's me," Rebecca answered, "at least I was the last time I looked in the mirror."

"I love your new look, especially your hair," the waitress added.

Rebecca felt good about it and looked at Gene when she replied to the waitress' comment, "Thanks, that's a nice compliment! At least somebody likes it!" Gene grinned after Rebecca made that comment, and the waitress then took their orders and walked away. As soon as the waitress was out of their booth, Rebecca started talking, "Gene, I have to be honest with you. Because of the way I felt when I failed to get into Kuttemopen Hospital, I decided to go out and find another job."

"Oh? That's a surprise!" Gene replied with a sad look on his face.

Rebecca then went on, "I got a tip from a friend about a job. I went to apply for it this morning, and I was hired on the spot. You have no idea, Gene, how happy I was when I was hired! That's the urgency that I told you about this morning that came up last night. Well, I'm hereby informing you that I will be starting my new job tomorrow morning at nine."

Gene was devastated and very disappointed with the thought of losing Rebecca, but he was happy for her. Before he had a chance to reply, their dinner was served. Unlike Gene, Rebecca started eating right away and very fast. After a short while, Gene finally replied to Rebecca's comments. By that time, he was eating, but very slowly. "Well, Rebecca, " he said, " what you have told me is shocking and extremely bad news for me, but I'm not going to try to stop you from doing what you think is best for you. I'm going to miss your great talents because I don't know anyone else who is half as good as you are."

"I'm sorry, Gene, but I had to do this," she replied.

"I understand, Rebecca," he said, but still with a sad look on his face, "and don't think for one minute that I'm holding anything against you. I wish you luck on your new job, and if you ever want to come back and do some more work for me, my door will always be open for you."

"Thank you, Gene," Rebecca responded while putting her head down. "I knew that you would understand."

Gene then said, "The only thing that bothers me is that you're a genius at what you do, and I hope that you don't waste your talents by doing something else."

"Gene," asked Rebecca, "do you think you can manage without me?"

"I would be lying to you, Rebecca, if I told you that I can manage without you," Gene answered, "but I don't want you to miss out on something that you want, just to keep you here. You go ahead and try your new job – you have my full support. If anything ever goes wrong, and you have to come back, please, do."

"Thanks again, Gene," Rebecca went on. "Well, let me tell you something – as far as wasting my talents, that wouldn't happen because I'll be working on an investigative case, just as I do here."

"Oh!" Gene exclaimed. "I didn't know that! Are you making the switch because your new client will pay you more than I'm paying you?"

"No, Gene," she answered, "as a matter of fact, my fee will be exactly one half of what you pay me."

"Now you have me totally confused!" Gene replied as he wondered. "I thought that we had a good working relationship, and I also thought that you were happy with that arrangement."

As their conversation continued, their dinner was totally consumed, and Rebecca called the waitress to order more coffee for both of them. After their coffee was served, Rebecca finally replied to Gene's comment, "Yes, Gene, I have been happy with our arrangement here, but wouldn't you like to know who my next employer will be?"

Gene answered, but he was still confused, "Okay, yes, of course, but it's not gravely important for me to know that, as long as you're happy there. I'm still in a daze after this bombshell, Rebecca!"

"All right, Gene, I'll tell you anyway," Rebecca continued. "I was hired as a private investigator to find out who is stealing drugs from – guess where!"

"Oh my God!" Gene exclaimed. "I can't even begin to think from where, but why are you acting so funny, Rebecca?"

"Okay, Gene," she said, "enough with this farce! I fooled you long enough already! Here it is – I was hired with full and unrestricted access to almost every corner of the facility, by none other than Doctor Butchar himself, to find out who's stealing drugs from Kuttemopen Hospital."

"Oh, wow!" Gene said very loudly. "Now I'm really shocked! Is this situation what I'm thinking it is?"

"Precisely what you're thinking it is," Rebecca replied as she read his mind.

"Rebecca," said Gene, "you have no idea what a relief it is to hear that you'll continue working on my case!"

"Gene," said Rebecca, "while I'm there, at Kuttemopen Hospital, investigating the drug theft, I'll be able to collect all the evidence that we need against the hospital and the doctors. I only have two weeks to do it, so we have to work very fast."

"Rebecca," said Gene, "you had me fooled there for a while. I guess you wanted to surprise me. I don't know how you did it – getting the job – but I imagine that your new hairdo and your sunglasses had something to do with it. No matter how you did it, great job!"

"Gene," said Rebecca, "after what happened yesterday, I was beginning to feel worthless, and let me tell…"

"Worthless!" Gene yelled as he interrupted her. "How can you possibly feel that way? There wasn't one single second when I thought that you were worthless."

"Well, thank you, Gene," Rebecca went on, "and let me tell you something else – I felt so bad while I was fooling you all along, but now I'm glad I did it, because I see that you're pleasantly surprised after you were almost ready to commit suicide. I didn't tell you anything when you called me this morning for two reasons. One reason was in case this didn't work out, and the other reason was because if it did work out, then I'd surprise you with the good news. However, when I was hired, I thought of an idea – to keep you in suspense for a while before telling you, and I see that it worked out just right, and I'm very happy about the whole thing now."

"You know, Rebecca," said Gene, "come to think of it, I was stupid to have been fooled by you so easily, because I know that you're a fighter – I remember how you persisted when I was employed by the Public Defender, and some of the defense attorneys there employed you – you never gave up and you always found the best way out of any tight spot that you were in until you produced marvelous results. I really don't know why I believed that you'd decide to get another job simply because you ran into some difficulties. I'll get my revenge against you some day for fooling me – don't worry, I'm just kidding, and I'm kind of glad that you did it this way, because now I'm really ecstatic after, as you said, I was ready to commit suicide."

"This really turned out to be God-sent" Rebecca went on, "and we should be glad now that I didn't get the janitorial position – imagine the advantages that I'll have now, working as a private investigator, with full and unrestricted access to almost everywhere in the hospital, instead of working as a janitor, with very little access to anywhere?"

"Yes, I agree," Gene replied, "and I can definitely see the difference, but I'm curious to know how you thought up such a plan that landed you right where we wanted you to be."

"Before we go into that, Gene," Rebecca replied, "let me tell you that I intend to deduct whatever payments I get from Doctor Butchar, for the investigation in the hospital, from your payments to me for the spy work."

"Oh, no, Rebecca," Gene insisted, "you keep it all, and don't deduct anything from my payments to you – you deserve it all. After all, without you in the hospital, I wouldn't know what to do right now. Besides, I was paid by my clients so well, that I can say now that I'm financially independent."

"Thanks again, Gene" said Rebecca while she smiled. "As always, you're very generous."

"Okay, Rebecca, I'm dying to hear how you got this job," said Gene with a curious look on his face.

"Okay, Gene," Rebecca began, "get ready for the longest story that I have ever told you. It goes like this – when I got home last night, after failing to get hired by Kuttemopen Hospital as a janitor, I was getting ready to come here to Gudphood to have dinner. As I was getting ready to walk out of my house, my phone rang – it was my best friend, Vivian Halpfall. She owns and operates an advertising agency. She told me that she was just about to go out to eat also, but something had just come up, and she thought that I'd be interested in it. We agreed to meet right here, and she'd tell me what it was that came up. When we met at the diner, she told me that when she was getting ready to leave her office, a last-minute call came in, asking her to place an ad for an investigative position. She copied down the information before she left her office and gave it to me. I nearly died of joy when I read the ad. I read it so many times, that I have it completely memorized. It said: 'Wanted: Kuttemopen Hospital is in urgent need of a top-notch private investigator to look into matters concerning the possibility of employee theft. Applicant must have extensive experience in the field. Apply in person at the personnel department at 944 Eezeemonee Street.' After that, we left the diner, and I went home.

"This morning, after breakfast, I had the intention of going to Kuttemopen Hospital to apply for the job, but then I remembered that the guard at the door, as well as the woman in the personnel department, might be there again and recognize me, because I had been there before when I went to apply for the janitorial job. However, I also remembered that no one even bothered to ask me what my name was. That's when I decided to change the color and style of my hair before going to apply for the job, so they wouldn't recognize me, or at least I hoped that they wouldn't. Can you see now why I changed my looks, Gene?"

"Sure!" Gene exclaimed. "Yes, I definitely see that, but I figured that there was a connection there somewhere. Please go on."

"Okay," Rebecca continued, "before I left my house to go to Kuttemopen Hospital, I was about to pick up the phone to call you to tell you that I wouldn't be able to meet you this morning, as we had planned to, but my phone rang before I had a chance to pick it up to call you – it was you. Remember, Gene that you called me this morning?"

"Yes, of course I remember," Gene answered, "how can I forget? But, please, go ahead. I want to hear the story."

"After our conversation," Rebecca went on, "I went directly to a nearby beauty parlor and changed my looks completely. After that, I stopped at a discount store to buy a pair of sunglasses because I didn't have any with me. After I put my glasses on, I went straight to Kuttemopen Hospital. Upon entering the hospital, I was again stopped by the same huge security guard who I had to go through when I went there yesterday. He was as rude as always and displayed the same serious and mean look on his face that he always had.'

"He asked me, 'What is your business here, Lady?'

"I then said to him, 'Good morning, Sir, I'm here about the investigative job.'

"He said, 'That's funny, I don't know anything about any investigative job here. This is a hospital, not a police station.'

"Then I said to him, 'Yes, I understand that, Sir, but there was an ad in a newspaper that clearly stated that they need a private investigator here. I have the ad here – take a look at it.'

"I then showed him the slip of paper that Vivian had given me. The guard glanced at it without even reading it, and then he said, 'Okay, let me find out what this is all about.'

"The guard then looked around to see if there were any other guards on the floor, but he didn't see anyone within sight, so he locked the main entrance door to the hospital and escorted me to the information desk. When we arrived, the guard told the receptionist to call the personnel department to see if they knew anything about a position for a private investigator. The receptionist did as the guard told her, and she was told that indeed they did place an ad in the newspaper. After a brief conversation, the personnel supervisor was told that the guard was there alone and couldn't leave his post unattended. The supervisor then said that she would be downstairs in a few minutes to escort me upstairs so I could apply for the job.

"Shortly after that, the supervisor arrived at the main lobby, and I noticed that it was the same woman that I had dealt with when I was there the day before to apply for the janitorial job. The woman escorted me to her office, and while we were walking away, I realized that neither the guard nor the woman had recognized me. As soon as we arrived at the personnel department, I was given a number of forms to fill out. When I completed all the paperwork, I was briefly interviewed by the same woman, and she happened to like the way that I had filled out the papers, so she said, 'Well, Miss Fynedzowt, everything here seems to be in order, but it's not up to me to make the decision – Doctor Butchar was the one who placed the ad in the paper. I'll have someone bring you to his office.'

"After I waited for a few minutes, an orderly walked in to bring me to Doctor Butchar's office. The supervisor gave him my papers, and he escorted me to the doctor's office. When I entered Doctor Butchar's office, the orderly gave him my application and walked out. Doctor Butchar started reading the forms. Then he looked at me and said, 'Wow! Those advertising agencies surely work very fast – it was only last night that I called in this ad to them. Miss Fynedzowt, my name is Doctor Butchar. In case you're hired, let me brief you on what's going on here – I have reasons to believe that one of our employees is stealing drugs from our hospital and selling them in the black market. Whoever is doing it is very clever and elusive, because I have reviewed all the tapes from our security cameras, and I haven't been able to see anything at all. It would be your job to find out who it is – that's all we need you for. Do you think you can handle that?'

"I said to him, 'That would be a piece of cake, Doctor Butchar. I don't think it would take me very long at all to get results. I can deliver very fast.'

"Then he said to me, 'I like your attitude, and I think that you're very qualified to fill this position, based on what I see here on your application. I actually do believe that you would get results very fast. By the way, I'm not too familiar with your work, Miss Fynedzowt, but I do know that private investigators work until their job is completed, and then they move on to another case. What time frame do you consider very fast?'

"Then I told him, 'Well, it all depends on how much you would like me to find out. If all you want is the name of the employee who's stealing the drugs, then a week would be sufficient, but if you want more information, such as other people involved, then it would take me longer. For instance, if you want to know who his accomplices are, where he's selling the drugs and who his customers are, then I think a month would be enough to thoroughly complete my job.'

"After a few more questions and answers, Doctor Butchar finally arrived at an offer and said, 'Well, I'm very pleased with what I see here on your application, and what I have heard from you. In spite of the fact that more people should be interviewed, I'm willing to gamble on you, because this is very urgent, but I was thinking more in terms of two weeks. How do you feel about that?'

"I was ecstatic and accepted immediately, but I had some conditions that would make my job easier. I was also able to keep a very serious look on my face without giving my enthusiasm away. I knew very well that I didn't need much time at all – perhaps even less than a week, but I wanted to make sure that I would remain in the hospital as long as possible to complete my spy mission for you, so I told him, 'Well, if I have complete and unrestricted access to every corner of the hospital, then I believe that I have a fighting chance to do it all in two weeks.'

"Doctor Butchar had no objections and said, 'There are certain areas where there may be some kind of restriction, such as operating rooms and the like, but even there, I'll get you some access. Miss Fynedzowt, we haven't discussed your cost, how does that work?'

"Knowing that money was so important to Doctor Butchar, important enough to butcher his patients for the sake of it, I didn't want to scare him off, so I asked him for an amount that was about one half of my usual fee. Gene, can you see now why my fee from my new client will be so low?"

"Yes," Gene replied, "I can definitely see that, and that was good thinking."

"After all, when I was there," Rebecca continued, "I thought that if I was hired, I would be under your expense account during my entire spy mission. Anyway, the doctor couldn't refuse such a reasonable amount after hearing me tell him what my fee was, so he said, 'Okay, you're hired. When can you start?'

"I did my best not to jump up and down when I was hired, and I managed to answer while maintaining that same stone-cold look that I still had on my face. My answer was, 'I just finished a case this morning before I came to apply for this one. I can start tomorrow morning if it's okay with you.'

"The doctor was just as anxious to have me start as soon as possible. He took a tag out of his desk drawer and wrote my name and an expiration date on it. He then said, 'That'll be fine. Here's a temporary employment tag, which expires in two weeks. Come back tomorrow morning at nine with the tag on, so Curtis Hewgegaard will let you in. Report directly to my office. I'll be here to give you more details so you can begin working as soon as possible. Good bye, Miss Fynedzowt.'

"I said, 'Good bye, Doctor Butchar, I'll see you tomorrow,' and then I walked out of his office. I was thrilled when I stepped out of the hospital, and the first thing that I did was to call you. And tomorrow, first thing in the morning, I'll be reporting to Doctor Butchar at Kuttemopen Hospital to begin my investigation. Here's my employment tag, Gene – take a look at it!" Rebecca then proudly showed Gene her temporary work tag.

"Wow!" Gene exclaimed. "That certainly was a long story, Rebecca, and you have done something that not too many people have been able to do – you had me almost totally speechless for a long time." Following that long story, Gene and Rebecca chatted a little while longer. They then concluded their dinner and went their separate ways.

The following day, Rebecca Fynedzowt reported to work at Kuttemopen Hospital as both a spy for Gene Lissenzwel, and a private investigator for Doctor Butchar. She was wearing a miniature camera disguised as a decorative hairpin. She was allowed to pass through the watchful eyes of Curtis Hewgegaard as soon as he saw the expiration date on her name tag, which she had pinned onto her blouse. She went straight to Doctor Butchar's office without any hassle from anyone. A few minutes later, she arrived at his office and said, "Good morning, Doctor Butchar, how are you?"

"Good morning, Miss Fynedzowt," the doctor replied, "fine, thank you, and how are you?"

"Fine, thank you, Doctor," she answered. "Well, here I am, ready to expose the culprit or culprits."

"Well, Miss Fynedzowt," said the doctor, "I've been anxiously waiting for your arrival, because a massive amount of drugs was stolen again last night. We can't waste any more time. I have to know who's doing it. Please have a seat."

"Thank you, Doctor Butchar," Rebecca replied as she sat down. "I'm sorry to hear that you had another robbery. I'll find out who's doing it in no time."

"I have full confidence in you, Miss Fynedzowt, let's get to work," said the doctor. "By the way, it is very crucial to your investigation that no one knows why you're here. I haven't told anyone, and I don't want you to tell anyone either. Is that a problem, Miss Fynedzowt?"

"Don't worry, Doctor Butchar," Rebecca responded, "I have been in this business for quite a while, and I had that angle covered even before you hired me. If anyone becomes overly concerned about my presence in the hospital, I'll tell them that I am an Environmental Expert, but if they want to know more, then I'll tell them that they can ask you all about it."

After a while, Doctor Butchar finished telling Rebecca what he expected from her and where she could and couldn't go during her entire operation in the hospital. "Okay, Environmental Expert, go do your thing," the doctor concluded. From that moment on, Rebecca had total freedom to go almost anywhere in the hospital at anytime. She left Doctor Butchar's office and started looking around and exploring every corner of the hospital to prepare to plant her numerous bugging devices.

At about two in the afternoon, Rebecca finally had a chance to go to lunch. She decided to take a chance and have lunch in the hospital's cafeteria, because she thought that that it would be a good way to learn as much as she could about the hospital and the people who worked there. After all, Rebecca was legitimately hired to do a job in the hospital. In spite of the fact that she was spying on them, she also felt that she had an obligation to do the job that she was hired to do. She was trying to kill two birds with the same stone – to get information for Gene Lissenzwel, and to expose the people involved in the drug theft. She thought that the hospital employees would be more likely to talk to her during their lunch breaks, rather than while they were on duty. She felt that they would be more relaxed at that time, but even then, she wasn't able to get anything out of anyone.

Right after lunch, Rebecca started going all over the hospital again and planting her devices at numerous locations. She wasn't even worried about removing the devices at all after the spy job was completed. It didn't matter if anyone found them, because they were planted with authorization. Besides, the devices were so small and innocent-looking, that no one would ever suspect anything. Before leaving for the day, Rebecca planted all the devices at all the locations that she wanted to monitor. She was so good at doing her job, that even with the hospital's extensive surveillance system and heavy security, no one noticed her activities.

Before going home, Rebecca reported to her boss and said, "Doctor Butchar, I'll have the culprits delivered to you very soon. I feel sure, because I have accomplished a lot today. I'm going home now and I'll be here first thing tomorrow morning. Is it okay, Doctor Butchar, if I don't report to you here in the morning, and instead, I can get to work right away?"

"Absolutely, Miss Fynedzowt!" he replied very loudly. "No problem, and thank you for keeping me informed. Good night."

"Good night, Doctor Butchar," Rebecca concluded as she walked out of the doctor's office.

As soon as Rebecca got home, she had plans to go to Gudphood Diner for dinner, but she decided to call Gene before leaving. She dialed his number, and he answered, "Gene Lissenzwel."

"Hi, Gene, it's me, Rebecca. Have you eaten yet?"

"Oh hi, Rebecca, no, I haven't eaten yet, and if you haven't either, let's go to Gudphood and have dinner, so we can talk. How does that sound?" Gene asked.

"That's exactly what I had on my mind," Rebecca answered. "I'll meet you there in about twenty minutes. Okay, see you there, Gene."

"I'll be there. See you, Rebecca."

Gene and Rebecca met at the diner in a little less than half an hour. As soon as they arrived, Gene began the conversation, "Okay, Rebecca, I'm dying to hear what happened in the hospital on your first day on the job. How did it go?"

"Wow!" Rebecca replied. "That was one of the easiest investigative jobs that I have ever had. I had complete freedom to do what I wanted, and in no time, I planted my bugs in every single location that I wanted monitored. After we finish here, I'm going to begin watching some good stuff from my computers at home. If there's anything hot, I'll call you at home and tell you all about it."

"Great!" said Gene. "I'll be home, waiting for your call." With that, they continued chatting a little while longer, and then they left the diner after they finished their dinner.

As soon as Rebecca got home again, she turned on her computer monitors, and Lo and Behold, the first thing that she saw was Curtis Hewgegaard turning off the power to the camera that was pointing towards the entrance to the hospital pharmacy. She then saw him taking a box that seemed to contain drugs from a medicine storage bin. After he took the box, he walked away with it. In a few minutes, he went back to turn the power to the camera back on. Rebecca called Gene at home, but there was no answer, so she left a message in his machine and waited for his call, because they preferred not to be called on their cell phones unless it was urgent. Besides, most people are unable to conduct business while in transit, especially while driving. Before Rebecca was able to change her clothes, her phone rang – it was

Gene. He had gotten home a little later because he lived somewhat farther from the diner than Rebecca did. She then told him all about the theft, and Gene was amazed after Rebecca told him what she had seen. He then said, "Wow! It only took you one day to deliver! You're terrific! As I told you before, you're the best there is."

"Keep complimenting me, Gene – I love it!" Rebecca exclaimed with a big smile on her face. "I'll continue going over my equipment, and if I see something else interesting, I'll call you, but if I don't see anything, then, good night – I'm too tired to continue much longer. Oh! Wait a minute, I forgot to tell you, yesterday when I went to apply for the investigative job at Kuttemopen Hospital, I showed the ad to the same security guard who steals the drugs. It was a good thing that he was too lazy to read it, because he would have seen that Doctor Butchar needed a private investigator to find out who was stealing drugs, and it was him. If he had read the ad, we'd be back at the beginning now, or even worse, because he probably would have taken me as a prisoner, or at least he wouldn't have stolen the drugs while I was there."

"Wow!" Gene replied. "You're absolutely right – if the guard had read the ad, you'd be totally out of the picture as far as Kuttemopen Hospital goes. That would have been a great loss and a major setback – we were lucky. Okay, good night, Rebecca, and keep up the good work."

"Okay, Gene, good night," she said as they concluded and went to their homes.

Rebecca was getting sleepy, but when she got home, she continued monitoring her equipment, off and on, while tending to numerous other domestic activities. When she stepped out of the shower, she was drying her hair while watching the monitors. After a few minutes, she was extremely excited when she started witnessing Doctor Manypewlatar and other surgeons preparing for surgery. To her amazement, she saw and heard how the surgeon spelled out numerous operations that they had planned for the patient. As he finished reading the list, Rebecca heard the patient say, "Wait a minute! I'm only here because I have a grain of sand in my right eye, and I went to Doctor Sayahagain's office because I wanted him to remove it. What are you going to do to me? I'm getting out of here!" Rebecca also saw the patient attempting to get up, but he was instantly overpowered. She saw and heard the surgeon say that the patient was hallucinating, and Doctor Manypewlatar anesthetized him.

Shortly after that, the doctors made a mess out of the poor victim by cutting him open in various places. Rebecca then saw several organs being removed. She then heard one of the doctors say that the patient was dead, and Doctor Oargandeelar then told Doctor Manypewlatar to make sure that he manipulated the next of kin into having the body cremated. She also saw Doctor Oargandeelar placing all the parts that they removed from the victim into a cooler. A little later, she saw him take the cooler, walk over to a large refrigerator and place the cooler in it. She was totally horrified when she saw the entire event. After that, she was too tired and sleepy, and decided to go to bed without calling Gene.

The next morning, as soon as Rebecca got up, she called Gene to give him the good news. She also told him that she wasn't going to work until a little later, so they decided to have breakfast at the usual diner. While at the breakfast table, Rebecca gave Gene a copy of the video containing the complete operation performed on the poor victim – that video alone was enough evidence against Kuttemopen Hospital as well as Doctor Manypewlatar to proceed with the lawsuit, but they decided to continue their monitoring. Besides, they still had to get evidence against Doctor Butchar and Doctor Oargandeelar. After breakfast, they left the diner. Rebecca headed to Kuttemopen Hospital, and Gene headed to the office.

On her way to the hospital, Rebecca thought that she should wait before giving Doctor Butchar the results of her drug theft investigation. She decided to hold back in case Doctor Butchar felt like dismissing her after having that information. She couldn't take any chances of being let go before getting evidence against Doctor Butchar and Doctor Oargandeelar. Besides, that's what she had agreed to do when she was at the diner with Gene. A short while later, Rebecca finally arrived at the hospital and reported directly to the doctor's office. "Good morning Doctor Butchar," she said.

"Good morning, Miss Fynedzowt," the doctor replied, "we had a…"

Rebecca interrupted him as he started talking – she was prepared for such a situation, "Yes, I know, you had another robbery last night, and I have the culprit exposed. That's precisely why I came here to your office this morning."

"Very good," said Doctor Butchar, "let's have the information, so I can go to work on it right away."

Rebecca was too smart to do as he demanded. She knew that she had to continue being present in the hospital in order to complete her work. She still had to unmask Doctor Butchar, as well as other doctors in the hospital, so she told him, "With all due respect, Doctor Butchar, I have to do my job the proper way. Let me complete all the details and try to get the names of other people involved, instead of providing you with an incomplete report. Please, let me do a little more before I give you what I have. The only thing that I can tell you right now is to post a guard from a private security company, only for a short time, at the medicine storage bin at the pharmacy. You should call them immediately and have a guard sent right away."

"Okay," the doctor agreed, "but we have to put this matter behind us very soon, because I can't afford to continue losing money."

Following that, they both went about their own affairs. Rebecca went to check on her bugging devices. After she left, Doctor Butchar made arrangements for a security guard from a private company to be posted later on at night at the medicine storage bin. After he finished with that, he went to the operating room.

Rebecca didn't have much to do at that point of her investigation because she had already planted all the bugging devices that she was going to plant, and there was really nothing more for her to do in the hospital. She spent a great amount of time in the cafeteria, talking to as many people as she could, but it turned out that she was unable to get anything out of anyone. After a while, late in the afternoon, she went home.

As soon as Rebecca got home, she started watching her equipment again. To her amazement, she uncovered who the huge guard's accomplices and customers were. After a while, she decided to look at some of the information recorded earlier that day during Doctor Butchar's shift. After skipping over lots of footage of insignificant events, Rebecca couldn't have been more shocked when she saw a similar series of unnecessary operations being performed by Doctor Butchar and other surgeons on an unfortunate victim. She felt that she had to call Gene right away, and she did. After they talked on the phone, they agreed to meet the next day for breakfast at the usual place. Then Gene called it a night, but Rebecca continued going over the live and prerecorded information on her monitors.

The next morning, as Rebecca was getting ready to go meet Gene, she turned on her computer monitors to see if she could see anything new. After a few minutes, she saw Doctor Oargandeelar come in through a rear door. He was accompanied by two men in black suits. One of the men was carrying a cooler, and the other man was carrying a briefcase. Rebecca was surprised to see that Doctor Oargandeelar was already in the hospital so early in the morning. She saw the doctor open a big commercial refrigerator and pull out the same cooler that she saw him place there before. The doctor then opened the cooler and took a human heart out of it. Rebecca stopped what she was doing to devote her full attention to what she was seeing. As soon as Doctor Oargandeelar took the heart out, one of the men opened the cooler that he was carrying, and the doctor filled it with several organs and other human body parts. When the cooler was full, the doctor went through several motions as he figured out the total value of all the organs and the other items. The other man opened his briefcase, and Rebecca noticed that it was completely filled with several large stacks of one-hundred-dollar bills. Doctor Oargandeelar took the briefcase and closed it. He then led the men out of the building through the same rear door that they came in through – an organ transaction had just been executed by the organ dealer. Rebecca then realized that that's why that door wasn't monitored by any security cameras – because they wanted to keep their business of selling human body parts a secret. She then made copies of Doctor Oargandeelar's organ transaction, Doctor Butchar's operation, and all the activities of the drug theft team. After a little while, she left her home to go meet Gene.

When Rebecca arrived at the diner, Gene was already there. She gave him a tape revealing the entire operation performed by Doctor Butchar on a poor victim. She also gave him a tape containing the organ transaction executed by Doctor Oargandeelar. During their breakfast, Rebecca told Gene all about the operation and the organ transaction. They then decided that it was time to turn over to Doctor Butchar all the names of the drug robbery team, because they already had all the evidence that they needed for the lawsuit. After they finished their business in the diner, Gene went to his office, and Rebecca went back to the hospital.

After a while, Rebecca reported directly to Doctor Butchar's office. At that point, she didn't worry about being dismissed, because she had already collected enough evidence against all the doctors and the hospital. Besides, the bugging devices were still planted and sending plenty of information back to her computers. Soon after she arrived at the hospital, Rebecca entered Doctor Butchar's office. He saw her come in with a big smile on her face. "Good morning, Miss Fynedzowt," he said.

"Good morning, Doctor Butchar," Rebecca replied.

"I'm glad to see that smile, because I also have something to smile about," the doctor went on. "I'm glad to inform you that nothing was stolen last night. I guess the posting of the guard was a good idea. Anyway, what do you have for me today?"

"Well," Rebecca answered, "I have even better news for you. I have a complete list of all the culprits and a detailed explanation of their actions. The first name on the list is the head of the entire drug theft ring. I also have a tape that reveals their complete operation." Rebecca then handed a sheet of paper containing a list of names to the doctor. She also gave him a few other sheets of paper detailing everything, and a tape containing their entire operation in action. She felt that her presence at the hospital was at risk at that moment, but she wasn't overly concerned about it because she had enough evidence against everyone, and her devices were still planted throughout the hospital.

Doctor Butchar looked at the tape, took the papers and started reading the list of names. After a moment, he finished reading the list, and was satisfied, so he let out a big sigh of relief. He also complimented Rebecca and told her what she expected to hear. "This is great!" he said in a rather loud voice. "You did a terrific job, and it only took you two days to do it. I guess I don't need you anymore, and I don't need the security guard that I hired yesterday either. I'll call the company and tell them not to send him tonight. After I watch the tape, I'll also call the police department to tell them to come and arrest the culprits. I looked at the list of names, and I never could have imagined that Curtis Hewgegaard would be the mastermind behind all this. You may go now – your job is done. Let me have your admittance tag, Miss Fynedzowt, please, and good bye."

"Okay, Doctor Butchar," Rebecca responded, "I'll take a check for my services now."

"Well, now, Miss Fynedzowt," the butcher added, "I also do things my own way. You can't expect me to give you a check right here and now – just like that. This situation has to go through the proper channels. We'll send you a check in the mail. Good bye."

"Okay, Doctor Butchar, have it your way, good bye," Rebecca replied as she gave him the name tag and started walking out.

After leaving the hospital, Rebecca went straight to Sam's office to meet Gene. Upon her arrival, Gene was surprised to see her there so early in the day. She started talking as she sat at the conference table near a window, "The butcher fired me when I gave him the tape and the list of all the culprits. He even refused to pay me on the spot for my work. He told me that they'll send me a check in the mail, but I knew that he was lying and had no intention of paying me at all. Good thing that we still have the bugging devices planted there. They'll continue running and sending information back to my computers for a long time before the batteries die."

"Well, that's okay," said Gene, "because even though you have already delivered, you're still on my expense account for the duration of the lawsuit."

"Wow!" Rebecca exclaimed. "Thank you, Gene, that's wonderful. I really didn't expect any more financial compensation after completing the job."

"The spy plan went so well," said Gene, "that you accomplished both tasks in only two days. You amaze me more and more and day after day as we work together. I have to say again that you're a pure genius. By the way, I was reviewing the tapes you gave me containing those operations and the organ transaction, and I think we have enough evidence against Doctor Butchar, Doctor Manypewlatar, Doctor Oargandeelar and Kuttemopen Hospital to begin the lawsuit. However, I also think it's a good idea to continue collecting as much new evidence as we can with your bugging equipment, in case we need it. Oh, I meant to ask you before you started the spy work, did you use self-destructing bugging devices at Kuttemopen Hospital?"

"No," Rebecca answered, "because I was authorized to spy on the employees there, I used regular bugs because they cost less. Anyway, Gene, I have been falling behind on a lot of errands, so, if you don't mind, I'd like to call it a day."

"No, not at all, Rebecca" Gene replied. "As a matter of fact, I have also been falling behind on a lot of stuff. I was just getting ready to finish up something I was doing regarding another case, and then call it a day, too."

"Oh, Gene," Rebecca went on, "I just remembered something – as it turned out, we didn't really need to hold back on Doctor Butchar. We could have given him the information as soon as we found out who the thief was, because my presence in the hospital wasn't needed anymore after I planted all the devices there. I actually accomplished everything from home after they were in place."

"You're absolutely right," Gene replied, "and that makes me realize that we don't need Maria's presence at Deprivayshun Psychiatric Hospital anymore either, because of the same reason. Besides, we don't need anything from there anymore. I'll call her right away and tell her to get out of that place. Okay, bye, Rebecca, talk to you later."

"Bye, Gene." Following that, Rebecca left the office to take care of her personal things. Gene stayed in the office for another few hours, and after he finished what he was doing, he also left to take care of his errands.

Later on that evening, Gene called Maria Jannytarboz to tell her to quit her job at Deprivayshun Psychiatric Hospital immediately, to prevent her from being exposed to any danger there. He also told her that he had enough evidence against Deprivayshun Psychiatric Hospital and Doctor Ryppemuff at that point. "You'll remain as my employee with the current salary that I'm paying you now," Gene told her. "Even if this case goes belly-up, and I'm financially ruined, then I'm sure that one of the others would gladly hire you with at least the same salary. Anyway, that wouldn't happen because I'm also working on numerous other cases, and new cases keep popping up almost every day – that's another reason why I need you here."

"Thank you, Gene," Maria responded with a great sense of relief. "I am really extremely grateful to you, and totally ecstatic to hear that I'm finally freed from that diabolical place. I'm so happy that I'm not even going there tomorrow, and instead, I'll report to you to start my duties as your secretary and assistant – I'm looking forward to working for you. Many times I felt like walking off the job, and now I'm actually doing it. Oh, wait a minute, Gene, what about the bugging devices that I planted? Don't I have to remove them to make sure that no one finds them?"

"No, not really," Gene answered, "they'll continue sending information back to Rebecca's computers – we may need it. Besides, she told me that she used self-destructing bugging devices at Deprivayshun. I don't remember what she told me about their life expectancy, but I think they self-destruct thirty days after she gave them to you." Following that, Gene Lissenzwel went about his business. Maria Jannytarboz stayed home extremely happy with the thought that she didn't have to go back to Deprivayshun Psychiatric Hospital ever again.

Maria reported to Gene first thing in the morning the following day, ready to go to work. Two days later, she signed up for a four-credit legal course at night at a local community college. From that moment on, her life completely turned around for the better. She liked her new life so much, that she decided to register for a regular college degree after completing the legal training, which would be used as part of the credits that she would need for her degree. She would be attending college at night and knew that she would be very busy for a few years while working and studying. She looked forward to it anyway because she saw Gene as an inspiration due to the fact that he finished law school at a young age because he worked hard at it.

Meanwhile, Gene set up a meeting for everyone involved with the lawsuit to take place the following Monday. Martha's parents, Mark and Julie Innaddayze, participated in every meeting very effectively, and they were there that day. Rebecca Fynedzowt had been an active and important member at almost every single meeting, and she was also there. Anna's three children were able to attend some meetings, and that day, all three were present. With such a successful investigation and everyone in attendance, the meeting was conducted very effectively and lasted several hours. After they discussed everything, Gene told everyone that the case was ready to go to trial.

As soon as the meeting was over, Sam Towhertz invited everyone to have dinner in his penthouse, which was on top of the same building. Everyone willingly accepted and left the office immediately. When they arrived at Sam's home, his chef had already prepared a wonderful dinner, which was tremendously enjoyed by everyone. During their dinner, they didn't talk business at all. Instead, they socialized. After several hours, they concluded their get-together and everyone went home with full stomachs.

The following day, the lawsuit was finally filed. All summonses, subpoenas and notifications were sent out. All the defendants, namely, nine doctors and the two hospitals, retained counselors. When their attorneys heard that Gene Lissenzwel was representing the plaintiffs, and also because they had read all about Gene's trial during which he defeated Ralph Byggshatt, every one of the lawyers wanted to see the evidence that Gene had against their clients before proceeding with the case. The counselors knew that Gene was good at obtaining evidence. One by one, they contacted Gene, and he told each one that he would get back to them. When Gene finally heard from every one of the attorneys, he called them all back and told them to meet him at Sam's office the following week. Gene also called Rebecca to ask her to be present at the meeting. She told him that she wouldn't miss it for anything else.

Martha Innaddayze mysteriously went into a coma shortly after her inclusion in the lawsuit with the others. Luckily, Rebecca's bugs recorded Doctor Ryppemuff injecting Martha, causing her to pass out. She would not be able to provide any testimony whatsoever. However, the evidence obtained during the many weeks of hard work was so overwhelming that her testimony wouldn't be necessary.

Another lucky break was that Rebecca's bugs also recorded Doctor Oargandeelar as he visited Doctor Ryppemuff at Deprivayshun Psychiatric Hospital. With the help of several orderlies they overpowered a very large male patient, who seemed to be in his twenties, and sedated him. Doctor Oargandeelar then paid Doctor Ryppemuff for the patient and took him away. Later on the same day, at Kuttemopen Hospital, Doctor Butchar himself dismembered the patient, and Doctor Oargandeelar placed all his parts in the refrigerator. Doctor Oargandeelar later sold the parts.

The Settlement

A WEEK LATER, ALL the attorneys finally had a meeting with Gene. As soon as they sat at the table, every one of them wanted to see the evidence that he had. Gene didn't want to show them everything that he had, but he showed them a small sample of some very incriminating evidence. Rebecca assisted Gene with the presentation of the evidence. Some of the attorneys were speechless when they saw some of the material that Gene and Rebecca showed them.

It took several hours, with the questions and answers, for Gene Lissenzwel and Rebecca Fynedzowt to show the eleven attorneys, representing the nine doctors and the two hospitals, some of the evidence that Gene had against their clients. Following that, they decided to end the meeting. Rebecca and the eleven attorneys left the office. Gene and Maria Jannytarboz remained in the office and continued working on the lawsuit and several other cases. After a while, they also decided to call it a day.

The evidence that Gene had against the doctors and hospitals was so overwhelming that all the attorneys started thinking about a settlement. In view of the fact that Gene recently had such a huge victory against Ralph Byggshatt, and also because the evidence that he had was so overwhelming, the defendants' attorneys highly advised their clients to settle out of court. It took a lot of convincing for some of the defendants to agree, but some others agreed right away.

A few days later, the final defendant, Doctor Butchar, finally agreed to do as his attorney advised him, and everyone settled out of court. The amount that they settled on was undisclosed, but it was so substantial, that the plaintiffs who were poor became rich, and those who were rich, became richer. Of course, the malpractice insurance paid for most of it, but it did cost the defendants a substantial amount.

Gene knew all along that it was illegal to collect evidence by planting surveillance equipment without authorization from the parties under surveillance or a court order, but he expected the defendants to settle out of court because he didn't think that they would take a chance by being exposed of doing all the horrendous things that they did to their patients. If the defendants had not agreed to settle out of court, Gene would have told them that he would go to the media and show it all to them. The defendants, of course, wouldn't let that happen because they would have a lot more to lose then. First of all, they wouldn't be able to rip off their victims anymore. Secondly, there would be a question as to whether or not the DA would have been able to use that evidence against them in a criminal case – in that situation, the DA would have obtained that evidence from the media, making it legal, and then the defendants would definitely have gone to jail if the evidence had been accepted in court. All the defendants' attorneys knew that as well, so, when they discussed with their clients the option of settling out of court, they felt compelled to tell them that. Gene never mentioned anything about the legality of the evidence-gathering method to anyone because he didn't want the facts to leak out.

When the plaintiffs collected their shares of the settlement, everyone involved gave Maria Jannytarboz and Rebecca Fynedzowt very generous bonuses for their effective participation before and during the lawsuit. Although Gene Lissenzwel received a percentage of the settlement as his fee for representing the plaintiffs, they also gave him a generous bonus because they felt that his fee was more than reasonable. Everyone involved in the lawsuit, including Gene, Maria and Rebecca felt as though they had just hit the jackpot.

Gene went a step further and managed to convince a judge to issue court orders demanding that the seven fake patients, the ones that he sent to see all the doctors involved, should get reimbursed, with interest. After he served the court orders, the doctors complied immediately to prevent any further lawsuits. He let all the fake patients keep the money in payment for their participation.

District Attorney Gudgovaygint brought charges against the nine doctors and the two hospitals involved. He obtained court orders to try to get his own evidence against them. The nine doctors knew one another and got together to discuss their defense. During one of their many meetings, they decided, for the first time in their medical careers, to practice medicine the right way on a full-time basis until they were acquitted, which they felt sure would happen. Because of that, the DA didn't get any evidence at all. Instead, he made another attempt to use the incriminating evidence that Gene had illegally obtained, but he was unable to use any of it, and the case was thrown out of court. In spite of the overwhelming evidence that Gene had been able to produce during his preparations for the lawsuit, the DA was unable to prove that the doctors did anything medically or criminally wrong, because without Gene's evidence, he had no proof of any wrongdoing. At that point, even if Gene had gone to the media with the sole purpose of introducing the illegally obtained evidence, he and the DA knew that no court would have accepted it. Ultimately, the DA was once again unable to strip them of their rights to continue practicing medicine.

The nine doctors continued having discussions after the trial, and they decided to guard themselves against any future attempts by anyone to trap them again. They installed equipment all over their facilities to detect any and all bugging, recording and photographic equipment, hand-held or planted anywhere.

Robert Berndhend eventually married Carmen Pynkeehertz. They have two children and to this day, they still live in his original house.

Gene's father, Anthony Lissenzwel, was hired by Robert Berndhend to be the foreman of the maintenance department in his chemical plant. Eventually, with the proper training, Anthony was promoted to work in the chemical department as a formula specialist. One day, Robert asked him to look into the mixture that turned mortar into powder – it was the mixture that Robert had put together while he was a prisoner at Deprivayshun Psychiatric Hospital. Although Robert had invented that mixture before he was a prisoner in the hospital, he wasn't quite happy with it, so he told Anthony to see if he could improve the mixture. After many months of various futile attempts to improve it, Anthony finally came up with a very powerful blend that safely and rapidly turned mortar, brick, stone and much more, into powder. It was far faster and more effective than the original formula. It was a clean and safe way to demolish buildings. It could also be used for all types of excavations. It would be a very effective way to free trapped miners, earthquake victims and many others, without the possibility of any cave-ins caused by heavy objects falling or sliding, because everything would be completely turned to powder by the mixture. After obtaining a patent, Robert opened a new plant to specialize exclusively in that formula. Robert made Anthony a partner in his new venture. Anthony's wife and son were extremely proud of him. Anthony Lissenzwel had finally accomplished his second big achievement in his life – his first was to raise Gene with the help of his loving wife, Annette.

Anna Lyphesayvar eventually married a good man, and they have two children, in addition to Anna's three children. Her new husband treated her three children as his own. To this day, they still live in the spacious condominium that Sam Towhertz donated to her.

Gene Lissenzwel became one of the most successful attorneys in the nation. He became associated with Sam Towhertz and Robert Berndhend. He finally opened his own law office in one of Sam's commercial buildings not too far from Doctor Sayahagain's medical practice. Sam did charge him market value for the rent because at that point, Gene was very well-off. In addition to his exposure, due to his great success, Gene was getting far more clients than he ever dreamed of when he moved to such a busy area. Shortly after moving to his new location, he had to rent additional space from Sam to expand his practice by hiring some experienced attorneys. He also hired some inexperienced attorneys that he recruited from the law school that he attended. He hired them solely based on their grades and on his feelings about them after he interviewed them. Gene eventually married Anna Lyphesayvar's oldest daughter, Christine, and they have two children. They moved into a condominium, also donated to them by Sam Towhertz, right next door to Gene's parents. To this day, Gene continues running his law firm with the total support of his loving wife. She eventually became a lawyer and works for the firm.

Rebecca Fynedzowt became a full-time private investigator for Lissenzwel & Associates, as Gene's law firm was called. Later on, Gene had an entire section in the firm that was called "The Investigative Department," and Rebecca was the head of it as one of the Vice Presidents of the firm. She's still as good as she always was and enjoys every minute of it. She married an associate attorney at the firm, and they have two children.

Vivian Halpfall was kept up to date during the entire investigation, evidence-gathering and lawsuit, as Rebecca had promised her. She handled all of Gene Lissenzwel & Associates' advertising from that point on. She often got together, on a social basis, with Rebecca and some of the other people associated with the law firm, including Gene and his family.

Martha Innaddayze was eventually rescued from Deprivayshun Psychiatric Hospital and put under a rehabilitation program at Gud Hospital under the care of Doctor Honnastt. The medication that Doctor Ryppemuff was using on Martha Innaddayze was flushed out of her system. In a few days, she was totally cured and released immediately. She regained her memory and all her faculties and went back to live with her parents, who were extremely happy to see that she had her memory back. After a few months, she went to work as a doctor. She was employed by Gud Hospital under the supervision of Doctor Honnastt.

Everything happened due to Anna's willingness to help the prisoners escape from Deprivayshun Psychiatric Hospital, as well as Gene's willingness to listen to what the prisoners had to tell him in the jail cell the first time that he met them.

Some Doctors Know How to Lie

IN VIEW OF THE growing number of people talking about their bad experiences with doctors and hospitals, as well as the growing number of complaints filed by patients, the government once again wanted to get involved. A woman named Melissa Jernolrytar was assigned to write a journal about the medical profession. Melissa was a very naïve young woman, but she had extensive experience as a writer of medical documents. Therefore she was selected for the task of writing the journal. On a Friday afternoon, Melissa was briefed by her superiors on what they wanted in the journal, and she was ready to begin her project. She picked a familiar area not far from Gene Lissenzwel's office to conduct her studies. All the doctors that she had chosen to interview were within a short proximity from each another and from her home.

First thing the following Monday, Melissa started her long and difficult task by attempting to interview a well-known and respected doctor with many years of experience – she picked Doctor Sayahagain. Melissa walked into the doctor's office and approached the receptionist. Betty Whilling saw a young and attractive woman with long, black and shiny hair standing in front of her. She immediately remembered Carmen Pynkeehertz, because they were very similar in appearance. Since Carmen was a rich woman, Betty erroneously thought that she saw dollar signs all over Melissa. She then asked her, "How can I help you, Miss?"

"My name is Melissa Jernolrytar," she answered, "and the government has assigned me to write a journal about the medical profession. I've heard a lot of good things about Doctor Sayahagain, and he happens to be my doctor. I'd like to interview him if I may."

Betty was somewhat disappointed that Melissa wasn't going to leave her money behind. She didn't even remember seeing Melissa there before. She then shrugged as she said, "Well, the doctor is very busy at this time of the day. He's seeing a patient as we speak. Perhaps if you make an appointment to see him after business hours, he might be able to give you an interview then."

"I'm willing to interview the doctor at anytime," Melissa replied, "even if it means that I have to do it late at night. When can I make an appointment?"

"I'll see if I can interrupt him now and ask him. I'll be right back," Betty replied as she left her enclosure. She then walked into the examining room and explained the situation to the doctor.

When Betty finished telling Doctor Sayahagain why Melissa was there, his eyes became wide open because he was only thinking of what he was interested in – making money. He then said, "Ask her if my name will be in the journal."

"Okay, I'll be right back," said Betty as she started walking back to her desk. "Doctor Sayahagain is wondering if his name will be in the journal," Betty said after she returned to the enclosure.

"Absolutely!" Melissa responded. "All my sources will be revealed in the journal. That really will be good and free advertising for the doctor." Betty went back to the doctor and told him what Melissa said, and he told her to go ahead and make an appointment. Betty went back to her desk and scheduled a meeting between Melissa and the doctor for the following day after business hours. Melissa then left and went home.

When Melissa got home, she decided to use a different approach while attempting to make appointments with all the other doctors that she had on her list to interview. As soon as she made herself comfortable, she started calling the other doctors to try to schedule appointments with them, instead of walking in on them. After she had made some appointments with some of the doctors on her list, she stayed home until the next day. All the doctors with whom she had made appointments were very happy with the idea that their names would be mentioned in the journal, because they knew that it was a good and free way to get publicity.

The following day, while Melissa waited to go to her interview with Doctor Sayahagain, she went over her appointments very carefully and continued booking more until she had called everyone on her list. After a while, she had scheduled all her meetings with all the doctors that she had selected. She was scheduled to interview Doctor Sayahagain at six P.M. It was still very early, so she decided to go shopping for a while. After she got home, Melissa already had everything ready for her first interview, so she left her home after she had her dinner.

Just before six o'clock in the evening, she arrived at Doctor Sayahagain's office. He had just finished seeing all his patients that day as she walked in, and he was waiting for her in the waiting room. His receptionist was just walking out of the office. Melissa had no intention of telling the doctor that she was his patient, because she imagined that he would recognize her as soon as he saw her. Doctor Sayahagain greeted Melissa as soon as she walked in, "Good evening, I assume that you're Miss Jernolrytar. I'm Doctor Sayahagain."

"Good evening, Doctor Sayahagain," Melissa replied and was somewhat surprised that the doctor didn't recognize her, "yes, I am, glad to see you, and thank you for waiting for me. The government will be very grateful to you for making this interview possible."

"Very well, Miss Jernolrytar," Doctor Sayahagain replied, "let's use this waiting room for the interview. We have a nice table here and plenty of comfortable seats."

"Thank you," Melissa replied as she placed her material on the table. They both found convenient seats for the interview. Melissa was still a little surprised that he hadn't recognized her yet, but she decided to ignore it. "Doctor Sayahagain," she said, "let me start by asking you my first question – why did you become a doctor?"

"My dear," Doctor Sayahagain answered, "there's no greater pleasure for me than helping people – that's my one and only reason for practicing medicine. When a patient walks into the examining room, the first thing that I ask him is why he's visiting me. As soon as he tells me the reason for his visit, I make sure that he repeats his answer, so I can go to work on that problem immediately, and nothing else."

Melissa then had a very good question, which she thought about at that very moment, based on the doctor's answer. She already knew the answer because she was his patient, but she decided to go ahead as if she didn't know anything about it, "Do you provide your services for free or do you charge your patients a fee?"

"I do charge them a fee for my services," the doctor answered, "but I always try to take as little as possible from them. The only reason why I do take a small amount from them is because I provide the best of care, and my overhead is very high."

"Do you make a profit, Doctor Sayahagain?" she asked.

"I barely make a profit, Miss Jernolrytar," he answered, "but I'm so happy helping my patients that I make sure that I only make enough money to pay for my bills in the office, plus a tiny amount of profit for my own personal expenses."

"Do you mean to tell me that you have no money leftover after you pay for the business expenses plus your personal expenses?" Melissa asked.

"That's correct," he lied again. "Let me tell you what happened last year – I made the mistake of charging my patients too much, and I had over $2,000 saved just before the end of the year. Before the year was over, I made sure that I donated $2,000 to the poor to correct my mistake."

Doctor Sayahagain did make a donation of $2,000 – that was the only thing he said that was true, but what Melissa didn't know was that he didn't make a donation to correct his mistake – what the doctor failed to disclose was that the $2,000 that he donated brought his income to a lower tax bracket, and he saved money on his income taxes. Another lie was that he donated the $2,000 to the poor – he actually donated it to a hunting club, of which he was a member. All the members of the club were doctors, and the club pretended to be a conservation club, instead of a hunter's club – that way, all the donations it received were tax-free, and the donors were able to claim their donations as income tax deductions. The club was also exempted from paying real estate taxes. The most important reason for the donation was that the club needed some improvements to make the doctors' lives more pleasant when they were there. It was a wonder how anyone could be such a big liar as Doctor Sayahagain was. He surely deserved an award for being the biggest liar in town, and Melissa, of course, was totally fooled by the doctor.

After a while, she had asked him everything that she could think of, and then she concluded her interview in good faith by making one final remark, "Well, Doctor Sayahagain, I think I have enough information about your practice. I can see now why you're so well-known and respected. Thank you for your time and cooperation. I'm sure that you'll be reading this journal when it's published." The doctor was very pleased to know that the information that he had given Melissa was going to be read by millions. After concluding the interview, they both left the office and went to their respective homes.

The next day, Melissa left her home to go to Doctor Louzi's Office for her interview with him, which was to take place at seven in the evening. When she walked in, the doctor was there alone, waiting for her. He stood up with some difficulty, due to his weight. "Good evening Doctor Louzi," she said, "I am Melissa Jernolrytar. Thank you for waiting. How are you?"

"Very well, thank you, and how are you, Miss Jernolrytar?" he asked.

"Fine, thank you," she answered.

"Please, make yourself comfortable," the doctor added. "Let us use this table. It has ample room, and there are plenty of chairs here. Just pick one."

"Doctor Louzi, I understand that you're a very good psychiatrist, and you come very highly recommended," Melissa said as she placed her material on the table and sat down.

"I am one of the best – who knows? Maybe I am the best!" Doctor Louzi replied as he also sat down.

"Doctor Louzi, can you please tell me something about your medical practice?" Melissa asked.

"Of course, Miss Jernolrytar," the doctor responded with a sense of confidence, "I'll be delighted to tell you anything that you want to know. I am a professional, and I know what I'm doing. I only treat people who need treatment and I only provide the care that is needed for each patient – no more and no less. I would never send a patient to another doctor unless I have already done my best to cure him. There are extremely rare occasions when I do have to send a patient to another doctor, but that happens only once in a blue moon. I always try to charge my patients as little as possible, while providing the best of care for them. My fees are so low, that I barely make a living."

"I will now ask you the same question that I asked another doctor before you – why did you become a doctor?" Melissa asked.

"The answer is simple and obvious – I care for people," the liar answered. "I want to help those who are in need. Many times I don't even charge them anything at all, because the satisfaction that I get out of helping them is enough compensation for me."

Melissa very gullibly spent a long time asking Doctor Louzi several questions, and then she concluded the interview, "Well, Doctor Louzi, it seems like we have a lot of very nice people in this world of ours. I will not take any more of your valuable time. Please read the journal when it becomes available."

"Very well, Miss Jernolrytar," the doctor concluded. "You did a marvelous job, and thank you for choosing me to be part of your study. Good night."

"Good night, Doctor Louzi," she replied.

The next day Melissa's appointment was with Doctor Louziar. She arrived at his office at six in the evening. The interview with Doctor Louziar was almost a carbon copy of the other two interviews with Doctor Sayahagain and Doctor Louzi. The next two evenings, Melissa interviewed Doctor Byggliar and Doctor Sharlottan. It was an amazing coincidence that those two interviews were almost identical to those with the other three doctors previously interviewed – it seemed as though they had rehearsed their answers to Melissa's questions – maybe they did!

When Melissa left Doctor Sharlottan's office, she realized that she spent too much time writing down everything that she was told by all the doctors. Therefore, she decided to bring a tape recorder for her next interview.

The following day, Melissa's appointment was at ten o'clock in the morning with Doctor Butchar, at Kuttemopen Hospital. As soon as she walked into the main lobby of the hospital, at about nine thirty, an alarm went off. A guard who was very similar to Curtis Hewgegaard immediately walked towards her. As soon as the guard got close to Melissa, he held her arms and handcuffed her. He was so rude and sloppy, that he made Melissa drop all her material on the floor. "Who are you, Miss?" he asked as he finished handcuffing her. "That alarm indicates that you're carrying electronic recording equipment. What is your business here? Are you a spy?"

Before Melissa had a chance to reply, several other guards went running from all over the hospital and surrounded her and the big guard. "My name is Melissa Jernolrytar, and I have an appointment at ten with Doctor Butchar," she answered. "I have a tape recorder because I'm here to interview the doctor, but he knows about it, and I'm not a spy."

The big security guard told another guard to escort Melissa to the information desk. He also told another guard to pick up all of Melissa's belongings and follow them. Upon arriving at the desk, Melissa spoke with a receptionist, who had already been notified that Doctor Butchar had an appointment with her. As soon as Melissa introduced herself, the receptionist called Doctor Butchar and told him that Melissa was there, and also that she had a tape recorder with her. Doctor Butchar told her that it was okay to allow recording equipment that time. Melissa's handcuffs were removed, and she was escorted by the same two guards to Doctor Butchar's private office. A few minutes later, they arrived at the doctor's office. The guards remained outside of the office. Melissa went inside and said, "Good morning Doctor Butchar. I am Melissa Jernolrytar, how are you?"

"Good morning, Miss Jernolrytar. I'm fine, thank you, and how are you?" he asked.

"I'm fine, thank you," she replied.

"Miss Jernolrytar, I have been very anxiously waiting for you, and I'm looking forward to helping you in every way that I can. Please make yourself comfortable. Is this table good for your interview?" Doctor Butchar asked as he pointed at a large table in a corner of his office.

Melissa was overwhelmed by the warm reception, not knowing that it was all a faked attitude by the doctor. "Oh, yes it is – it's perfect," she replied as she placed her material on the table, while they both got ready for the interview. "Okay, Doctor Butchar, I would like to begin by asking you the same question that I have asked everyone else that I have interviewed thus far – why did you become a doctor?"

"My dear young lady," the butcher answered, "I have been around a long time, and I have done many things in my life, but nothing that I have ever done gives me more pleasure than helping people. That's the answer to your question – I became a doctor to help people, and nothing else."

"Thank you, Doctor Butchar," Melissa went on. "It seems like all doctors are very kind and helpful. I haven't met a single one who's in it for the money yet. It gives me great pleasure to see that such professionals take time out to help others. Can you please tell me what your duties are, here, at Kuttemopen Hospital?"

"Of course," the butcher answered, "I am the director of the entire hospital, and I am also in charge of all surgeries. I decide what operations are to be performed on what patients. I also assign the surgeons to particular procedures, and I occasionally perform operations as well."

"Now, I would like you to tell me a little about what this hospital does, if you don't mind, Doctor Butchar," Melissa went on.

"This hospital has been in operation for over fifty years," he answered. "It has always done a brilliant job, due to the high-caliber professionals that we employ. We handle all illnesses, but we put a strong emphasis on surgery. We always try to avoid it, but it isn't always possible. However, when we decide that surgery is the only way, we perform those surgeries that are absolutely necessary, and nothing more."

"Have you ever ordered an operation that wasn't necessary?" she asked.

"Absolutely not!" the liar answered. "We're the best there is, or, I should say, I am the best there is, at diagnosing patients, and nothing escapes me. When I say that an operation is needed, it is indisputably necessary. In all my many years here, I have never failed to make a proper diagnosis."

Melissa spent over two hours with Doctor Butchar. With the aid of the tape recorder, she asked him far more questions than she had asked all the other doctors combined. Doctor Butchar didn't tell the truth about any of her questions, except the question about his duties in the hospital. Of course, she didn't know that he had lied to her about all her other questions. Melissa then decided to conclude her interview, but she continued talking while putting her things away simultaneously, "Based on everything that I have heard from you and all the other doctors that

I interviewed, I don't see why anyone should complain about doctors. I can see that you and the others are a group of highly respectable and efficient professionals. I think that I have wasted enough of your time. I'll make sure that I emphasize in the journal that you're the best, as you told me you are. Thank you Doctor Butchar. I'll be leaving now. Please read the journal when it's available. Have a nice day."

"No, don't thank me – thank YOU, Miss Jernolrytar," Doctor Butchar concluded. "I'll make sure to read the journal. Good bye."

Melissa walked out with a sense of accomplishment. As soon as she stepped out of the doctor's office, the two guards made sure that she went directly to the exit door of the hospital. When she got home, she started going over her material and getting ready for her appointment with Doctor Ryppemuff at Deprivayshun Psychiatric Hospital, which was scheduled for four in the afternoon the same day. After Melissa put her work in order, she had something to eat. After she finished eating, it was about half past three, and time for her to go to the hospital for her final interview. She left after tidying up a bit.

When Melissa arrived at Deprivayshun Psychiatric Hospital, the alarm went off. She was put through a very rigorous security check before she was permitted to even enter the main lobby. When she was finally allowed to proceed, she went to the information desk, accompanied by a guard. As soon as Melissa introduced herself, the receptionist told her that Doctor Ryppemuff was expecting her. The same guard was assigned to escort her directly to the doctor's office. In about two minutes, they arrived. The guard remained outside near the door when Melissa walked in to see the doctor. He greeted her as soon as he saw her, "Good afternoon, Miss Jernolrytar. I am Doctor Ryppemuff, and I'm very happy to meet you."

"Good afternoon, Doctor Ryppemuff. The pleasure is all mine," she replied.

"I have been desperately waiting for your arrival," said the doctor.

"I am also very excited about this interview Doctor," said Melissa, "and thank you for allowing me to interview such a giant in the medical profession."

"Please make yourself comfortable and sit anywhere you want," he said.

"Doctor Ryppemuff," Melissa said as she placed her material on a table and sat in a chair next to it, "I must thank you once again for making this interview possible. It is such an honor for me to be sitting next to someone like you. I read about that Peter Emppostar, who drugged and impersonated you for a long time, and also that he was sent to spend the rest of his life as a patient here in this hospital. Thank God that it's all over, and you're all right."

"Why, thank you, Miss Jernolrytar, but, please, feel free to begin the interview," said the doctor.

"Before we begin, Doctor Ryppemuff," Melissa asked, "did you retaliate against Peter Emppostar for everything that he did to you?"

"Oh, no! My goodness!" the doctor exclaimed. "I'm here to help people – not to harm them. He was extremely mentally confused and didn't really know what he was doing, so I did my best to cure him."

"What happened with him after he became a patient here?" she asked. "Did you cure him?"

"The poor fellow couldn't take it anymore and died of a heart attack not long afterwards – just before his final treatment that would have cured him," Doctor Ryppemuff answered.

"Oh, well, maybe he deserved it!" Melissa added. "Okay, Doctor Ryppemuff, let me begin by asking you the same question that I asked all the other doctors that I have interviewed – why did you become a doctor?"

"It was a lifelong dream for me to take care of people who need help," the doctor answered. "As I started growing up, I wasn't financially able to help people with money or material things, so I thought that I had to try to find some other way to help them – that's when I decided to

313

become a doctor. I struggled for a few years, but here I am today, doing what I always wanted to do – to help people. Here at Deprivayshun Psychiatric Hospital, we treat our patients with love, tenderness and care. We do our best to make their stay as short and comfortable as possible. Our fees are so low that they don't make a significant impact on our patients' financial positions."

"Well, I think that's wonderful, and you're a very kind man. Okay, Doctor, what is the average time that your patients remain in this hospital?" she asked.

"I don't have any statistics to give you an average of how long my patients remain here, Miss Jernolrytar," the doctor answered, "but I can tell you that we release them as soon as they get well. With our excellent care, they recover from their mental illnesses very fast."

"Can you tell me if you know what the longest time that anyone ever stayed here as a patient has been?" Melissa asked.

"Yes, that I do remember," he replied, "we had a lady here once who was so mentally disturbed, that she stayed here for a very long time – two months I believe, but that was the absolute longest time for anyone."

"Okay," Melissa went on, "it sounds like you're a great psychiatrist. Do you remember the shortest time that anyone ever stayed?"

"Yes, of course," he answered, "we have had many patients who came here with problems that were taken care of in less than a day. They were discharged, completely cured, the same day they came in."

"Why do so many people complain about the quality of the medical services that they receive from doctors?" Melissa asked.

"I don't really know," the liar responded, "but I can only imagine that they have nothing else better to do, or perhaps they want to maliciously extort money from unsuspecting good doctors – such as me."

"That's terrible," Melissa sighed, "and I agree with you – many people are greedy, and they want to make money the easy way, even if it means harming other people. Doctor Ryppemuff, I understand that this is not only a hospital, but also a senior citizens home – can you elaborate on that?"

Doctor Ryppemuff was taken by surprise when Melissa asked him that question. He hesitated momentarily, and after a moment, he answered with another lie, "Yes, of course, I have clearly defined the boundaries between the hospital and the senior citizens home. I make sure that the hospital patients are completely separated and away from the home residents, to avoid confusion and the possibility of any mishaps."

After several more questions and answers, Melissa then believed that she had enough information from the doctor. She then decided to conclude the interview, "Well, Doctor Ryppemuff, I think that I have wasted too much of your wonderful and valuable time. The government and I appreciate the tremendous cooperation that you have given us. Thank you, and don't forget to read the journal, I will personally bring you a copy when it's ready. Is that okay with you?"

"Yes, please," the doctor replied, "and I'll read it as soon as you bring it to me. Okay, I guess we're finished now. Have a nice day. I'll be looking forward to your return with the journal. Good bye." He let out a sigh of relief because he was glad that it was all over. He knew that he had completely fooled Melissa.

"Good bye, Doctor Ryppemuff, and thank you again," Melissa concluded as the doctor summoned the guard outside of his office to take Melissa to the main lobby. She left the doctor's office, and the guard escorted her directly to the exit door of the hospital.

After Melissa walked out of the hospital, as she was walking on the sidewalk, someone approached her from behind. When she heard the steps, she turned around to see who it was. When she looked behind her, she saw a tall, frail and elderly man, who had a slight forward lean. "Excuse me, Miss," said the man, "aren't you the lady who's writing a journal about the medical profession?"

"Yes, Sir, I am. My name is Melissa Jernolrytar, but how did you know that?" she asked.

"I heard it from some of the doctors at Kuttemopen Hospital when I was there for my treatment, and I saw you talking to Doctor Butchar," he answered. "My name is Doctor Telsdetrooth. I used to work there once as a surgeon. If you're interested, I can tell you the real truth about our profession, instead of all the lies that you probably heard from all those doctors. I am terminally ill, and I have a very short time to live, so now I'm ready to admit the truth."

Doctor Telsdetrooth was the same doctor that the personnel manager at Kuttemopen Hospital told Rebecca Fynedzowt that he had contracted terminal cancer and quit the hospital as soon as he found out.

"Well, Doctor Telsdetrooth," Melissa replied with a baffled look on her face, "this is very confusing to me, because I was under the impression that everything that I heard from all the doctors that I interviewed was true."

"Don't believe a word of it," he added. "I know what I'm talking about because I was once one of those doctors at Kuttemopen Hospital. Don't trust either Kuttemopen Hospital or Deprivayshun Psychiatric Hospital, and don't trust any of the doctors in either hospital."

"Well, this is very shocking to me! I really don't know what to say," said Melissa, still with a confused look on her face.

"You don't have to say or do anything right now," Doctor Telsdetrooth went on. "I suggest that you take one of two options. Your first option is to go ahead and publish your journal and forget about me, but in that case, you'll be publishing a pack of lies. Your second option is to make sure that you check me out thoroughly, so you can see that I was a doctor at Kuttemopen Hospital. Before you publish your journal, I suggest that you should go home. When you're ready to interview me, you can call me, but don't take too long because I don't have much time. When you check my credentials, you'll find out that I am telling the truth. You can always take the first option, because that would make your job a lot easier, but no one will ever know the truth then. Here's my number." Doctor Telsdetrooth gave Melissa a piece of paper with his home number written on it.

Melissa took it and said, "I'll do just that – I'll check your credentials and call you as soon as possible. You'll hear from me. Thank you and I'll call you. Here's my number also, in case you wish to call me for any reason. Okay, Doctor Telsdetrooth, have a nice day."

"Okay, Miss Jernolrytar," he said as he took Melissa's card, "I'll be waiting for your call. So long."

Melissa started heading home with her head down. She was planning to take option one and go ahead and publish the journal with the information that she had, but she was so confused, that she was wondering if she should take option two instead. After a while, she got home and spent the next couple of days putting her work in order. Most importantly, she was thinking of changing her mind about taking option one.

After another couple of days, she decided to switch to option two and started looking into Doctor Telsdetrooth's story. After a careful and thorough investigation, she confirmed that he was indeed a doctor, and that he had been a surgeon at Kuttemopen Hospital. Her investigation also revealed that Doctor Telsdetrooth left his job due to his terminal illness. After she was satisfied that he had told the truth about what she checked out, she finally called him to arrange an interview.

"Hello," the doctor answered.

"Hello, Doctor Telsdetrooth," she said, "this is Melissa Jernolrytar. I checked out everything that you told me, and I was wondering if we could meet at Gudphood Diner. Do you know where that is?

"Of course!" he answered. "Everyone knows where Gudphood Diner is."

After a brief conversation, they agreed to meet at Gudphood Diner. In a way, Melissa felt that she was back at square one, because she thought that if Doctor Telsdetrooth was right, then what the other doctors told her was all false and practically worthless.

Confessions of a Doctor

THE NEXT DAY, MELISSA and Doctor Telsdetrooth met at the diner at nine in the morning. They ordered breakfast, for which Melissa insisted that she should pay and charge it to the government. She began questioning the doctor as they waited for their breakfast. She had a question for the doctor, which she thought was extremely important, "Doctor Telsdetrooth, shortly after you introduced yourself to me the other day in front of Deprivayshun Psychiatric Hospital, you told me that you learned about my writing of the medical journal because you were at Kuttemopen Hospital when I was interviewing Doctor Butchar. You said that you saw me in the hospital while you were getting your treatment there, and you also told me not to trust any of the doctors at Kuttemopen Hospital – okay, if Doctor Butchar and Kuttemopen Hospital are so bad, why did you go there for your treatment?"

"Miss Jernolrytar," Doctor Telsdetrooth explained, "even though Doctor Butchar is a butcher, and the hospital employs many others like him, they do know how to correctly treat patients, but they only do it for their friends and family members. I am a doctor, and they know me, and I know what treatment I should be receiving, so they actually do treat me properly, instead of butchering me."

"Okay, Doctor Telsdetrooth," Melissa went on, "in that case, let us begin. I'm going to start by asking you the same question that I have asked all the other doctors that I interviewed – why did you become a doctor?"

"My dear," the doctor answered, "before I contracted terminal cancer, I would have told you that I became a doctor for the benefit of others, followed by a vast amount of baloney, but now I'm going to tell you the truth – I became a doctor for the money and prestige. I didn't care about what happened to any of the patients. If any of the doctors that you interviewed told you otherwise, they were lying. They don't care for any of their patients. They're only interested in extracting as much money as they can from their unsuspecting victims."

"That seems to be very dishonorable!" Melissa exclaimed with a sense of disgust that could be seen all over her face. "Have you ever known of any doctor who actually cares for his patients?"

"Maybe!" the doctor answered in a rather loud voice. "They do exist, and I imagine that there are many of them, but I can't recall right now meeting any. Perhaps some of the women doctors that I have met actually care for their patients. They seem to be more compassionate with them than men doctors, and most of them refuse to join us in our cruel practices. All we wanted to do at Kuttemopen Hospital was to rip off all our victims, but many women doctors actually wanted to cure them. Because of that, we had a lot of problems with women doctors when I was there."

At that point, their breakfast was served, and they continued talking while they ate it, very slowly. Melissa then asked, "Doctor, do you remember any particular incident that you would like to tell me about women doctors?"

"Oh, yeah," Doctor Telsdetrooth responded, "and I was very happy at that point to participate in that case! The biggest incident that I remember was an historical event, and we were proud of it at Kuttemopen Hospital. This is what happened – once I was in my office, training a young woman doctor named Martha Innaddayze to do what I did – to rip off people by butchering them. She refused to do it because she wasn't interested in harming anyone, and instead, she wanted to help the patients. That's when I went to my boss, Doctor

Butchar, to tell him to fire her. He called both of us into his office. Doctor Butchar and I spent several hours with her, trying to convince her to join us, so she could become very rich, very fast, as we had become, but she refused. After realizing that we couldn't convince her, Doctor Butchar told her that he had no choice but to fire her. He also told her that he'd give her a bad recommendation so she wouldn't be able to practice medicine as long as she lived – he only told her that, so she would reconsider and join us in our evil ways. She then threatened to expose him and the rest of us. She was about to walk out of Doctor Butchar's office, but we immediately overpowered and sedated her. Luckily, no one else in the hospital had seen Doctor Innaddayze that morning, because she and I walked in together, and we didn't run into anyone else. Besides, we walked in through a rear door that only a few of us had keys to. We knew that that door wasn't monitored by the security system because Doctor Butchar himself made sure of that by having a maintenance man remove the camera that was mounted there when they first installed the system – later I'll tell you why he didn't want a camera there. After we sedated her, we sent her to our buddy, Doctor Ryppemuff, at Deprivayshun Psychiatric Hospital. He knew exactly what to do with Doctor Innaddayze – he turned her into a zombie-like prisoner. Doctor Ryppemuff had no intention of ever letting her out again. After…"

"Oh!" Melissa interrupted Doctor Telsdetrooth. "I read about her being wrongfully held in the same mental institution where a man named Peter Emppostar impersonated Doctor Ryppemuff, but I missed that she was also a doctor."

"Yes, she was a doctor, and a good one at that," Doctor Telsdetrooth replied. "Anyway, after a while, just before her body and mind had fully recovered from the initial drugs that made her lose her senses, Doctor Ryppemuff painted a good picture of himself and gained her trust. He then started giving her a daily dose of some medication, which turned her into a zombie. The new drug kept her in a daze and in a state of almost total confusion and partial memory loss. She thought that she was taking the medicine so she didn't get worse, but it was just the opposite – to keep her from getting better. Doctor Butchar is very clever, because right after he sent Doctor Innaddayze to Doctor Ryppemuff, he called her home to ask her parents why she didn't report to work that day. With that information, her parents reported her as missing from that day on. Let me tell you something else that Doctor Butchar did – when the authorities went to the hospital to investigate, they couldn't find anyone who had seen Doctor Innaddayze that day. They reviewed all the surveillance tapes in the hospital, and they didn't see her at all – bear in mind that there was a camera in Doctor Butchar's office, recoding the entire kidnapping, but Doctor Butchar destroyed that tape within minutes after the kidnapping. When they went to his office to check his tape, he had already replaced it with another tape containing events that took place on a day that Doctor Innaddayze wasn't in the hospital. I don't know how he did it, but he was able to change the date on the tape. And let me tell you something else that Doctor Butchar did – he changed his clothes to the same clothes that he was wearing on the date of the tape, because the two detectives watched it right in his office. They could have found out that the tape was a fake, by looking at what other people were wearing, but because they didn't suspect anything, they didn't think of it. Both Doctor Butchar and I knew that that was the only camera that filmed Doctor Innaddayze that morning, and we totally got away with that crime. After that, Doctor Butchar made it a rule never to hire women doctors again. He always found a way to turn them down in a way that they wouldn't press charges against him for sex discrimination."

"All this sounds very weird and terrifying, Doctor Telsdetrooth," said Melissa. "Thank you for telling me about it. Can you please tell me why you're doing this – I mean, telling me something so contrary to what all the other doctors have told me – including Doctor Butchar?"

"Sure," the doctor answered, "I'm all alone in the world, and I have no relatives or heirs, so I am now willing to say things that I would never have said before. It doesn't matter to me anymore if people know the truth. I was part of the corrupted system until I contracted a deadly form of cancer."

"When and how did you get sick?" Melissa asked. "I hope you don't mind my asking you."

"I don't mind at all, Miss Jernolrytar," Doctor Telsdetrooth replied, "in fact I'm glad you asked me that question, because it reminded me of another horrible thing I did at Kuttemopen Hospital – God punished me while I was ripping off an unsuspecting cancer patient when I was still practicing. The patient had a very small mark on his skin, right on his elbow, which was honestly found to be malignant. It was an easy thing to remove, and the cancer would have been totally gone. Instead of just removing the malignant spot, I was going to remove his prostate, which was in perfectly good health. I was also going to remove half of his stomach and three quarters of his large intestine, which were also in perfectly good health. Another surgeon was going to remove his left kidney and his right ear, which, again, there was absolutely nothing wrong with them. A third surgeon was about to remove his arm from his elbow down, and he started cutting it right where the cancerous mark was. As soon as he made the first incision, he severed an artery right on the malignant spot. The patient's blood started shooting up, and it went right into my left eye. I washed it off as soon as possible, but it was too late, because it had gone right into my blood stream very rapidly. It spread all over my body in seconds. I was instantly infected with his cancer, but I didn't know it until sometime later. We then proceeded with the removal of everything that we had planned to remove from the victim. The poor guy died, because his system was unable to endure the surgery. We told his wife that his cancer had spread all over his body and killed him."

"Oh my God!" Melissa exclaimed. "I'm totally horrified now, after hearing about all the parts that were removed from the patient, when there was nothing wrong with them. Anyway, how long did it take you to find out that you had cancer?"

The doctor put his head down momentarily and replied, "It didn't take long for me to find out that I had caught it, because I, as a doctor, had a lot of experience in the symptoms of cancer. Shortly after the eye incident, I was experiencing all the symptoms that cancer patients felt. I had Doctor Butchar diagnose me right away. When he told me that I had cancer, I immediately realized that I caught it from that victim."

"Did you continue practicing after you contracted it?" she asked.

"Oh, no!" he answered. "I stopped practicing medicine as soon as I learned that I was terminally infected with this malignant disease – I didn't see any sense for continuing to accumulate money, just to leave it behind to the state, because I have never thought of making a will to leave my money to anyone."

By that time, they had finished their breakfast, but they ordered coffee several more times while they continued the interview. "Now that you're no longer a surgeon at the hospital, is that practice still going on there?" Melissa asked.

"Oh, yeah" Doctor Telsdetrooth responded, "I was one of the best at performing operations that people didn't need, but I wasn't the only one. The same practice still continues at Kuttemopen Hospital today, and it will never stop."

"Why is it being done?" she asked.

"We did it all for the money," he replied. "All the doctors involved are very wealthy, the same as I am, because of those unnecessary operations."

"What about everything that the other doctors told me?" Melissa asked. "I know you said that it was all a bunch of lies, but isn't there any truth in what they told me?"

"Well," he answered, "it all depends on who you talked to. I know all the doctors in the area – tell me the names of the ones that you interviewed, to see if I know them. If I do, I'll tell you plenty about them."

"Yes, of course," Melissa said, "Doctor Sayahagain, Doctor Louzi, Doctor Louziar, Doctor Byggliar, Doctor Sharlottan, Doctor Butchar, Doctor Ryppemuff and now, you."

"Aha!" he exclaimed. "A bunch of bad ones! No exceptions! I know them all. Therefore, I can tell you that there was no truth at all in what they told you. Well, let me tell you exactly what they do, which is the truth, and then you can answer your own question based on what they told you. Are you ready for a long story, Miss Jernolrytar?"

"Yes, Doctor, I'm all ears, and I have plenty of blank tapes," Melissa answered. "I also have plenty of time, so go ahead."

"Hmm! I wish I could say the same thing about the time that I have," the doctor continued. "Well, let me tell you about Doctor Sayahagain first – as patients walk into his examining room, he tells them to open their mouths and say, 'Ah' regardless of..." the doctor told Melissa everything that Doctor Sayahagain does in his office. He then concluded, "Okay, Miss Jernolrytar, I just told you what Doctor Sayahagain does. Before I tell you about Doctor Louzi, do you have any questions at this point?"

Melissa was quite disturbed about what Doctor Telsdetrooth told her that Doctor Sayahagain did, because he was her doctor. She didn't want Doctor Telsdetrooth to know that, so she said, "Well, no, I don't have any questions. If all that is true, I'm shocked, because Doctor Sayahagain painted a completely different picture – he told me exactly the opposite of what you just told me about him. Oh! Yes, I do have a question – why does Doctor Sayahagain always send his patients to see a psychiatrist?"

"You see, Miss Jernolrytar," the doctor answered, "the easiest and cheapest way for a medical doctor to wash his hands is to refer his patients to a psychiatrist. Besides, he gets a referral fee from the Rigmarole Specialist anyway." By that time, both the doctor and Melissa had already ordered several cups of coffee each, and the doctor continued his accusations of the doctors that Melissa interviewed, "Okay, Miss Jernolrytar, let's talk about Doctor Louzi and the others now – when the unsuspecting patients go to…" the doctor told Melissa everything about Doctor Louzi and Doctor Louziar, and then continued, "Doctor Louziar then sends them to Doctor Butchar at Kuttemopen Hospital, telling them that they'll get an evaluation there, knowing very well that the butcher will make sure that the patients get cut open unnecessarily."

"Geez!" Melissa exclaimed with a sad look on her face. "Cut open unnecessarily! I'm shocked! Please, Doctor Telsdetrooth, explain that one to me."

"I'll be more than happy to," the doctor went on. "At Kuttemopen Hospital, the victims will undergo several operational procedures to remove parts of their bodies that are in perfectly good health. After the victims are cut open, unnecessarily, they will be in terrible pain for a long time. I know what I'm talking about, because I was one of those doctors, and I did it numerous times every day when I was there."

"My God! What a horrible thing to do!" Melissa said while still shocked.

"That's nothing, Miss Jernolrytar," the doctor continued. "There's plenty more, and much worse than that, too. From Kuttemopen Hospital, most victims are sent to Doctor Ryppemuff, at Deprivayshun Psychiatric Hospital, where they'll spend the rest of their lives. Once there, they're doomed to die broke, because Doctor Ryppemuff will make sure that he takes all their money. At Deprivayshun Psychiatric Hospital, they're totally deprived of…" the doctor told her all he could about Deprivayshun Psychiatric Hospital.

"Doctor Telsdetrooth," said Melissa, "those are the most horrible thing that I have ever heard! I don't know how they get away with that, because there are laws that protect people."

"There may be laws, Miss Jernolrytar," he replied, "but physicians and psychiatrists have too much power in our society. According to the laws of our court system, what doctors say is sacred, and they have the right to decide what's best for their patients."

"Okay, Doctor, what about the other two doctors that I mentioned – Doctor Byggliar and Doctor Sharlottan?" she asked.

"Doctor Byggliar sits in his office, waiting for Doctor Sayahagain to send him patients for a second opinion, and…" Doctor Telsdetrooth told Melissa all about Doctor Byggliar, and then he said, "This is what Doctor Sharlottan does – he waits for Doctor Byggliar to send him patients for a third opinion. Then he…" the doctor told her all about Doctor Sharlottan, and then he concluded, "His presence is just another leg of the victim's journey to doomsday. Of course, chances are that the poor victim will end up at Deprivayshun Psychiatric Hospital, one way or the other, to spend the rest of his life there as a prisoner."

"And there," Melissa added, "I imagine that he gets the royal treatment, as all the others do, huh, Doctor Telsdetrooth?"

"Oh, yes, he does," the doctor replied, "and you have no idea what Doctor Ryppemuff charges the poor victims there."

Second Opinions

"Doctor Telsdetrooth, you mentioned second opinions before. Is there anything wrong with sending a patient to another doctor for a second opinion?" asked Melissa.

"Well, Miss Jernolrytar," the doctor answered, "the best thing that I can tell you about a second opinion is that it's one of the biggest farces in the medical profession. The only second opinion that I know is one where a doctor sends his patient to another doctor. Right there, the first doctor is already making some more money, because he'll get a referral fee from the second doctor. The first opinion doctor tells the second opinion doctor what his diagnosis of the patient was. Of course, the second doctor never goes against what the first doctor tells him. However, he may put the patient through some rigmarole, nonsense and gibberish, simply to make believe that he's doing something constructive and to take the patient's money – thus, the diagnosis is always the same in every case. A real second opinion would be one where the patient goes to a second doctor, who knows absolutely nothing about the patient or the first doctor's diagnosis – in that case, the second doctor would have to truly try to find out what's ailing the patient, and you'd have an honest second opinion then. People don't do that because they only go for a second opinion when a doctor sends them. Besides, they don't want to spend the extra time and money that a second opinion costs. If you don't believe it, you try it – go to a doctor and tell him that you have a headache. Then go to a second doctor, far away from the first doctor, but don't tell him that you had already seen a doctor. Then tell the second doctor the same thing that you told the first doctor – you'll be amazed to hear the differences in the diagnosis."

"Hmm, maybe I ought to try that," Melissa replied after thinking for a few seconds.

"I forgot to tell you," Doctor Telsdetrooth continued, "all the doctors in the hospitals spend far more time writing useless information than treating patients. The only reason for all the rigmarole that doctors write is for them to get good reviews from their bosses, not for the benefit of the patients. We all know very well that the patients never know what the doctors write. I remember all the lies that I used to put down on those logs, and I also remember all the lies that other doctor wrote down as well."

"That's very interesting," she said.

"It sure is," he agreed.

Medical Cures Kept a Secret by Doctors

"DOCTOR TELSDETROOTH, ACCORDING TO what you have told me that doctors do, it's a wonder how some people do get cured when they go to doctors when they're sick. Can you tell me anything about that?" asked Melissa.

"Well," the doctor went on, "there are good doctors around, and they do cure sick people, but not all doctors do that! Besides, many times it isn't the doctors who cure sick people – it's their own immune systems that cure them. Remember that Doctor Sayahagain prescribes useless placebo medicine to all his patients, and most of them get cured from whatever they have. The patients who don't get cured by their own immune systems return to Doctor Sayahagain for another dose of his 'Ahs.' Other patients go to other doctors. Still others become worse and are taken to hospitals. Some of them decide to live with their problems. Of course, some of them die. There are some who commit suicide when they simply give up, because they don't trust doctors anymore after visiting Doctor Sayahagain. Most of Doctor Sayahagain's patients – a great majority to be exact – actually get cured by their own immune systems, and they think that the placebo cured them – those patients will highly recommend Doctor Sayahagain, thinking that he's a good doctor. There are millions of people out there recommending doctors to people they know, not knowing the facts."

"If there are good doctors, then, how come there are so many diseases that doctors don't cure?" asked Melissa.

"Okay," Doctor Telsdetrooth answered, "let me tell you my opinion about many known ailments, such as cancer, diabetes, arthritis, AIDS, the common cold and many others – I have reasons to believe that the cures have been found for many so-called 'Incurable' diseases, because I have spoken with hundreds of doctors regarding research that they have been conducting. Every time that I talk to someone working on finding the cure, I always get evasive answers. It is my opinion that with the tremendous advancements that science has made, the cures for many ailments have been found, but the doctors involved simply won't release the cures because they'd be out of a job. Not to mention that many doctors and hospitals would also have to find something else to do."

"Okay, Doctor Telsdetrooth," Melissa went on, "now that you're talking about medical cures kept a secret by doctors, even though you said that that's only your opinion, I need at least one reason why you feel that you're right."

"Okay," he replied as he hesitated for a few seconds, "a long time ago, I heard about the cure for the HIV virus. A doctor friend of mine – he's dead now – once told me that the blood of an HIV patient can be removed from his body and heated to about one hundred and eleven degrees to kill the virus – the blood can't be heated in the patient's body because brain tissue cooks at about one hundred and nine degrees. Anyway, after the blood is cooled off again, it can be put back into his body, and the patient would be free of the virus. After talking to many other doctors who have done experiments on that, I understand that it works, but it isn't being done. Of course, there's only one reason why it isn't being done – because there wouldn't be any need for doctors and hospitals that treat AIDS patients on a continuing basis. Besides, pharmaceutical companies would lose billions if they didn't have to produce the drugs that doctors use to treat AIDS patients."

"Well," asked Melissa, "how come they don't tell the public all this – I mean that they can kill the HIV virus by heating the blood?"

"No!" he answered. "You're wrong, they do tell the public – I even saw it on television when it happened, but that was after my friend had already told me. What happens is that people forget very easily once the media puts the issue to rest."

"The whole thing sounds so gruesome that I can't even think what to say about it. Now that you're terminally ill, Doctor, why don't you try to find out if anyone has found the cure for cancer, so they can cure you?" asked Melissa.

"Aha! I beat you to it, Miss Jernolrytar," Doctor Telsdetrooth replied with a smile on his face. "Now that I'm doomed, I have been doing a lot of research on what has been done to find the cure for cancer. I have contacted many research groups and spoken with many of the doctors involved. In every case, I found them to be very evasive, as though they were trying to hide something. The last group that I contacted was Ghetrychkwik Cancer Research Center. I spoke with the five doctors involved in cancer research in the center. After listening to their story, I was one hundred percent sure that they had found the cure. I'll tell you why I feel this way – once, I went to a private office in the center and tried to pay them to cure my cancer. I offered them my entire lifesavings, and I'm talking about many millions – in the tens of millions – close to one hundred million to be exact. They asked me to let them have a private talk, and I stepped outside of their office. After about ten minutes, they opened the door to let me in again. I was very hopeful at that point, but they only let me in to tell me that they had nothing to offer me because they hadn't found any cure yet. I'm sure that they had found it, but they wouldn't release it because they'd be out of a job. I guess the money that I offered them was insignificant compared to the amount of grants and donations that they're getting to continue their research. Therefore, it was more advantageous for them not to cure me, in fear that the information could leak out, and their research would have to end, together with their tremendous income."

"My God!" she exclaimed. "Doctor Telsdetrooth, you're filling me with fear, more and more, as you continue telling me all theses horrible things. I can't imagine how anyone can hide the cure for diseases that are killing people every day!"

"It isn't my intention to fill you with fear, and I'm sorry if I did," he replied.

Cholesterol Checks

"LET ME ASK YOU something different now," Melissa continued. "Is it true that cholesterol can cause heart attacks?

"Miss Jernolrytar, you're absolutely right!" the doctor answered. "Cholesterol can kill you. Have you ever had your cholesterol checked?"

"Yes, I have, why?" she asked.

"Because I'd like to know what the doctor told you after he drew your blood – what did he tell you?" the doctor asked.

"He told me to go back the following week to get the results," Melissa replied.

"Okay," Doctor Telsdetrooth went on, "and what did the doctor tell you when you went back?"

"Well," Melissa replied, "actually I didn't go back because I was too busy that week."

"Aha!" Doctor Telsdetrooth exclaimed. "That's precisely what I was waiting to hear. Okay, did you ever go back at all to get the results or to have you blood checked again?"

"Well, yes," Melissa answered, "I went back several months later to start all over again. He took my blood and told me to go back the following week for the results, and I actually did go back the second time."

"Okay, let me guess what he told you when you went back for the results – he told you that your cholesterol was okay. Is that correct, Miss Jernolrytar?" the doctor asked.

"Well, yes, Doctor, but what's wrong with that, if my cholesterol was okay?" she asked.

"What's wrong is that your doctor shouldn't just have told you that your cholesterol was okay," Doctor Telsdetrooth answered. "Instead, he should have given you a detailed report. Let me tell you what a well-stated cholesterol report is – the doctor should have told you what your total cholesterol count was, followed by your bad cholesterol, or LDL count, and then your good cholesterol, or HDL count. At that point, he should have told you whether those numbers were within the guidelines that are considered to be safe or unsafe."

"Well!" Melissa yelled. "He didn't do his job then, because he never told me anything about any of those numbers or letters that you mentioned."

"Of course he didn't tell you anything about any numbers or letters," the doctor said and then explained, "I'll tell you a little bit about them – LDL are the initials for Low-Density Lipoprotein, which is your bad cholesterol. HDL are the initials for High-Density Lipoprotein, which is your good cholesterol. You want to keep your bad cholesterol low, while keeping your good cholesterol high. There have been many differences in opinions among many doctors, as far as what the numbers should be considered to be safe – some doctors tell you that you want to keep your total cholesterol below two hundred and your bad cholesterol below seventy five, while some other doctors give you other numbers that are much lower – for instance, I heard of a doctor who wants his patients to have their total cholesterol no higher than one hundred and fifty, and their LDL, or bad cholesterol, no higher than twenty five. If you follow some guideline, you'll be much better off than simply knowing that your cholesterol is okay, even if the numbers vary among doctors."

"Well! How come my doctor never told me that?" Melissa asked.

"There are many reasons why he didn't tell you that, Miss Jernolrytar," the doctor answered, "but the most popular one is to make his job easier. What is your doctor's name?"

"I was really hoping that you wouldn't ask me that question," Melissa answered as she showed a sad face. "I'm so ashamed to say that my doctor is Doctor Sayahagain, but I won't go to him anymore after everything that you have told me about him."

"Oh my God!" the doctor yelled. "You're lucky to be alive, or at least to be here, talking to me! I guess that was one of the very rare occasions when Doctor Sayahagain actually did something contrary to his normal cruel practices, if he actually drew your blood – maybe he was under surveillance or something that day, and decided to practice medicine the right way. What was your reason for choosing him and for going there to begin with?"

"Ah," Melissa hesitated for a moment, and then went on, "I had just moved into the neighborhood, and I specifically wanted to have my cholesterol checked because I heard a lot about that in the news – that's why I asked you if cholesterol can cause heart attacks. I chose him because he was near my new apartment. He did ask me to say, 'Ah' four times before I told him that I wanted my cholesterol checked – even though I told the receptionist, and I also stated it on the form that I filled out – he seemed not to know, or not to care, why I was there. I guess I was lucky that he didn't send me to a psychiatrist. He did draw my blood and told me to go back in a week for the results. I did notice that my bill was extremely high after he finished with me. I thought it was because he was an extremely good doctor. I actually felt good about having found such a good physician, and so close to my home. After I didn't go back in a week, I let several months pass by before going back to start all over again. The second time, he put me through his 'Ahs' again before I told him why I was there. I was such a fool because I thought that he put me through his 'Ah' routine because he was so good that he didn't want to let anything go past him. I was lucky the second time again because he didn't send me to a psychiatrist, and he did draw my blood again – maybe he was still under surveillance, as you said he might have been the first time.

Even when I went back for the results a week later, he again put me through seven 'Ahs' before I told him why I was there, and he didn't even seem to know who I was. My three visits to him cost me $4,965 just to find out that my cholesterol was okay, or at least he told me that it was okay."

"Oh my God!" Doctor Telsdetrooth exclaimed. "$4,965 just to have your cholesterol checked! He probably didn't even bother to send the blood specimen to be checked anyway. Okay, Miss Jernolrytar, let me tell you why the doctor tells you to go back to get the results about a week after he draws your blood – first of all, many people won't go back for one reason or another – just like you didn't go back the first time. The doctor knows that very well, that you probably won't go back. In the event that you do go back for the results, he'll tell you that your cholesterol is okay, and he wouldn't give you any numbers or explanation. After hearing that your cholesterol is okay, thinking that you're in good health, you would be very happy to pay his inflated bill – as you did. I'll..."

"You're absolutely right, Doctor," Melissa interrupted him, "that's exactly what happened – that I felt good when he told me that my cholesterol was okay, and I was happy to pay the big bill, thinking that I was in good health. Hmm, I'm beginning to believe everything that you're telling me now."

"Well," the doctor continued, "I'm glad to hear that. Anyway, I was about to tell you why he never said anything about the numbers or the letters that I mentioned, or why he didn't explain anything to you – the truth of the matter is that, to save money, he probably never sent your blood to the laboratory for testing – he either threw the specimen away or sold it to a blood bank. Besides, he also made his job easier by not saying anything."

"But, Doctor," Melissa asked, "what about when he's dealing with someone who has some knowledge of what you're telling me that the cholesterol level should be?"

"That's very simple," he answered, "in a case like that, he'll make believe that he's looking at the information on a computer monitor, and he'll give him some numbers that are favorable to the patient – of course, the doctor always makes sure that the patient can't read what he has up on the screen – either because the monitor is turned away from the patient or because the letters are very small and hard to read, or perhaps the information is all camouflaged among a lot of other garbage on the screen. The doctor will look and sound very convincing, but either way, the patient will be very happy to pay that astronomical bill, thinking that he's in good health."

"What if the patient's cholesterol level is dangerously high, and he's never told anything about it, and something happens to him as a result of that?" she asked.

"Miss Jernolrytar," Doctor Telsdetrooth went on, "an entire journal can be written in response to that question. First of all, the chances of that happening in a short period of time are extremely slim, if not impossible. Even if something bad does happen to the patient immediately after he leaves the doctor's office, as a result of having a dangerous level of cholesterol, the doctor won't be held liable for several reasons. Chances are that no one else knew that the patient had his cholesterol checked by that doctor on that day. If someone did know it, and the doctor was questioned about it, he can always say that he told the patient the danger that he was in because of his high level of cholesterol. There are many levels of culpability that could be claimed against the doctor, but very difficult to prove, and no lawyer would want to handle a case like that anyway. The worst scenario would be that the doctor is accused of misdiagnosing the patient, in which case, it would be extremely difficult to prove that misdiagnosing the patient caused his death or decline in health. Even if he did misdiagnose him, that is not a crime, and I can guarantee you that the doctor would find the way to fix it, by writing some kind of false information on the report so that he's on the safe side. The bottom line is that the chances of anything happening to the doctor are so slim, that he's not concerned about it. Of course, Miss Jernolrytar, there are thousands of doctors that will give you a true, detailed and honest cholesterol report. On the other hand, there are also thousands of doctors that will simply tell you that your cholesterol is okay, and nothing else – whether it's okay or not. All you have to do is to go to the right doctor."

"I'll try to choose the right doctor from now on, but I really don't know how. Do you, Doctor Telsdetrooth?" asked Melissa.

"Choosing the right doctor is a very difficult task, and a subject that I really don't want to talk about," the doctor responded.

"Okay then," said Melissa. "I don't really know what I'm going to do from now on about going to doctors – maybe I won't go at all."

"That's your own decision to make, not mine," he replied.

Cured Patients Don't Need Doctors

"ANYWAY," MELISSA WENT ON, "you said some horrible things about the cholesterol doctor – doesn't he care about what happens to his patients?"

"Caring for the well-being of the patient is the last thing on that doctor's mind," he answered. "He's only concerned about removing as much money as he can from the patient, and with the slightest amount of difficulty."

"But doesn't he want to cure his patients?" she asked.

"A cured patient has no need to go to a doctor," he replied. "Does that answer your question, Miss Jernolrytar?"

"I guess you're right, but what else can you tell me about that?" she asked.

"Would you like to hear another long story, Miss Jernolrytar?" he asked.

"Definitely, Doctor – that's what I'm here for! Go ahead!" she answered.

"Okay," he went on as he took a deep breath, "let me tell you what happened to a doctor friend of mine – oh, you mentioned him before, and I told you a little about him – his name is Doctor Sharlottan. He once had a steady patient who was suffering from severe headaches for years. The patient was a woman, about forty years old, and he had been treating her on a weekly basis for over ten years for the same ailment. He had her under medication, which gave her slight relief. He grabbed tens of thousands of dollars out of her bank account. Once, he took a vacation for about a month. His son wasn't a doctor yet, but he was studying to become one, so Doctor Sharlottan allowed him to take over his patients and practice in his office while he was away. It so happened that the first patient that his son treated was the woman with the headaches. As soon as he started talking to the woman, he noticed that she was constantly squinting every time that she had to read something. After he examined her, he told her that her problem was probably with her eyesight, because he was unable to find anything wrong with her. He then sent her to an eye doctor after charging her only a small amount of money for the examination that he gave her. Well, Miss Jernolrytar, he never saw the woman again during the four weeks that he was in his father's office.

"When his vacation was over, Doctor Sharlottan returned to his office to begin working. One day, he noticed that the woman wasn't going back for her weekly visits anymore. He checked her record to see if there was anything on it that revealed why she wasn't visiting him any longer. When he looked at the records, he noticed that she had been there the first week after he went away on vacation, and she never returned again. He called his son to ask him what happened, and his son told him that he had sent her to an eye doctor because he felt that she needed glasses when he couldn't find anything wrong with her. He told his son that he knew perfectly well that there was nothing at all wrong with the woman, except that she had a vision problem and probably needed glasses, but he didn't want to send her to an eye doctor because he'd lose her as a victim.

"Doctor Sharlottan told me that after that, he had a long talk with his son to set the record straight on how to make a good living as a dishonest doctor. After that, he had his son practice, side by side with him, until he learned all the dirty tricks. Sometime later, his son moved to another city, down south, to begin ripping off unsuspecting people as another Doctor Sharlottan."

"My God!" Melissa yelled again. "That's really disgusting. I'll really have to watch out for that kind of doctor from now on, but I can't tell a good one from a bad one. Maybe what I should do is stay away from all doctors. Doctor Telsdetrooth, I know that you said that you didn't want to talk about this, but how can I make sure that I pick the right doctor then?"

"You know, Miss Jernolrytar," the doctor answered, "you seem to be hungry for long stories, because this one is also very long. You're right – I didn't want to talk about this because I really don't know how you can pick the right doctor. Remember that some of the bad doctors that we have talked about are very highly recommended by others, so, a recommendation is not always the best way to choose a good doctor – the bottom line is that I don't know.

"Oh, you just reminded me of something we spoke about a while ago when you asked me if I had ever known of any doctor who actually cares for his patients – well, the only thing that I can tell you right now is that there's only one doctor that I would highly recommend, and that would be Doctor Honnastt, at Gud Hospital – she's very good. It's too bad that she's not a cancer specialist, so at least she could prolong my life somewhat, but I'm going to visit her soon, so she can treat me anyway, because I won't be going back to Kuttemopen Hospital in case they hear about what I'm telling you.

"Ah, there's another doctor who is also a good one. His name is Doctor Guddok – I accidentally met him at a convention about two years ago. He works at Gud Hospital, but he's thinking of opening his own private practice not too far from here. At least, that's what he told me when I met him. Maybe he has already opened his private practice, but I don't know whether he did or not. The reason why I know that he's good is because of the things that he was telling me, which were totally contrary to what all the bad doctors do.

"Those are the only two good doctors that I know. Martha Innaddayze was probably also going to be a good doctor, but we stopped her path that would have turned her into one – oh, wait a minute! I think I read in the papers that she was rehabilitated by Doctor Honnastt, and she's now practicing at Gud Hospital. I'm still planning to go there for my cancer treatment, because I don't think that she'll retaliate against me for helping to put her in a ward at Deprivayshun Psychiatric Hospital. Even if she does, I deserve it, but I don't think she will because she's a good doctor, and good doctors don't harm people in anyway, even after what I did to her. This is something that doctors, such as the bad ones that we have been talking about, would never do – to recommend a good doctor to any patient, except Doctor Guddok and Doctor Honnastt. Of course, those two doctors do recommend their patients to other good doctors. Maybe Doctor Innaddayze does the same because when she was practicing at Kuttemopen Hospital, she actually wanted to cure people, instead of butchering them. Actually this is the very first time in my many decades as a doctor that I have ever recommended a good doctor to anyone.

"Okay, now I can give you an accurate answer to a question that you asked me a while ago – yes, I have known of doctors who actually cared for their patients – Doctor Honnastt, Doctor Innaddayze and Doctor Guddok, but I still don't know the answer to your question about how to go about choosing the right doctor– all I did here was to recommend three good doctors to you, but I didn't tell you how to go about choosing one from the general public, because I don't know how. I don't think that you'll be knocking on Doctor Honnastt's, Doctor Innaddayze's and Doctor Guddok's doors anytime soon to be their patient, because it was I, a butcher doctor, who recommended them to you."

"Well!" said Melissa. "Doctor Telsdetrooth, for a change you didn't say anything scary this time. Okay, what else can you tell me? Or is this the end?"

"Not really," the doctor answered, "and we can sit here forever talking about the things that go on in my profession on a daily basis. If I had twenty years to live, I wouldn't have enough time to tell you everything that I have seen and done. Even if we only talk about the bad things that I have experienced during my long career as a butcher doctor, I wouldn't be able to tell you the entire story.

"Oh, I forgot to tell you, I have already told you plenty about each doctor that you interviewed, except one – me – but I think I have already told you some 'Wonderful' things about myself. I'll tell you a little more about my side of the story now. I was one of the biggest rip-off doctors involved with Kuttemopen Hospital. The unnecessary surgeries that I performed on my victims were numerous and very expensive. No one passed through me without getting at least three or four unnecessary operations, and I was proud to be one the best at butchering victims. The more I deceived and butchered them, the more money I extracted from their pockets. What's more important, I never inquired about their original problems because I didn't care less what ailed them to begin with. I wasn't interested in curing them – all I wanted to do was to get huge sums of money out of them. Doctor Butchar loved the tons of money that he took to the bank every day, just because of the unnecessary operations that I performed. I'll tell you something else, Miss Jernolrytar, there are plenty of other doctors like me out there – not only at Kuttemopen Hospital, but in many other hospitals as well."

Psychiatrists

"Doctor Telsdetrooth, what else can you tell me about all the wonderful things that those doctors told me that they do?" Melissa asked.

"All lies!" the doctor replied. "They do absolutely nothing good for their victims. On the contrary, everything that they do is detrimental to the patients' physical and mental health and their bank accounts. I even heard, as I mentioned before, that many of Doctor Sayahagain's patients – the ones who survived after visiting him – committed suicide, but no one knew why – well, I shouldn't say that no one knew, because we knew exactly why they did it – because they gave up after being emotionally slaughtered by him."

"Oh my God!" Melissa exclaimed. "Imagine that – committing suicide after seeing a doctor because you're hoping to get better! I guess I was lucky to run into you, Doctor Telsdetrooth, because, as I said before, I won't go to Doctor Sayahagain anymore. I don't know if the same thing could happen to me if I continue visiting him! The more I listen to you, the more shocked I become! You're frightening me so much now that I don't even know if I ever want to go to a doctor or hospital again as long as I live! Okay, is there anything that you can tell me about psychiatrists?"

"I can tell you plenty about psychiatrists," the doctor went on with another long explanation. "In my many decades as a doctor, I have never known of a mental patient who was ever cured by psychiatrists. Their patients are always put through a great deal of

347

rigmarole, when the psychiatrists know very well that the patients will not be helped by it. The psychiatrists do prescribe tons of medication to their patients – that way, they make loads of money from the kickbacks that they get by dishing out the prescriptions. Not to mention the money that they make in the stock market by investing in the companies that manufacture the medicines that they prescribe. They usually watch their drug stocks skyrocket. They know very well that those drugs that they prescribe to their patients will only keep them in a state of numbness, and won't cure them anyway.

"A psychiatrist is just one more tool that the medical doctors use to get rid of their patients when they can't, or don't want to, find the patients' physical problems. The medical doctors send their patients to psychiatrists so they can get ripped off some more. Of course, the medical doctors don't do it for nothing, because they get kickbacks from the psychiatrists. Sending patients to psychiatrists is the easiest way for medical doctors to wash their hands. They find it much easier to make that extra amount of money by sending their patients to the psychiatrists than by making honest efforts to find out what's ailing them.

"You see, Miss Jernolrytar, in our society, psychiatrists have too much power, and once a patient has been diagnosed to be crazy, no one will listen to anything that he says regarding a physical problem that he may be suffering from and complaining about. Even some good doctors will ignore his complaints, and dismiss any possibility that he may be suffering from a legitimate physical ailment.

"There are millions of patients in The United States who visit psychiatrists on a regular basis. After many money-losing visits, the patients are just as crazy as they were before their first visits to the psychiatrists. They never get cured, and the psychiatrists know that very well, but they keep dispensing their cruelty so they can watch their own bank accounts grow larger and larger. One thing for sure, Miss

Jernolrytar, a patient is definitely lighter in weight when he walks out of the psychiatrist's office."

"Really?" asked Melissa. "I'd like to know why, because I want to lose some weight myself."

"Oh, no, Miss Jernolrytar," said Doctor Telsdetrooth with a smile on his face, "you don't want to lose the kind of weight that I'm talking about – I'm referring to the weight that the patient loses because he walks out of the psychiatrist's office with a lot less money in his pockets than he had when he first walked in. Believe me, when it comes to psychiatrists, you're talking about great amounts of money that are lost by people who get absolutely nothing in return."

"But, Doctor," said Melissa, "I have heard many times that people committed crimes that were proven in court that they committed them because they were insane. They were put through rehabilitation programs by psychiatrists in mental institutions and released to society. They never committed other crimes. That should be proof that they were cured by psychiatrists. Isn't that true?"

"Well," the doctor answered, "there have been many cases also where such criminals were rehabilitated, and shortly after they were released, they committed similar crimes again. The reason why some of them don't commit other crimes is not because they were helped by the psychiatrists, but because of some other reason. Remember that criminals who serve their prison sentences because they were found guilty after committing crimes are released to society without any psychiatric rehabilitation. Many of them don't commit any more crimes either. Besides, when criminals get away with committing crimes because they are proven in court that they are insane, that's only because they have good lawyers who convince the jury that their clients are insane – of course, the biggest factor here is that the defense attorney introduces a few psychiatrists as witnesses for the defense. As I told you before, psychiatrists have too much power in our society, and when they testify in court, whatever they say, is considered to be sacred. Criminals get away with their crimes that way."

"I guess that makes sense," Melissa agreed. "Doctor, you have said on several occasions that doctors put their patients through a great deal of rigmarole, nonsense and gibberish. Isn't it a lot easier for the doctors to skip all that garbage and get right to the point?"

"My dear," the doctor replied with still another long story, "doctors would rather get right to the point, as you put it, and simply say, 'Pay this amount' and, 'Good bye' as soon as their patients walk into their examining rooms, but the doctors know that the patients wouldn't quite be that stupid, so the doctors feel that they have to say something to impress the patients. They know very well that if they use proper medical terms, the patients wouldn't understand them anyway, so they use rigmarole instead, which they find more adequate and much easier to say.

"I'll give you an example – 'Helicobacter Pylori' is a real medical term – it's a bacterium that attacks the gastric system, especially the stomach, and many doctors refer to it as a 'Bug.' If the doctors have patients suffering from the effects of the Helicobacter Pylori bacterium, they would probably tell their poor victims that they're suffering from 'Bugosis' if they intend to send them to psychiatrists, but if they intend to send them to other physicians, they would tell them that they're suffering from 'Bugitis.' They would use one of these two bogus names or something similar because it's a lot easier for the doctors to say, 'Bugosis' or 'Bugitis' rather than 'Helicobacter Pylori,' and the patients wouldn't understand either one anyway. Therefore, the doctors stick to whatever makes their jobs easier. They probably would use a different spelling to try to disguise their phony diagnosis – they would probably spell them 'Bawggosis' and 'Bawggitis' or something close to that."

That sounds very interesting," she said. "I don't really know what else to ask you about Psychiatrists."

"Well, he replied, "there's plenty more, but I think you got the picture by now."

Medical Insurance

"WHAT CAN YOU TELL me about other medical issues or problems in our society?" asked Melissa.

"Let me help you as much as I can, Miss Jernolrytar," Doctor Telsdetrooth continued with yet another long story. "Here's another subject on which you can write a complete journal – when the patients have medical insurance, we make sure that we do all the tests that are approved by the insurance companies. We take as many specimens from the patients as the insurance companies allow us to take, and many times we don't even bother to send the specimens to the laboratories so we can save money. We bill the patients for taking the specimens from their bodies, and also for sending the specimens to the laboratory, even if we don't send them. Many patients don't even bother to return to the doctor's office for the results anyway. Even if they do go back, we will tell them that everything was all right. In that case, we charge them extra because we had to speak to them again – we charge them a consultation fee when they return. Of course, when the patients hear that they're all right, they're very happy to sign all the insurance forms that we put in front of them, without even reading them or complaining about them. Many times they sign blank forms, which we fill out later. If they insist and want to hear more, we put them through a little more rubbish to sooth them. If they're not happy with our findings, then we send them to a psychiatrist. The rigmarole process continues at the psychiatrist's office, and, as you already know, the patients will lose a lot of weight after paying the psychiatrist's fee, but actually, they'll probably get reimbursed by the insurance companies."

"Doctor Telsdetrooth, you said that doctors do all the tests that are approved by the insurance companies, and also that the patients sign blank forms – how do you know that?" asked Melissa.

"Everything that I have told you I personally know about because I have seen it done, or I have done it myself – the answer to your question is that I did it many times. I remember one particular case when a woman came to my office with nothing other than an ingrown toenail. Miss Jernolrytar, I simply applied an ointment on her toe and sent her home – by the way, that was before I joined Kuttemopen Hospital. Anyway, before she left, I gave that woman a number of blank forms to sign. She had very poor eyesight and forgot to bring her glasses that day, and of course she signed all the forms without reading them – she probably would have signed the form either way, with or without her glasses. I filled out the forms later, and I stated that I gave her every kind of test that I could possibly give her – including a colonoscopy. I sent the forms in, and they sent me a big check for thousands of dollars, simply because I applied an ointment on her toe. The ointment wasn't going to help her anyway, but I was hoping that she wouldn't come back, and I was right because I never saw her again – she probably went to another doctor or simply gave up and decided to live with her ingrown toenail."

"Wow! I guess you're very dishonest then, aren't you, Doctor?" Melissa asked.

"Yes, I guess you can say that," he answered.

"Doctor Telsdetrooth," asked Melissa, "when a doctor refers a patient to a psychiatrist, does he charge the patient for that?"

"No," he answered, "but as I told you before, he makes sure that he gets a referral fee from the psychiatrist, which is usually twenty percent of what the psychiatrist charges the patient – well, in a way, the doctor actually charges the patient indirectly, because that extra twenty percent means that the psychiatrist has to rip off the patient more severely to cover the doctor's referral fee. By the way, nobody ever disputes the cost of medical care – doctors can practically charge whatever they want. The more the doctors charge the patients, the better the patients think that the doctors are. By the way, the physician knows very well that the psychiatrist rips him off also, because the psychiatrist never tells him what he actually charges the patient. Of course, that is something that the doctor has no control over, but he still gets a nice kickback from the Rigmarole Specialist anyway."

Public Assistance

"Doctor Telsdetrooth," said Melissa, "what you told me about patients who have medical insurance is quite similar to stories I've heard about Public Assistance. Isn't that so?"

"You're absolutely right, Miss Jernolrytar," the doctor went on, "let's talk about that then – any patient on Public Assistance, or on Welfare, as some people prefer to call it, is a sure way for doctors to make big money. They rip off Uncle Sam every time without anyone ever suspecting anything. Doctors charge their victims as much as they can, and force taxpayers to pay for it. When it comes to patients on Public Assistance, doctors try to get as much as possible out of them because the patients don't care and they'll sign anything that the doctors put in front of them without even reading it – exactly like patients covered by insurance. Many times the patients sign blank papers, which are filled out later by the doctors – again, exactly as patients covered by insurance.

"Here's something else that doctors do – they fill out prescriptions using the names of Public Assistance patients. Huge amounts of drugs are ordered that way. The prescriptions are usually filled by someone at the pharmacies who the doctors can trust. The doctors then sell those drugs to patients who are not on Public Assistance for many times the amount that they paid for them. Of course, there's plenty more that I can tell you about illegally bought and sold drugs, but I don't think that that's very important for your journal.

"Many times the pharmacies are owned by relatives of the doctors. In some other cases, the doctors themselves actually own the pharmacies, but they have them under the names of other people because the doctors are not allowed by law to own pharmacies."

"But aren't there any laws against that?" asked Melissa. "How do the doctors get away with it?"

"My dear," he answered, "of course there are laws against that, but the doctors get away with it because no one checks. Most doctors are considered by society to be 'Gods,' so they're free to do whatever they want. However, there have been some very rare cases when doctors were actually caught ripping off Uncle Sam, by abusing the system, but they don't get caught very often.

"I'll tell you another secret about Doctor Sayahagain – he told me that he owns the pharmacy across the street from his office, but he has it under his brother's name, who happens to be the pharmacist there, and Doctor Sayahagain always sends his patients there to have their useless-medicine prescriptions filled. He also told me that he and his brother invest very heavily in the company that manufactures the useless medicine – Plasseebow Pharmaceutical Corporation."

"Oh," said Melissa, "so I guess Doctor Sayahagain doesn't get a referral fee when he sends patients to his own pharmacy to get their prescriptions filled. Am I Right?"

"Oh, no, you're wrong," Doctor Telsdetrooth replied, "Doctor Sayahagain still gets a twenty percent kickback for every patient he sends to his brother, but that's because his brother sends him cash – that way the doctor doesn't report that amount on his income taxes. His brother enters the twenty percent as an expense of another kind – perhaps as payment to a floor sweeper or something like that. I got news for you, his brother once told me that he rips off the doctor, because he also takes cash out of the cash register and enters it as other expenses as well. Many times he doesn't ring up some of the sales he makes so he can pocket the money."

"Doctor, you said before that you ripped off insurance companies many times by having patients sign blank forms that you filled out later. Have you done the same with Public Assistance patients?" asked Melissa.

"Oh, yeah," the doctor answered, "I did exactly the same thing with those patients, and I found it easier to rip off Uncle Sam than the insurance companies, because the government employees seemed to care much less than employees of the insurance companies.

"Now, Miss Jernolrytar, let me tell you an interesting story about a particular Public Assistance patient. She was a single mother with three children. She came into my office with a severe case of sunburn, and I applied a lotion all over her body. The woman had a very pleasant-looking body, so I made sure that she would go to my office again for a follow-up visit. Before long, she became my lover. We worked out a scheme where she would sign blank forms every week, which I filled out later stating that she came to my office for cancer treatment. I was supposed to give her half of the money that Uncle Sam sent me, and she was very happy with that arrangement. Shortly after I gave her the first check, she even bought herself a brand new luxury automobile with the thousands of dollars that I was giving her every month. Of course, the woman didn't know that I was ripping her off because I was only giving her one fourth of the checks that I got from Uncle Sam, but I told her that I was giving her the entire check because she was so good to me. I even claimed the money that I gave her as salaries, cleaning and maintenance expenses on my business income taxes. So you see, Miss Jernolrytar, I was getting something from her, and she was getting something from me, while we were both getting money in return from our rich uncle. It was a perfect case of one of the many Public Assistance rip-offs, and I had quite a few other different schemes going simultaneously with other patients."

"Well!" Melissa exclaimed. "I guess there are fringe benefits all over. Aren't there, Doctor?"

"Yes, definitely," he answered.

Senior Citizens

"Doctor Telsdetrooth," Melissa continued, "since you're talking about things that didn't occur to me, I'll ask you a different question now – I don't know if you know the answer, but what is the quality of the services that are provided by doctors for senior citizens?"

"Years ago," the doctor answered, "we let old people die, but for a long time now, they have been a gold mine for the medical profession. We keep them alive as long as possible. They provide a nice income for us. We don't care about how bad they feel or how much they suffer. We simply want to keep them alive. The worse their condition, the more we treat them, thus making us very rich. Old people are usually sent to homes by their own relatives who want to get rid of them. Many times we are the ones who advise their families to send them to homes, so we can continue treating them there. Once they end up in homes, we charge them more for the same useless services that we provide, which will not help them anyway, except to keep them alive as long as possible and as sick as possible. Old people's bones are so loaded with medication, that they can't do much with their bodies. That's good for us, because that way they stay indoors, where they get more and more useless as time passes, thus needing more and more medical attention."

"Doctor," said Melissa, "I remember my poor grandmother, who was taking eleven different medications, and she didn't seem to get any better – on the contrary, her health kept getting worse and worse.

They kept prescribing one medication after another, and she complained about new problems every time the doctor gave her a new medicine. When she passed away, not too long ago, she was almost a vegetable. Let me ask you something about that – why do they keep prescribing so many drugs when they don't seem to help at all?"

"Let me repeat one thing that I have already mentioned," Doctor Telsdetrooth replied, "but I'll also tell you something new about this issue. I have prescribed tons of medications to patients who didn't need them, so I could watch my drug stocks go through the roof. Many other doctors do the same. Okay, another reason for prescribing one medication after another is because almost all medicines have negative side effects. Doctors prescribe one drug to counteract the effects of the previously prescribed medicine. Of course, the doctors don't tell their patients to stop taking the one before. They know perfectly well that the newly prescribed drug will also cause negative side effects, which will need another drug to fight off – meaning that another medication will have to be prescribed later. Your grandmother was taking eleven different medications. Well, I remember when I had some old people taking as many as thirty five different drugs. I remember some doctors who had some of their patients on many more than that. There's plenty more that I can tell you about this, but I think you probably have the picture by now."

"Oh my God!" Melissa exclaimed. "Maybe my grandmother would have been better off not taking any medicine at all."

"Well, Miss Jernolrytar," said the doctor, "whether or not she would have been better off without taking drugs is difficult to say, because the probabilities are debatable. I'd be inclined to believe that you're right – that she would have been better off without taking them."

"Doctor Telsdetrooth, getting back to the issue about senior citizens – what happens to them when they're sent to senior citizens homes?" she asked.

"Okay," he responded, "once they end up in those homes, they're doomed to stay there for life. They get very few visitors, and when they do, the visits are short. The doctors can do to them whatever they want, and nobody cares, or at least, nobody knows about it. The doctors get away with anything there, and they keep taking the senior citizens' money very fast. Another thing, Deprivayshun Psychiatric Hospital has a very lucrative home called 'Diebroak Senior Citizens Home.' All the patients who end up there die broke because the director of the home, Doctor Ryppemuff, makes sure that he takes all their money. The senior citizens home is at the same location as the hospital, but it has no definite boundaries separating it from the rest of the hospital – that way..."

"Wow!" Melissa exclaimed as she interrupted the doctor. "Doctor Ryppemuff told me a completely different story when I interviewed him – he told me that he clearly defines the boundaries of the home and keeps it completely separated from the hospital."

"Don't believe a word of it," Doctor Telsdetrooth continued. "I had numerous conversations with him about that. He boasted about keeping the victims together and classifying them differently. That way, he could juggle them around, only on his records, but not physically, so he could make more money. By switching them around, Doctor Ryppemuff can juggle the patients back and forth between the hospital and the home. He does that because there are certain medical procedures that the insurance companies will not pay for when the patients are assigned to the hospital, but they do pay for them when the patients are assigned to the home, and vise versa. There is also a limit to the length of time that patients are covered under certain insurance plans when they're assigned to the hospital. Usually when they're assigned to the home, the coverage is unlimited. Another reason for the juggling of patients is because Doctor Ryppemuff can make far more money for hospital care than for the care in the home – which is the same place anyway, but whoever is supposed to check on that, is either not doing his job or is being paid off to look the other way. The patients there get astronomical bills every month, whether they're hospital patients or home residents.

Doctor Ryppemuff assigns them to the hospital, as soon as they're admitted, to make sure that he takes all their savings as very high medical bills. After they go broke, he assigns them to the home, and then he can only charge whatever the insurance covers. Now, when he gets wealthy victims, he assigns them to the hospital and keeps them as hospital victims, because he gets huge amounts of money out of them every month. Many of his wealthy victims are paying millions of dollars per month. By the way, we also invest in the growing number of senior citizens homes that are springing up all over the nation every year as the senior citizen population increases."

"Okay, Doctor, all this sounds like a horror story. Forgive me for my doubts, but how can I find out if any of what you have told me in the last few hours is true?" she asked.

"It's very simple, Miss Jernolrytar," he answered, "do some research on that famous trial that took place sometime ago, in which a young inexperienced lawyer named Gene Lissenzwel defeated the most successful attorney in the nation. The defeated attorney's name was Ralph Byggshatt. The trial was plastered all over the news when Gene defeated Ralph. Have you heard about this case?"

"No," Melissa answered, "but as I said before, when you told me that Martha Innaddayze was a doctor, I did read about someone named Peter Emppostar, who impersonated Doctor Ryppemuff at Deprivayshun Psychiatric Hospital, and there was a big trial – is that the same case?"

"Yes!" the doctor quickly replied. "That was it! A patient named Sam Towhertz, and some other victims, who passed through my hands before they ended up at Deprivayshun Psychiatric Hospital, were also involved in the trial. I personally performed some of their unnecessary operations at Kuttemopen Hospital."

"Okay, I'll do that," she agreed, "I'll research the case on the internet."

"Very well," he said.

Cremated Human Remains

"BEFORE WE FINISH, IS there any more to this horror story?" asked Melissa.

"Oh, yeah, there's plenty more, Miss Jernolrytar," Doctor Telsdetrooth answered, "as a matter of fact, something just popped into my mind – it is an almost daily occurrence at Kuttemopen Hospital – when someone passes away, one of the doctors in the hospital, Doctor Oargandeelar, talks to the next of kin of the deceased to have the body cremated. He's not good at convincing them to do it, so he always calls his buddy, Doctor Manypewlatar to persuade them to do it. Doctor Manypewlatar does it in such a way that he almost always convinces them to do it right away. After the next of kin agrees to have the body cremated, Doctor Oargandeelar takes the body and does something else with, it and he never cremates it, but he charges the next of kin a hefty price for cremating it."

"Good grief!" Melissa yelled. "Doctor Telsdetrooth, I was never aware that these things could possibly happen, but now that you told me, what do they tell the next of kin about the body, if they don't cremate it?"

"Well," he answered, "I'll tell you about one particular incident at Kuttemopen Hospital that took place sometime before I quit my position there – a patient named James Syckcolun was told by Doctor Manypewlatar that he had the possibility of the onset of colon cancer. Of course, we all knew that Mr. Syckcolun was in perfectly good health, and there was absolutely nothing wrong with his colon, but we were greedy and wanted more business. We were actually amazed to see that James Syckcolun was in such good health, because he was past his retirement age. Less than two months after we performed numerous unnecessary operations on him, he died. We got over a million dollars out of James in medical bills for killing him. Doctor Oargandeelar then had Doctor Manypewlatar talk James' wife into having his body cremated. After she agreed, Doctor Oargandeelar let a couple of days go by, while he went around the hospital, collecting cigarette ashes from several ashtrays. He filled an urn with the cigarette ashes and called James' wife to go pick up James' ashes. She took the urn, containing the cigarette ashes, home and placed it on her mantelpiece, thinking that it contained James' ashes. Of course, Doctor Oargandeelar kept James' body because it was never cremated."

"My God!" Melissa yelled again. "I'm horrified! That's terrible! Wow! I can't get over it! Now I have to ask you another question about that – how can people be sure that they actually have their loved ones' ashes then?"

"People who have the ashes of their loved ones, don't know for sure that the ashes actually came from their deceased," Doctor Telsdetrooth answered. "In my opinion, the probability is very low. Even when they do have the actual ashes, they can't be sure that some of the ashes of other corpses in the crematory didn't get mixed in with the ashes of their loved ones."

"Doctor Telsdetrooth," asked Melissa, "how do you know that James Syckcolun's wife put the urn containing cigarette ashes on her mantelpiece?"

"Well," the doctor replied, "I could have guessed that she did that, because that's what most people do, but I wasn't guessing when I told you – actually Doctor Oargandeelar told me that that's what Mrs. Syckcolun told him that she was going to do when she picked up the urn. She was so appreciative, not knowing that she was taking home cigarette ashes to put them on her mantelpiece! Another thing, there were times when Doctor Oargandeelar couldn't find enough ashes in the hospital's ashtrays to fill the urns that he needed to satisfy all the relatives of the people they killed in the hospital. To fix that problem, he went to the city incinerator and told them that he wanted a barrel of ashes to use as fertilizer in his garden. From then on, he had a never-ending supply of ashes, but for some reason – which didn't occur to me to ask him – he continued collecting cigarette ashes because that's what he preferred to use. He only used the ashes from the incinerator when he was out of cigarette ashes."

The Sale of Human Body Parts

"Okay, Doctor," Melissa went on, "why did Doctor Oargandeelar pretend that the patient was cremated, when he actually kept the body, and why did he keep it anyway?"

"That's very simple, Miss Jernolrytar," he answered, "I know exactly why, because I was there when it happened – he wanted to use James' body parts."

"He wanted to use his body parts! What for?" She asked in a loud voice.

"There's a huge market for human body parts all over the world," he replied.

"What in the world can anyone do with human body parts?" Melissa asked.

"Such parts are in great demand," the doctor answered. "There are plenty of legitimate people and organizations that use human body parts for research and other purposes. There's also a huge demand for human body parts in a seemingly endless black market. James Syckcolun's body parts were sold by Doctor Oargandeelar at Kuttemopen Hospital. He's a very timid man, but he's an extremely good businessman. He has a lot of connections in the trade of human body parts, not only in legitimate markets, but also in the black market. A huge fortune was made by the hospital by selling James' body, piece by piece. Perhaps by now you can understand why so many people undergo numerous unnecessary operations at Kuttemopen Hospital – because they remove many of their healthy organs to sell them.

"Let me tell you how the system runs at Kuttemopen Hospital – Doctor Oargandeelar keeps a log of what organs and other body parts are on order by his numerous customers. He makes sure that Doctor Butchar always has on his desk a current list of parts that are needed to fill the outstanding orders. Before a victim is brought into the operating room, Doctor Butchar fills out a chart listing numerous operations to be performed on the victim to remove parts that are on order. Believe it or not, Doctor Oargandeelar even has customers who buy brain fluid and the fat and other fluids that are extracted when a liposuction is performed. I'll tell you later why they buy this material. He also has unlimited customers who buy blood, and that's why the doctors at Kuttemopen Hospital perform unnecessary blood transfusions – because they take out the good blood from the patients and put back a water-downed solution into their bodies to imitate their own blood. Of course, many times the victims become anemic or develop other health problems as a result of the transfusion, but whatever happens to the patients has no meaning to the doctors there.

"By the way, now you can see why Doctor Butchar had the camera removed from the rear door that I told you about – because that's where Doctor Oargandeelar conducts his sales of human body parts."

"Okay, I think I'm getting the picture now, and I think the whole thing is just horrible. Anyway, who usually buys human body parts that are not organs?" she asked.

"As I told you before," the doctor answered, "there are numerous legitimate organizations that buy human body parts. They're doing research on finding the solutions to certain human disfigurements and many other problems. They use human tissue and other parts to create artificial solutions to some of these problems. They also use almost any part of the human body for transplants – it isn't just organs that are transplanted, but many other parts as well, including bones. This is only a drop in the bucket compared to the many other uses for human body parts.

"Miss Jernolrytar, there's something else that I wanted to mention, but I kept forgetting it because of all the good stuff that we're talking about – sometime after we killed James Syckcolun, we gave his wife, Elizabeth, an annual checkup, and we found out that she was in perfectly good health. We started wondering why she was so healthy, because she was also past her retirement age. Doctor Butchar told Doctor Manypewlatar to write Elizabeth a letter telling her that she had advanced colon cancer. All he wanted to do was to operate on her and remove all her good organs to sell them. Well, he goofed because she never answered the letter, and she never contacted the hospital again. I can only imagine the devastation that we put her through, especially after we killed her husband. Of course, she didn't know that we killed him, because she thought that he had cancer and died from it."

"My God, the horrible stories that you're telling me seem to be endless!" Melissa exclaimed.

It is a wonder why Peter Emppostar didn't dispose of Doctor Ryppemuff with the help of the malicious doctors at Kuttemopen Hospital, because the doctor's body would have yielded a great fortune in the black market – the answer is not that Peter's reign was short while he impersonated Doctor Ryppemuff, because he got away with that crime for about sixteen months – the real answer was that when Peter took over, Doctor Ryppemuff stopped paying his cousin, Doctor Butchar, his kickbacks for sending him patients. Doctor Butchar noticed at the same time that his cousin wasn't calling him at all. At that point, Doctor Butchar didn't trust, who he thought was his cousin, anymore, and he didn't talk to him about the macabre activities that took place at Kuttemopen Hospital. When Doctor Ryppemuff stopped paying Doctor Butchar, the butcher continued sending patients to Deprivayshun Psychiatric Hospital, but he didn't talk to his cousin until the time he sent him Sam Towhertz – when Peter had already been there impersonating Doctor Ryppemuff for about a year, but even then, Doctor Butchar didn't tell Peter anything because he still didn't trust him.

The Biggest Shockers

"MISS JERNOLRYTAR," SAID DOCTOR Telsdetrooth, "here's another shocker for you – there have been numerous times when corpses, or pieces of corpses, were stolen from morgues or funeral parlors to be used for transplants and other purposes. In many cases the corpses were people who died from infectious diseases, and of course, the recipients of their body parts contracted whatever the deceased people had."

"Geez! Now I have to worry about receiving infected parts if I ever need a transplant!" said Melissa as she moaned.

"Okay, Miss Jernolrytar," the doctor continued, "there's something that I didn't want to tell you because it will probably kill you. The issue is very shocking, so, prepare yourself for it, because even I was shocked when I learned about it. Here it..."

"Doctor Telsdetrooth," said Melissa as she interrupted him, "I have already been horrified by you numerous times, so it doesn't bother me anymore if you continue telling me shocking stories. Please go ahead, I want to hear it."

"Okay," he said, "here it goes now, and this is the biggest shocker – there's also a big market for human body parts for human consumption. Believe it ...:

"Human consumption?" she yelled as she interrupted him.

"Yes, human consumption," he answered. "Believe it or not, as I told you before, Doctor Oargandeelar even has customers who buy brain fluid and the fat and other fluids that are extracted when a liposuction is performed. His customers use this material for soup and other dishes."

"Oh my God! No! That can't be real!" Melissa exclaimed as she nearly fell off her chair. "I thought I was going to handle this somewhat better! Cannibalism is a thing of the past, and only practiced by primitive people. Am I wrong, Doctor?"

"Yes, you were wrong," he answered, "you'll be surprised to know that cannibalism has never died."

"You mean to tell me that there are still people today who actually eat people?" she asked.

"There are thousands, if not millions, of cannibals throughout the world today," the doctor answered. "There are plenty of them right here in this great city of ours. There have been numerous headlines where the police found human meat in people's freezers, and soup or other dishes made with human flesh. Of course, the reasons for their cannibalism are not because they're hungry – they have other reasons."

"Doctor Telsdetrooth," said Melissa, "I don't get it – what other reasons could there be for eating human flesh?"

"Well," he answered, "one reason is that the members of certain groups want to achieve a certain status, and they have to do something drastic. Another reason is that there are people who consider the consumption of human flesh to be a delicacy. I even heard from Doctor Oargandeelar that he has a customer who buys a whole body of a dead old person almost every month. He's the minister of a local church and uses the bodies to make soup and stew for the whole group every time they get together. The customer..."

"Oh, my God!" Melissa yelled as she interrupted the doctor again. "That tops it all! I thought I heard everything, but this is totally sinister! Imagine that – a church minister making soup from the bodies of deceased old people! What is this world coming to?"

"Miss Jernolrytar," the doctor went on, "this is the real world around us. You just haven't been exposed to as much as I have been exposed to. There are even far more sinister things that go on in our society."

"Wow!" she shouted. "I'm not sure that I want to be exposed to anything more sinister than what you just told me. You started saying something about Doctor Oargandeelar's customer – please go on."

"Yes," Doctor Telsdetrooth continued, "his customer, the minister, Reverend Stoomaykar, only accepts bodies of people who are from seventy and up, because he says that they have the most delicious flavor. He does have to boil the flesh for hours to soften it – at least that's what Doctor Oargandeelar told me that the reverend told him. As a matter of fact, during the time that James Syckcolun was being butchered, Reverend Stoomaykar made a deal with Doctor Oargandeelar at Kuttemopen Hospital in the presence of Doctor Butchar to supply him with old people's bodies. I even heard from Doctor Butchar that the minister wanted James' wife, Elizabeth to join his congregation. I don't know if she ever did. Anyway, all the members of that church have been eating old people for years. What I don't know is whether they know that it's human meat or not, because Doctor Oargandeelar never told me, and I never asked him – I don't even know if he knows that. Reverend Stoomaykar notifies Doctor Oargandeelar when he's running low, so the doctor has time to get him another body before the minister and the church members meet again. Doctor Oargandeelar has never had a problem filling the reverend's orders right away because he has access to plenty of dead old people, and there isn't much demand for their organs or other parts. Doctor Oargandeelar told me that the minister told him that he even charges his members for their human meat meals. They gladly pay for what they eat because they find it to be delicious and unique. He says that the members can't wait to meet again so they can eat some more. That way, Reverend Stoomaykar keeps them going to church – I think it's a very interesting way to maintain his religious attendance."

"I guess you're right," Melissa added, "but if that's what it takes for him to force them to go to church, well, let it be. So, what other reasons are there for people to eat people?"

"There are numerous other reasons that I know why people eat human flesh," the doctor explained. "I'm sure that there are other reasons that I don't know about. Another reason that I do know is that some people want to go against society in general. Still another reason is that it may taste good. Of course, believe it or not, some people find it cheaper and easier to dispose of a deceased loved one by eating the corpse, rather than going through the usual process to dispose of it. Another..."

"Oh, my God!" Melissa exclaimed while interrupting the doctor once again. "I can't imagine anyone eating the corpse of a loved one! Imagine me, eating my grandmother's body! Oh no! Wow! You sure are good at shocking me, Doctor Telsdetrooth! Anyway, how do you know that anyway? And how do you know that some people eat people just to go against society?"

"I know a police captain," the doctor answered. "He's a corrupt cop, and that's why he's my friend. He tells me a lot of what goes on in this city. He once told me that he arrested a whole group of people who engaged in eating human flesh just to be different. He also told me that throughout his career as a cop, he has arrested several people who ate family members because they couldn't afford to bury or cremate them."

"That's awful!" Melissa exclaimed. "What other uses are there for human body parts, and don't tell me anymore about eating human flesh, please!"

"Another use for human body parts is that certain people use human bodies or parts of them as human sacrifices," the doctor went on, "but many times they use people who are still alive for those sacrifices. Of course, that's another story, because they usually use missing people, and some other times they use babies that have been bred specifically for such uses. That's something that has nothing to do with a medical journal, so it wouldn't be of any interest here, except when they use such babies for medical reasons. Let's not get into that subject because even I think it's too gruesome for a mother to have her baby specifically bred to kill it, or to have someone else kill it, no matter what the reason is."

"Yes," Melissa agreed, "that I have heard about — that there are certain religious cults that practice those horrible things, and I agree that it's too horrible to even think about it."

"Yes, I agree," he said.

Missing People

"Okay, what else can you tell me that I haven't heard yet?" Melissa asked.

"Miss Jernolrytar, why do you think that there are so many people missing every year, and they're never found?" Doctor Telsdetrooth," asked.

"I don't know," she answered, "but I guess they're kidnapped."

"Oh, sure, many of them are kidnapped," he replied, "and there are many reasons why people kidnap them, but one of them is that they're used for food by others. Another reason is that they're used for transplants. Still another reason is that people are used for human sacrifices."

"How do you know that they're used for sacrifices, transplants and human consumption?" she asked. "Oops, we're talking about eating people again – well, that's okay! That wasn't too gruesome this time."

"Well, now, of course, not everyone who's missing is used for those purposes," the doctor answered. "There are numerous other reasons why people are missing – such as drowning in the ocean, missing in jungles, murdered for other reasons, kidnapped and used for other purposes, voluntarily disappearing to hide from someone and so on. The number of people missing every year in The United States alone is somewhere in the neighborhood of half a million. The number of missing people every year throughout the world is in the millions.

"I wasn't going to tell you, but now that you asked me, let me tell you some things. Well, here's another shocker – the doctors at

Kuttemopen Hospital are responsible for hundreds of those missing people every year. When I was there, we actually had some people that we called 'Harvesters,' who went around kidnapping children for us to dismember their bodies and sell their parts. Of course, the term 'Harvester' is only used for such people in our group – those of us involved in the illegal business of selling human bodies and their parts. I personally got a hold of several of those missing people throughout my years as a butcher at Kuttemopen Hospital. I dismembered their bodies and watched Doctor Oargandeelar sell their parts, mostly in the black market. The doctors at Kuttemopen Hospital are still doing that today. Doctor Oargandeelar has various types of customers from all walks of life – cannibals, religious cults, crazy people, curious people and many others.

"Of course, he also has legitimate concerns as well, such as doctors, hospitals, clinics, laboratories and the like, and he makes millions from that alone. All the money that is received from the sale of human body parts in the black market is in cash, and that money is spread among all the doctors involved, but Doctor Butchar always gets the lion's share, mostly because he's the mastermind behind it all. We all have millions in cash in safety deposit boxes in various banks."

"Oh my God! Wow!" Melissa exclaimed as she yelled once more. "Doctor Telsdetrooth, you mentioned that Kuttemopen Hospital had, and still has, harvesters who go around kidnapping children, so the hospital can dismember their bodies and sell their parts – isn't that murder?"

"Of course it's murder," he answered, "but why are you so surprised? Don't you know that there are people in all walks of life who commit their murders just for the Almighty Dollar? Besides, many of the other things that I have told you that we did were also murder, such as the killing of James Syckcolun. And don't forget about the various other people who died after we cut them open to remove their perfectly healthy organs at Kuttemopen Hospital."

"Okay, I guess you're convincing me," Melissa said as she finally accepted the doctor's theory. "Anyway, you mentioned a while ago that bones are also used for transplants. Now I can understand why I heard in the news last week that some people were steeling bones from cadavers in funeral parlors and replacing them with plumbing pipes. They also said that many other parts were removed from those corpses and sold for big profits. Did you have anything to do with that?"

"I definitely had nothing to do with it, because you only heard about it recently, and I have been out of that business for quite some time now," Doctor Telsdetrooth replied. "Kuttemopen Hospital has nothing to do with it either because they always have a good supply of fresh bodies to use their parts. We did know about similar incidents when I was there, because some harvesters offered such parts to us, but we turned them down because we preferred fresh bodies."

"All this is so horrible!" said Melissa. "Okay, let me ask you a question pertaining to the kind of murder that we're talking about here – what are the categories of people that are most likely to become victims of kidnapping for such purposes?"

"I specialized in children," the doctor replied. "They were, and still are, in great demand, both for transplants and for human consumption. Oh, and also for sacrifices, but they usually want them alive for that."

"I'm ready to begin crying for those children and their families. What you're telling me is that you're a murderer. Isn't that true, Doctor Telsdetrooth?" Melissa asked.

"Of course I am," he answered, "well, at least I was, and I don't care if the whole world knows it now. I got huge sums of money by removing children's organs and watching Doctor Oargandeelar sell them to the rich parents of sick children who needed organ transplants. Many of those rich children would have died if they had to wait for organs to be donated. I was happy to destroy other people's lives for the Almighty Dollar. In a way, we actually saved some people from dying by killing others – is that so bad?"

"Well!" Melissa replied as she hesitated for a few seconds. "Ah, it's not only bad, but it's horrible – imagine being the parent of one of those children who were killed and cut up – how would you feel if that happened to you?"

"I wouldn't know, Miss Jernolrytar," Doctor Telsdetrooth answered. "Not being a father, I don't know what it feels like to love your own children. Besides, we can analogize to that by thinking of a war – where many young men die to save others. Don't get me wrong, I know it's murder, but at least it has some kind of justification. If you think I was the only one doing that, think again – children are still being missing every day, and in big numbers, even though I'm not doing it anymore. The practice of abducting children is not only being done by doctors like me, but also by people who are not doctors at all, but in every case, there's at least one doctor involved when they use the missing children for medical purposes.

"Miss Jernolrytar, you mentioned before that Doctor Ryppemuff was impersonated by Peter Emppostar. Well, let me tell you how that happened – I know the story because Doctor Ryppemuff told me all about it a few days ago, and Peter was actually the intended victim. What happened was that Doctor Ryppemuff tried to kidnap Peter to sell him to Doctor Oargandeelar so he could dismember his body and sell his parts – Doctor Ryppemuff was actually one of the harvesters, but Doctor Oargandeelar had to pay him a lot more than he paid other harvesters. Peter turned the table on Doctor Ryppemuff – one day, late in the afternoon, Peter Emppostar met Doctor Ryppemuff in the hospital's parking lot when the doctor was going home after work. Doctor Ryppemuff wanted to bring Peter into the hospital right there and then, but Peter told him that he was in a hurry. Peter then asked the doctor to give him a lift, and the doctor drove away with Peter sitting next to him. After they crossed a bridge, Peter told the doctor to let him off there. At that point, Doctor Ryppemuff wanted to use an alternative plan to trap Peter, but Peter beat him to it – he injected

Doctor Ryppemuff with a drug that made him pass out. Peter then took over the doctor's identity until Gene Lissenzwel unmasked him during that famous trial that I told you about. It was discovered, during Doctor Ryppemuff's rehabilitation, that the drug used on him to make him pass out and to keep him in that condition for more than a year, was bear tranquilizer."

Organ Transplants

"Doctor Telsdetrooth," said Melissa, "this story is really wearing me down emotionally. Because of that impersonation, I even felt sorry for Doctor Ryppemuff when I interviewed him. I guess he deserved it, because if his plan had worked, Peter Emppostar would have been cut up into pieces, because you told me that Doctor Ryppemuff wanted to sell him to Doctor Oargandeelar for that purpose."

"Oh, boy!" the doctor exclaimed. "I guess I have to tell you something else about Doctor Ryppemuff and Peter, now that you said that! Okay, here it is – Doctor Ryppemuff told me that when the media stopped talking about the case, and the issue was completely forgotten, he decided to retaliate against Peter Emppostar for drugging and impersonating him for over a year. Doctor Ryppemuff called Doctor Oargandeelar to tell him to go to Deprivayshun Psychiatric Hospital to get Peter and sell his body parts. The organ dealer gladly went there, and they drugged and transferred Peter to Kuttemopen Hospital for immediate dismemberment. Doctor Ryppemuff accompanied Doctor Oargandeelar to Kuttemopen Hospital because he wanted to see Peter being cut up into pieces. When they finally had Peter ready to be cut up, they made sure that he was awake, and Doctor Ryppemuff told him exactly what they were going to do to him. They started cutting him up without any anesthetics, and Doctor Ryppemuff started laughing when Peter started screaming. After they finished with Peter, Doctor Ryppemuff finally had his sweet revenge, and both he and the hospital made a lot of money. Ironically, Peter Emppostar finally did something that was beneficial to others – he unwillingly and unknowingly became an organ donor after his death. His organs were sold to various people who needed transplants, and many lives were probably saved because of his donations. Doctor Ryppemuff got away with everything that he has done, because as far as I know, he hasn't been punished for any of his crimes."

"Wow!" said Melissa in a very loud voice. "Doctor Ryppemuff told me that Peter couldn't take it anymore and died of a heart attack. Oh, well, let's talk about something else. I know that human organs are used for transplants legitimately. Can you tell me anything more about organ transplants?"

"Of course, Miss Jernolrytar," the doctor answered, "when I was a practicing butcher at Kuttemopen Hospital, I dealt extensively with organ transplants. Well, I can tell you plenty of stories about what went on when I was practicing there, and the same things still being practiced there today. I know, because I still talk to Doctor Butchar on a regular basis every time I go there for my treatment. He still tells me all I want to know, and we often talk about that. Is there anything specifically that you'd like to know, Miss Jernolrytar?"

"Well, I don't really know what to ask you. Okay, what are usually the organs that are used for transplants?" she asked.

"There's really no limit to the kinds of organs that are used, but some are more commonly used than others," he replied. "For instance, hearts, lungs, kidneys, livers and skin are…"

"Skin!" Melissa yelled as she suddenly interrupted the doctor. "Why did you mention skin?"

"Yes, skin," he answered. "The skin all around your body is an organ – it happens to be the largest organ in the human body."

"Oh, okay," she said.

"Anyway," he went on, "those are the ones that you hear about most frequently, but there are many other body parts that are used as well. For example, James Syckcolun's scalp and right ear were removed because, coincidentally, Doctor Oargandeelar had received an order that same morning for those two items. They were needed to be placed on a twenty-two-year-old firefighter who was a burn victim. James was in perfect health, so Doctor Butchar turned him into a donor after his operation by telling the recipient's hospital that he had a perfect match for the young firefighter."

"Oh, my God!" Melissa exclaimed. "Imagine removing someone's scalp to give it to someone else! Doctor Telsdetrooth, but if James Syckcolun was past his retirement age, doesn't that mean that he had gray hair, and if they placed his scalp on the head of someone who was only twenty two, then doesn't that mean that the young guy would have gray hair also?"

"Oh, yeah," the doctor answered, "it was quite a sight when the young fellow was fully recovered – I happened to see him on several occasions during his recovery, because I had plenty of business that I conducted with other doctors in that hospital, and I was there quite often – his hair was almost completely white, but he became an instant celebrity because of that – you see, Miss Jernolrytar, there are benefits in butchering people to death. Another thing that was very interesting was that the young guy's new right ear was a little wrinkled, but the same size as his left ear. The most interesting thing was that James Syckcolun was a black man, and the recipient was a Swedish fellow, with very light skin and blonde hair. You can imagine what he looked like with his new kind of hair and his black ear!"

"Oh my God!" Melissa yelled again. "But why did the doctors proceed with the operation if the parts weren't a perfect match?"

"When a nurse opened the cooler to hand the ear to the surgeon," Doctor Telsdetrooth explained, "she did noticed that it was black, but the doctor told her that she was wrong, and that it only looked black because it was almost frozen. The scalp had been shaven before they removed it from James' head. It was also black when the nurse took it out of the cooler, but she ignored it based on what the doctor had told her about the ear. Actually, the doctor told me sometime later that he knew that the scalp and ear were black as soon as he saw them. The real reason why they went ahead with the operation was because they had already removed what was left of the poor guy's scalp and ear, and his head was only a bare skull. They couldn't put back what they had removed from him because it was all shredded into pieces. That's the medical profession in action, Miss Jernolrytar!"

"I'm speechless," said Melissa. "Anyway, is that all they used from James Syckcolun's body?"

"Oh, no!" the doctor answered, "James Syckcolun's parts were used on many other people. Many lives were saved as a result of killing him. I think that this situation should fall into a popular phrase that says, 'The sacrifice of the few for the benefit of the many.' Again, as I mentioned before, the same thing goes on during a war. Besides, the doctors at Kuttemopen Hospital didn't care about any negative ramifications as a result of their cruel practices."

"Well," said Melissa, "even if there are positive ramifications, I still disagree with their practices! Besides, there are also negative ramifications that are too numerous to justify their crimes. I imagine that they probably used James Syckcolun's parts on other people who weren't black either, and they're walking around with mismatched parts all over their bodies!"

"I'm sure of that, too," the doctor replied, "but that only applies to parts outside of the body, because internal parts don't matter whether the donor and the recipient are of different colors or not."

"Doctor, where do most organs that are used for transplants come from?" asked Melissa.

"Are you kidding me?" he answered. "With all the good organs that are removed from perfectly healthy patients at Kuttemopen Hospital, there's no shortage of organs for transplants. There are many cases when someone alive actually donates an organ to someone else, but that's usually a kidney, because we have two of them and we can live with only one."

"Yes," said Melissa, "I've heard about people donating kidneys to others, but you said before that there is no shortage of organs – how come there's a waiting list for people to receive organs?"

"If you think that the waiting list applies to everyone, you're kidding yourself," the doctor answered.

"No? So, who does it apply to?" she asked.

"Well, think about it for a moment," the doctor replied, "I'm sure that you listen to and watch the news. Well, have you ever heard of a celebrity personality who was diagnosed with cancer or some other serious illness that required an organ transplant, and he had to wait at all to receive it?"

"Come to think of it," Melissa responded, "I was watching the news on television once, and I heard about a famous man who was diagnosed with some kind liver problem. I think it was Cirrhosis, but I don't remember, and he got a new liver immediately. He was even quite old, so I wondered why they got a new liver for him so fast – it was probably because he had plenty of money to pay for it, but I didn't know that then. After the transplant, he died anyway, and I then felt that the liver was wasted."

"There's your answer," he said, "money talks, Miss Jernolrytar."

"Okay," Melissa went on, "I'm going to ask you the same question that I asked you about other subjects several times before – are there any horror stories regarding organ transplants that you know and would like to tell me about?"

"Oh my dear," the doctor answered as he hesitated for a moment, "ah, an entire journal can be written about the horror stories that go on every day regarding organ transplants, but I'm only going to tell you about one situation – it happened shortly after I joined Kuttemopen Hospital. Prepare yourself for another shocker. Okay, here it is – once there was a patient who went to Kuttemopen Hospital because he had some pain in his abdomen. I personally examined him and found out that he had the West Nile virus. We cut him open and removed all his organs – of course he died, because his system couldn't function without organs. We told his next of kin that he died of complications. We knew that the liver was diseased, but we sold it to another hospital to be placed into the body of a poor woman – of course she also died, but she died from the effects of the West Nile virus, not from the operation. The hospital that performed the transplant didn't check the liver to see if it had the virus.

"After the hospital found out that the patient had the West Nile virus, they were required by law to report the problem to the Department of Health. As soon as Doctor Oargandeelar found out that the woman had died because of the bad liver, he told Doctor Butchar, and I was sent there to the hospital that performed the transplant to retrieve the liver before the Department of Health got a hold of it. We pretended that we wanted the liver back so we could destroy it. After we got the liver back, we needed to show proof to the Department of Health that we had destroyed it. Guess what we did instead of destroying the liver, Miss Jernolrytar."

"Well," Melissa replied, "I don't know, but I'm ready for a humongous bombshell now, so go ahead and tell me."

"Okay," the doctor continued, "I personally went to a butcher shop and bought a pig's liver. With Doctor Butchar's help, I incinerated the pig's liver while he filmed it. After the pig's liver was completely consumed by the fire, Doctor Butchar sent the video to the Department of Health as proof that the liver infected with the West Nile virus had been destroyed. Of course, the Health Department had no reason to suspect that the liver that was destroyed was a pig's liver. The bad liver was then resold to another hospital for another transplant, and, of course, the recipient also died. After that, the liver was no longer good to be resold, because it was all torn up, and the hospital that performed the last transplant with it sent it to the Department of Health. Many other people also died after receiving the West Nile virus victim's other organs, but we were able to make more money by doing the same thing that we did with the liver. So, as you can see, even good hospitals can also make fatal mistakes that cause many people to lose their lives. We, at Kuttemopen Hospital, didn't care about what happened to the victims. As I said before, we did it all for the Almighty Dollar."

"Doctor Telsdetrooth," she went on, "I really thought that I was going to be able to handle that, but now I think that I'm going to die of shock."

"Well," he said, "please, don't die on me."

Organ Dealers

"Anyway," Melissa continued, "you have been telling me all along that Doctor Oargandeelar sells organs, and that he sold the infected liver twice. I thought that enough people fill out organ-donor cards to supply all the organs that are necessary for transplants."

"Miss Jernolrytar," he replied, "millions of people fill out organ-donor cards every year, but there are people out there always making money from the tragedies that happen to other people. They always find the way to be financially compensated for their actions. People like that take organs that donors donate and give them to whoever compensates them the best – being financially or otherwise. Neither the donors nor their relatives have any control over who receives their organs – of course, the donors are dead anyway, so they definitely have no knowledge of what goes on.

"The only time when a donor has control over his donation is when he's still alive at the time he donates his organ, but, as I mentioned before, that's usually the case when someone donates a kidney to a loved one. There have been very rare occasions when people committed suicide to donate organs to their loved ones – in such cases the donors did have some control over who received their organs, providing that there were other family members to watch over those cases."

"Doctor Telsdetrooth," said Melissa, "I was always under the impression that organs were only donated and never sold, but now that I'm aware that they're sold, please tell me more about it."

"Miss Jernolrytar," the doctor explained, "I'll tell you about the biggest human organ dealer that ever lived. His name is Doctor Oargandeelar, and I have already told you plenty about him. As I mentioned before, he talks the relatives of deceased victims at Kuttemopen Hospital into having their bodies cremated, but of course, he doesn't cremate them. Instead, he uses their bodies for other purposes – to sell their parts. Now you see why he doesn't cremate the bodies, and instead, he fills urns with cigarette ashes or other ashes to give them to the relatives of the departed ones – it is because the bodies are dismembered and sold, piece by piece. James Syckcolun's body yielded Kuttemopen Hospital a great fortune. As I mentioned before, Doctor Ryppemuff is in cahoots with Doctor Oargandeelar in the business of selling body parts, and he supplies plenty of bodies from Deprivayshun Psychiatric Hospital, dead and alive.

"I know what I'm talking about because I personally accompanied Doctor Oargandeelar to Diebroak Senior Citizens Home – which is really Deprivayshun Psychiatric Hospital – several times to pick up bodies of old people who died and had no one to claim their bodies. I also accompanied Doctor Oargandeelar several times when he went there to pick up live people, but under sedation, so the organ dealer could kill them and sell their fresh organs. Doctor Ryppemuff only got rid of live patients when he had prisoners who were difficult to control and had no relatives and were poor. He wouldn't let go of any rich victims because he would get far more money from them while he had them as prisoners than selling them. Of course, while Peter Emppostar impersonated Doctor Ryppemuff, it wasn't done at all. They're still doing that today and making a fortune that way. Doctor Oargandeelar is not the only organ dealer in the country, but he's the biggest one, and his list of customers is endless."

"Oh my God!" Melissa exclaimed. "I had never realized that we live in such a murderous society. But, Doctor, isn't there a time when Doctor Oargandeelar has too many body parts and he can't sell them, or that the parts spoil and are no longer any good?"

"Of course!" the doctor replied, "supply and demand applies to everyone and everything. Doctor Oargandeelar has been in that position many times."

"So, what does he do when that happens?" she asked.

"Let me tell you something that you may find morbid, Miss Jernolrytar," Doctor Telsdetrooth went on, "but we did it for the Almighty Dollar. Several years ago, we contacted several pet food companies to sell them spoiled human body parts so they could use them for pet food. We only found a small company that bought them, because the rest of them didn't want to get involved. As soon as the owner agreed to buy the human body parts, he changed the name of the company to 'Humanfood Forpets' because he wanted to make people believe that the pet food was so good, that it was good enough for human food.

"After they started buying our spoiled human body parts, I remember that they used to advertise their high-protein all-meat pet food – it never occurred to me to pick up a can and read the ingredients. Dogs and cats were eating human flesh for years, and I don't know how many people probably ate some of that pet food as well, but that's another story.

"When Humanfood Forpets' owner died, the secret died with him because his family dissolved the company after he passed away. We were never able to find another pet food company to buy our spoiled human body parts."

"Wow!" Melissa yelled. "You're right, Doctor, I do think that the story about dogs and cats eating human flesh for years was very gruesome. I'm glad I never had a poor dog or a cat. It's also very horrific to think that some people may have also eaten some of the spoiled human flesh! So, when you couldn't find another company to buy the spoiled parts, what did you do with them?"

"When the supply was greater than the demand," Doctor Telsdetrooth continued, "I personally helped Doctor Oargandeelar, on several occasions, to put spoiled human body parts in bags, boxes and suitcases. We took them and dumped them along roads, into the ocean, into lakes and many other places. When..."

"Wow!" said Melissa as she interrupted the doctor, "now I know one reason why I've been seeing more and more reports about human body parts being found all over."

"Congratulations, Miss Jernolrytar," the doctor said, "now you know where most of those parts came from. Okay, what I was about to say was that when the supply was greater than the demand, Kuttemopen Hospital released all their patients – you see, occasionally, there were patients in the hospital during such times, and no one from the outside knew that those patients were there. The hospital even released them because there were too many body parts in stock. Otherwise the hospital would have dismembered such patients to sell their parts. They would have been dismembered if the supply had been low, because no one from the outside knew that they were in the hospital. I'll tell you the names of some people who were released, or sent to Deprivayshun Psychiatric Hospital for more cruelty, when the supply was greater than the demand – They were Carmen Pynkeehertz, Martha Innaddayze, John Suolenthom, Robert Berndhend and Sam Towhertz. Of course, there were plenty more, but the list is very long, and I don't remember them all. During lean times – that is when the demand was greater than the supply – we didn't release the occasional patients that I mentioned before, and we cut them up into pieces – because no one from the outside knew that they were in the hospital. We also had to send harvesters out to get bodies for us during lean times, and then the harvesters were very busy making small money and helping us, so we could make big fortunes."

"I imagine that you were not the only one doing that," said Melissa, "There must be many others who do the same."

"Precisely, Miss Jernolrytar!" he said. "Congratulations again, and welcome to reality."

Pharmaceutical Companies

"Doctor Telsdetrooth, there's one more thing that I'd like to see if you know anything about," said Melissa. "I've heard a lot about certain medications that are approved for doctors to use, and some of them are found to cause problems, even deaths, on some patients. What can you tell me about that?"

"Well," the doctor answered, "I only know a few things about that. Let me tell you what a doctor friend of mine told me once, not too long ago. Oh, you know him – Doctor Sayahagain. He once told me that a patient named Frank Icheethom went to his office because he had an itchy thumb. Doctor Sayahagain didn't bother to treat him, or even look at his thumb. Instead, he put him through his 'Ah' gibberish, and then gave him a prescription for useless medicine. Doctor Sayahagain..."

"Useless medicine!" Melissa exclaimed as she abruptly interrupted the doctor. "You keep talking about useless medicine, why did he give him useless medicine?"

"Doctor Sayahagain very rarely treats his patients," the doctor went on. "He only treats them whenever he feels like it. He mainly specializes in making his victims say, 'Ah,' and then he gives them a prescription for useless medicine – I'm even trying to avoid using the word 'Placebo,' but that's what I'm referring to. It doesn't matter to the doctor why his patients are there. He gives them all the same placebo medication – which is useless and will do absolutely nothing good for the patients. He doesn't even write the prescriptions himself because his receptionist pre-writes a bunch of them as soon as she walks into the office every day."

"That's a new one, Doctor," said Melissa, "you didn't mention that before. Well, okay, go ahead with your story about Frank Icheethom."

"Where did we leave off?" asked the doctor. "Oh, I remember now – okay, what I was going to say was that Doctor Sayahagain told me that the following week Frank Icheethom went back to the doctor's office because the medicine that the doctor had prescribed for Frank's itchy thumb caused fever, headaches, blurry vision, rashes and a few other problems. Doctor Sayahagain ..."

"Wow!" Melissa interrupted again. "That was terrible! Imagine that! Getting all those symptoms for taking a medicine that wasn't going to help him anyway! I'm sorry, Doctor, please continue."

"Okay," the doctor went on, "Doctor Sayahagain prescribes a placebo to his patients because he knows very well that in most case, the body's immune system takes care of most minor illnesses or injuries. The patients get better anyway, and then they think that the placebo cured them."

"Thank you, Doctor," said Melissa. "Now that we have this conversation going, what can you tell me about the pharmaceutical companies that manufacture those useless, or placebo, drugs and release them to the public when they can harm people?"

"I was just going to tell you about that in response to your original question," the doctor continued. "I'll tell you what I know about one particular drug manufacturer – Plasseebow Pharmaceutical Corporation is the company that manufactures all the useless medicine that doctors prescribe to their patients. I happen to know the president of Plasseebow Pharmaceutical Corporation. His name is Doctor Francois Phaykdok, and he told me that he bought his medical degree from a black market dealer who specialized in legal documents. He told me exactly what happened when they were developing that drug.

I shouldn't even call it a drug because it has no medicinal value. Well, okay, it is a drug because it does have negative side effects as most medicines do. Anyway, when they experimented with it, they found out that it had very severe side effects that could be very hazardous to many people and fatal to other people. Knowing that, Doctor Phaykdok released the medicine anyway, and it has been causing severe problems, as well as deaths, to many unsuspecting victims. It's really hard to understand, because all he intended to manufacture was a placebo, but he added some ingredients to it that actually caused the drug to be hazardous.

"Don't be surprised if you hear about others like Plasseebow Pharmaceutical Corporation that are manufacturing and releasing medicines that they know very well that those drugs are harmful to people."

"I had enough of that!" Melissa shouted. "Maybe we can talk about something else or just conclude now. What do you think, Doctor Telsdetrooth?"

"You're right," he replied. "There's plenty more, but I think that's about it for you to put that journal together, but if I think of something else, I'll give you a ring."

"Okay, Doctor Telsdetrooth," Melissa added, "and if I think of any other questions, I'll give you a ring."

"Oh, Miss Jernolrytar, I forgot something," said the doctor, "there's a little more that you should look into – Gene Lissenzwel spent many months preparing a lawsuit against all the doctors and hospitals involved. According to what I read in the papers, when he was ready to go to trial with the lawsuit, all the defense attorneys decided to throw in their towels because the evidence that Mr. Lissenzwel had against the doctors and hospitals was too overwhelming. The defense attorneys strongly advised their clients to settle out of court. The defendants decided to do as their attorneys had advised them, and the plaintiffs received a huge amount of money from the defendants. The fact that the defendants settled the lawsuit, instead of going to trial, should be enough proof that what I have told you is true."

"Thank you, Doctor," Melissa replied. "I'll definitely look into that. Another thing I have been meaning to ask you for a long time, but I kept forgetting – how do you know so much about all the doctors that you told me stories about? I hope you're not offended by my question, and think that I'm calling you a liar."

"That's quite all right, Miss Jernolrytar – no offense at all," he replied. "It's very simple – all the doctors that we spoke about – I'm talking about the bad ones – are my friends, and we still get together from time to time. We talk about everything that goes on in their practices. All they do is boast about how much they rip off their victims and how much they harm them. They make up bogus names for their diagnosis of their victims, so they can send them to other doctors and get kickbacks from the doctors that they send them to. We all laugh about it when we get together. During the time when Peter Emppostar impersonated Doctor Ryppemuff, the doctor stopped calling and getting together with us. We asked his cousin, Doctor Butchar, about ..."

"Oh!" Melissa interjected. "I didn't know that they were cousins."

"Oh, yes, they are," Doctor Telsdetrooth replied. "What I was about to tell you was that we asked Doctor Butchar why his cousin, Doctor Ryppemuff, stopped calling or seeing us. Doctor Butchar thought that the reason was because Doctor Ryppemuff owed him a lot of money for the kickbacks on the patients that Doctor Butchar sent him. At that point, none of the doctors trusted who we thought was Doctor Ryppemuff anymore, so the impostor was never able to get in on our little secrets. Doctor Butchar didn't want to press the issue, so he didn't call Doctor Ryppemuff at all for a long time, until he sent him a wealthy fellow by the name of Sam Towhertz. When Doctor Butchar told Peter Emppostar, thinking that he was Doctor Ryppemuff, about his kickback, Peter didn't know what Doctor Butchar was talking about, so Peter had to pretend that he had lost his memory for about a year. We only learned the truth when Doctor Ryppemuff was finally rehabilitated. As soon as that happened, he contacted us right away, and we continued our get-togethers with him again."

"Doctor Telsdetrooth, I'm beginning to be totally convinced now," said Melissa. "Anything else?"

"Yes, one last thing," the doctor responded, "if you want to hear about dentists, I'll give you the phone number of a dentist friend of mine, who's in the same position as I am. I met him in the hospital while he was getting cancer treatment – if he's my friend, you can imagine what kind of doctor he is, so I suggest you call him – his name is Doctor Molergryndar. Here, let me write his name and number down." The doctor wrote the dentist's information on a piece of paper and handed it to Melissa.

"Okay, thank you, Doctor Telsdetrooth," Melissa concluded as she took the paper from the doctor's hand. "It was quite an experience listening to you. I am very sorry about your condition, and I wish I could do something to help you. Well, thank you again, Doctor."

"Thank you, Miss Jernolrytar," Doctor Telsdetrooth also concluded, "I appreciate your offer to help me, but there's nothing that you can do for me. Well, it was also quite an experience for me to say things that I and my doctor friends kept a secret for a long time. I actually feel good now that I got everything out of my system. After I told you everything, there's no way that I'm going back to Kuttemopen Hospital for my treatment. As I told you before, I'm going to try to get my treatment done by Doctor Honnastt at Gud Hospital even though cancer is not her specialty. One last thing, if you contact Mr. Gene Lissenzwel, don't tell him that I know him, because I don't, and he doesn't know me – I only read about him in the paper, and saw him on television, but you can tell him about me if you wish. Good bye, Miss Jernolrytar."

"Good bye, Doctor Telsdetrooth," Melissa replied as they went their separate ways.

Confessions of a Dentist

THAT SAME DAY, DOCTOR Molergryndar was home watching television when he heard his phone ring. The dentist was surprised to receive a call, because he had been totally isolated from society after he contracted cancer. He thought it was either a telemarketer or a wrong number, but he answered it anyway, "Hello."

"Hello. Is this Doctor Molergryndar?" asked Melissa.

"Yes, it is, and who is this?" he replied.

"Doctor Molergryndar, my name is Melissa Jernolrytar," she said. "Doctor Telsdetrooth gave me your name and phone number and suggested that I should talk to you. The government has assigned me to write a journal about the medical profession. I know that you're a dentist, but I don't think that the inclusion of a dentist would be a detriment to the journal. Would you be kind enough to meet me, so I can interview you, Doctor?"

"No, not at all, Miss Jernolrytar," he answered, "but make it fast because I don't have much time. I don't know if Doctor Telsdetrooth told you that I have terminal cancer."

"Yes, he did. Ah, well," Melissa replied as she hesitated for a few seconds because she realized that she made a blunder – she was planning not to say anything about her knowledge of his cancer. "Ah, he told me that you're in the same position as he is." She then spoke very fast again to try to change the subject. "When and where can I meet you, Doctor?"

"You name it, and I'll be there," he answered without even realizing anything about Melissa's concern about knowing that he had cancer.

"Doctor Telsdetrooth told me that everybody knows where Gudphood Diner is. Can you meet me there tomorrow at nine in the morning?" she asked.

"Yes, everyone knows about Gudphood," he answered, "and yes, I'll be there. Good night, Miss Jernolrytar."

"Okay," she said, "I'll see you there. Good night, Doctor Molergryndar." When Melissa finished her phone conversation with Doctor Molergryndar, she was all excited about what he was going to tell her. She really wasn't prepared to interview a dentist, but because he was in the same situation as Doctor Telsdetrooth was, she thought that he would tell her the truth about his experiences as a dentist.

The following day, Melissa arrived at the diner just a little before nine in the morning. She asked a waiter if there was someone there waiting for her, but the waiter told her that there wasn't anyone, as far as he knew. She then asked him to be on the lookout for someone looking for Melissa, and then she went to a private booth at the rear of the dining area. Melissa waited and waited – it was almost half past nine, and the doctor hadn't arrived yet. She didn't know whether she should order breakfast or wait, so she decided to order coffee. Finally, at ten, she decided to go ahead and order something to eat. After all, she was starving and very disappointed that the dentist didn't show up. At about ten thirty, Melissa finished her breakfast and decided to go home.

Doctor Molergryndar walked in just as Melissa was going to get up to pay for her breakfast. The doctor was even frailer than Doctor Telsdetrooth, and besides being so frail, he was quite disheveled. The same waiter who waited on Melissa saw the doctor and, because of his appearance, the waiter thought that the doctor was a stray patient from Deprivayshun Psychiatric Hospital. The dentist asked the waiter if there was a Miss Jernolrytar at the diner waiting for him. The waiter said that he didn't know any Miss Jernolrytar, but there was a young woman named Melissa, about an hour and a half earlier, who had asked him if anyone was waiting for her. "I think she probably left by now. She was sitting in the last booth near the corner," the waiter concluded as he looked towards the rear of the dining hall. "Oh! She's still there, getting ready to leave."

"Thank you," said Doctor Molergryndar as he immediately went to Melissa's table. "Miss Jernolrytar," he said, "I am Doctor Molergryndar. I'm glad you're sill here. I'm sorry for my tardiness, but I had a flat tire while I was driving here, and my spare tire was without air. I never had a flat tire in my entire life before that, and it was a nightmare!"

"I'm happy to meet you, Doctor Molergryndar," Melissa replied. "I'm sorry about your trouble, and I'm very glad you made it. I was just getting ready to pay for my breakfast and go home, but now I'll stay. Please, sit down. Have you had anything to eat?"

"Yes," the doctor responded, "I always have my breakfast at home very early in the morning, but I can use some coffee." Melissa made a gesture to the waiter to bring two cups of coffee. Shortly after that, coffee was served, and as they started drinking it, the interview began. "Now, Miss Jernolrytar, what can I do for you?" the doctor asked.

"Well, Doctor Molergryndar," she answered, "I think this will take a while. I have many questions to ask you. First of all, I'll ask you the same question that I have asked everyone else when I started interviewing them. Why did you become a dentist?"

"Years ago," the dentist answered, "I probably would have told you that I became a dentist for the good of my patients, but now I'll be frank – I only became a dentist for the money. I always wanted to deal with the physical needs of people because they're willing to pay others a lot of money to take care of their well-being. At first, I wanted to become a physician, but later on, I thought dentistry would be simpler for many reasons. One of those reasons was that as a dentist, you don't have to make emergency calls in the middle of the night. Another reason was that there are far fewer complaints and lawsuits filed against dentists than there are against medical doctors."

"Are there any horror stories regarding dentists, Doctor Molergryndar?" she asked.

"Well, Miss Jernolrytar," the doctor answered, "I don't know what you mean by horror stories, but I know exactly what I used to do as a dentist. There are plenty of other dentists who do the same."

"Can you elaborate on some of the things that you did as a dentist?" she asked.

"Okay," he answered, "years ago, it was common practice for us dentists to drill perfectly good teeth to charge patients good money for filling the cavities that we created by drilling, but in modern days, we want to make more money. Today, instead of drilling, we do something else which is much more expensive. We give the victim the works – that means that we grind the tooth all the way down to make it flush with the gums. I personally specialized in grinding down molars because they're less visible than the front teeth, and when the patients look in the mirror, they can't see the damages as well. After grinding down the tooth, the dentist makes a hole in the root of it, so he can install a post with a cap on top of it that looks like a tooth. We refer to this procedure as a 'Root Canal, a Post and a Cap.' Even when the patient actually has a cavity that can easily and effectively be filled, the dentist never fills it. Instead, he does a 'Root Canal, a Post and a Cap' procedure on the defective tooth to make more money. Of course, the fake tooth will stand out among his other teeth, but the dentist shows the patient pictures of perfectly even-looking teeth before he does the work. The patient then thinks that his teeth would look the same, but they never do, because his fake tooth will be of a different color, and in most cases, of a different size. What's more important, you can tell that it's fake because the material looks different.

"Now, that opens the door to another big rip-off. As soon as the victim walks out of the dentist's office, he'll go home and he'll walk directly to the bathroom mirror to look at that tooth, time after time. Eventually, he realizes that he's not happy with it because it looks fake and different. Aha! That's where a bigger rip-off begins. Sooner or later, he'll want to have the rest of his teeth ground down to make them all the same. After the dentist makes huge sums of money doing his other teeth, all the patient's teeth do look the same, but in a negative way, because they all look fake, and then the patient goes home, thinking that he has good teeth with which to smile.

"When he gets home, he'll spend vast amounts of time trying to convince himself that his teeth look good, but that's where he will eventually be disappointed again because, as he smiles, he can see the dark discoloration and buildup of encrusted material that eventually accumulates at the point where the cap meets the gum, and that is something that never comes off, even if he goes back to the dentist so he can clean his teeth – that material that builds up is at a point where it can't be cleaned off. Of course, all that is of no significance to the dentist because, after he did all that, he nearly emptied the poor victim's bank account, and that was his only concern – to build up his own bank account."

"Geez!" Melissa exclaimed. "You're beginning to make me believe that it's better not to go to the dentist at all. Doctor Telsdetrooth had me believe that it's better never to go to the doctor. Okay, but don't the patients know whether or not they need the work that the dentist tells them that they need?"

"No, they don't know – they only know what the dentist tells them," Doctor Molergryndar replied.

"But, why are they visiting the dentist to begin with?" Melissa asked.

"Most times they visit the dentist for a checkup," he answered, "and not because they know that they need work."

"Okay, that's exactly what I do – I always go to the dentist for a checkup. Isn't that the way to take care of your teeth?" she asked.

"If you go to an honest dentist, it would be," the dentist answered, "but too many of us are not honest. Actually, Miss Jernolrytar, the best way to take care of your teeth is to stay away from the dentist, and at the same time, you'll be taking very good care of your bank account."

Dental X-Rays

"DOCTOR MOLERGRYNDAR, WHAT ABOUT x-rays? Don't they reveal if the patient needs work?" asked Melissa.

"Taking x-rays is the biggest rip-off in the dental profession," the dentist replied. "We charge the patients for taking the x-rays, and then we always find some work that has to be done as a result of viewing the x-rays – usually hidden cavities, or the need for a root canal, a post and a cap."

"You have me totally confused now, Doctor. What is wrong with that, if the dentist finds something wrong by reviewing the x-rays?" she asked.

"What is wrong is what the patient doesn't know or what he doesn't see," the dentist answered. "The truth of the matter is that there's nothing wrong at all with the tooth, but the dentist tells the poor victim that there was something wrong, so he can ruin it and charge him lots of bucks. You know that they never go for a second opinion when it comes to dental work, and of course, they tell us to go ahead and do the work. As far as a second opinion goes, that is one of the…" Doctor Molergryndar told Melissa all he knew about second opinions, both in the dentistry business and the medical profession.

"That's exactly what Doctor Telsdetrooth told me about second opinions. I guess it must be true then," Melissa added.

"It is very true, Miss Jernolrytar," Doctor Molergryndar agreed. "Anyway, all dishonest dentists tell their patients that the x-rays revealed some work that needs to be done – usually hidden cavities."

"You mean to tell me that the thirteen cavities that my dentist has filled didn't have to be filled at all?" she asked.

"Well," he went on, "you're very lucky, because you're an adult, and they have only ruined thirteen of your teeth! Let me tell you a story – I remember a young girl whose name was Francesca Rooindteath – she was my patient years ago. Her mother started bringing her to my office ever since she got her first tooth. I found the mother to be very naïve and easy to fool. By the time the girl was fourteen, I had drilled and filled every one of her teeth. I even filled some of her teeth several times on different spots. In reality, I never found anything at all wrong with her teeth, but I made a fortune by taking ex-rays and drilling and filling those healthy teeth. I actually made a mess out of the poor girl's mouth.

"As time passed, the girl was very unhappy with all the dark fillings that I had put into her teeth. When Francesca was about twenty years old, she appeared in my office one day and told me that she wanted to improve her smile. The 'Root Canal a Post and a Cap' routine was already common practice. I capped every one of her teeth. She didn't have enough money saved up to pay for all the work, so I did most of the job on credit, and she made monthly payments – of course, I charged her interest for financing the work. It took her many years to pay for my astronomical bill, which almost doubled, with the interest. Before she made her last payment, she was already very unhappy with the looks of her teeth, because of the dark spots where her teeth met the gums. Of course, at that point, her feelings were of no significance to me."

"I'm shocked! In that case, how can I be sure whether or not the work that the dentist is doing on my teeth is necessary?" Melissa asked.

"If you don't see anything wrong with your teeth, and if you don't have any pain, then you don't need any work," he answered.

"But my dentist always told me that I had a hidden cavity when he looked at the x-rays!" she exclaimed.

"That's the most commonly used method of ripping off our patients," he replied. "All cavities can be seen by visually inspecting your teeth. That is something that you can do yourself. A cavity that can't bee seen with the naked eye, with a simple inspection, is an extreme rarity – probably less than a million to one. Of course, you have to make sure that you look all the way around your tooth. You definitely have to use a dental mirror to look inside of your mouth, and make sure that you look very carefully around the area of the tooth that touches the gum."

"Are you telling me that all dentists tell you that you need work, when you don't?" she asked.

"Oh, no, but I think that an honest one is also an extreme rarity – again, in my opinion, probably less than a million to one," the doctor answered.

"Why are you making all these confessions, Doctor Molergryndar?" Melissa asked.

"My dear," the dentist went on, "at this stage of my life, I have nothing to lose by telling the truth, which is something that I always wanted to get out of my system. I have no relatives or heirs – I have no one. Doctor Telsdetrooth and I actually almost rehearsed this scenario, because we often spoke about ways to cleanse our souls by telling someone all this, and now, you have given me the opportunity to do it – I feel grateful to you. I imagine that Doctor Telsdetrooth also told you some things that are similar to what I'm telling you."

"Wow!" she replied. "Yes, he did, and now I can see why so many of your answers have been so similar to his answers."

"Anyway," he continued, "it was greed that drove me into doing all the things that I used to do. I really don't know why I did it, because most dentists have families to support, and they need the money, but unlike them, I didn't need it so badly."

"That's interesting," said Melissa. "How can I verify that all the things you're telling me are true?"

"I don't really think that you can verify it, because I have no proof to give you," the dentist said, "but you should be able to assume that what I'm telling you is true, because why would I be telling you all this, when I'm so close to the end of my life?"

"I don't know how to answer that question, Doctor Molergryndar," Melissa responded, "but I need more than my assumption to actually believe your story. I hope you can understand and help me with that."

"There is something that you can do to at least try to find out that some of the things I have told you are true," the dentist went on. "Go to a dentist. Have him take x-rays and give you an evaluation based on the x-rays. Regardless of what he tells you, don't let him do any work on your teeth, and then go for a real second opinion – go to another dentist, far away from the first dentist, but make sure that you don't tell him that you had already visited the first dentist. Also, don't tell the first dentist that you're going for a second opinion. If they're both honest, they'll tell you that you have no cavities. If at least one of them is dishonest, you'll be told by the dishonest one that you have a cavity or cavities. If one finds cavities, make sure that you tell him that you have no time at that moment to have the work done, and make an appointment with him to have the work done at a future time – of course, I advise you to cancel the appointment later, and don't go back at all. If they're both dishonest, you'll be told that you have cavities, but they will tell you that you have cavities on different teeth. With this last example, if it happens, you should then realize that I'm telling you the truth – bear in mind that that's probably what will happen anyway.

"By the way, there is a good reason to go see a dentist – to get your teeth cleaned, because that is something that requires the proper tools and experience, but make sure that you tell the dentist that that's all you want done, unless there's another reason for your visit."

"Doctor Molergryndar," Melissa continued, "when I interviewed a number of doctors regarding the medical profession, I was in total shock as I heard the confessions of a doctor – well, I am again in total shock now to hear your confessions about what goes on in the dental profession. I hope that you realize that I am compelled to fully state in the journal everything that you have told me."

"Of course, Miss Jernolrytar," he replied, "I want you to put it all on paper, and let me sign it in front of a notary public, if you want. That's the only proof that I can give you that everything I told you is the absolute truth. At least you can say that all the things that you wrote were the confessions of a dentist who practiced dentistry for more than forty years."

After a few more minutes of questions and answers, Melissa said, "Okay, Doctor Molergryndar, I thank you for your time. When I have everything in order, and on paper, I'll show you a copy so you can sign it, and we can have it notarized. Is there anything else that you would like to add?"

"No," he answered, "I think I said it all, and thank you for allowing me to get this load off my chest. Oh, wait a minute, would you like to know how I contracted terminal cancer?"

"Sure!" she quickly answered.

"It was my evil way of harming and ripping off people that cost me my life," the dentist began. "About a year ago, just before I stopped practicing, a victim came to my office for a checkup. I took ex-rays of all his teeth and I found absolutely nothing wrong with them. I told him that he had two extremely bad cavities on the roots of two of his upper molars, adjacent to each other. I told him that they couldn't be drilled and filled, and that they couldn't be repaired without a root canal, a post and a cap. I also told him that if he waited any longer, the infection could affect his brain. Of course he told me to go ahead and do the work right away. I had a small cut in one of my fingers, caused by some unnecessary braces that I improperly installed on a poor young girl.

"During my practice, occasionally I didn't wear surgical gloves, and that day was one of those occasions. As I started cutting his gums, some of his blood got all over my hands, and his blood penetrated my bloodstream through that little cut that I had. I finally finished the procedure, and everything went as planned. After almost emptying his bank account to pay for my bill, the patient went home, and I went about my business of ripping off other victims. A couple of days later, the victim went back to my office for a progress report. As soon as he walked in, I started giving him a small dose of rigmarole to make him happy and to show him that I was earning my fee – and of course, I took some more money from him, simply because I gave him some more gibberish, which I called a 'Consultation.' During our conversation, I found out that he had terminal cancer. Sometime later later, I started getting strange feelings all over my body. I then decided to go to a physician for a checkup, and I was diagnosed with terminal cancer."

"Wow! I'm sorry to hear that," said Melissa. "I guess that that was an unlucky thing for you – not to wear gloves that day."

"Yes," he agreed, "and it was greed and a tremendous lack of compassion that cost me my life."

"Doctor," Melissa went on, "it seems like bad doctors contract terminal cancer while performing unnecessary surgery on unsuspecting victims. If I ever hear that another doctor contracts terminal cancer, I'll think about you and Doctor Telsdetrooth. I'll also think that maybe he caught it the same way as the two of you did – who knows? I hope you don't feel offended because of what I just said, Doctor Molergryndar!"

"Not at all, Miss Jernolrytar," the dentist replied, "you're only saying something that's true – that we're both BAD doctors, and that you have to watch out because there are others like us out there."

Shortly after that, Melissa asked Doctor Molergryndar a few more questions, and after he answered them, she concluded by saying, "Okay, thank you, Doctor. It was quite an experience listening to you and Doctor Telsdetrooth! As I told him, I am very sorry about your condition also, and I wish I could do something for you that would help you. Well, thank you for everything, Doctor Molergryndar.

"Thank you, Miss Jernolrytar," the dentist replied, "I appreciate your concern, and I also wish there was something that you could do for me, but I doubt it. I also enjoyed saying things that I kept a secret during my entire career as a destructive dentist."

"If you ever need any kind of help, and you think that I can be of some assistance, please call me – you have my number," said Melissa.

"Well, that is very kind of you, Miss Jernolrytar. I will certainly keep that in mind. Okay, good bye," he concluded.

"Good bye, Doctor Molergryndar," Melissa also concluded. After they finished their conversation, they left the diner.

The Proof

THE FOLLOWING DAY, AFTER Melissa had the interview with Doctor Molergryndar, she started searching through the internet to see what she could find out about the trial that Doctor Telsdetrooth had mentioned. After several hours, she had all the information necessary to make her believe his story. That same day, she contacted Gene Lissenzwel on the phone. Gene was all alone in his office and getting ready to go home when he heard his phone ring. He picked it up, hoping that it would be the last call for the day. "Gene Lissenzwel," he answered.

"Mr. Lissenzwel, my name is Melissa Jernolrytar. I was assigned by the government to write a medical journal because of the growing number of complaints by patients about the medical services that they receive. I was wondering if you would be kind enough to allow me to interview you," she said as she hoped that he would accept.

"That would be an honor, Miss Jernolrytar, but why would you want to interview me, when I'm not a doctor?" Gene asked.

"Mr. Lissenzwel," she replied, "I interviewed a number of doctors, and they all painted a marvelous picture about the medical profession. Then I met Doctor Telsdetrooth – he told me a completely different story. Although he never met you, he mentioned reading about you and the trial, during which you defeated Mr. Ralph Byggshatt. He also mentioned Mr. Sam Towhertz. Doctor Telsdetrooth suggested that I should do research on the case. When I looked it up on the internet and found out that it was all true, I decided to contact you."

"Well, Miss Jernolrytar," Gene replied, "in that case, I think that it would help you a great deal if you can hear it all straight from the horse's mouth. Would you like me to contact all those people that were involved on my side during the trial, so we can all give you the complete picture?"

"Wow! That would be wonderful, Mr. Lissenzwel! Of course I'd like that very much," Melissa answered.

"Very well then, Miss Jernolrytar," Gene said, "I'll contact them all and try to arrange a meeting, so we can all be present. Leave your number, and I'll call you when it's all set." Melissa left him her number, and they ended their conversation.

Three days later, Gene phoned Melissa and told her to be at his brand new office the following day, first thing in the morning. At nine o'clock in the morning the following day, Melissa arrived at Gene's office. He was there alone, and said, "Good morning, Miss Jernolrytar, please call me Gene and have a seat."

"Good morning, Mr. Lissenzwel, I mean, Gene, thank you, and please call me Melissa," she replied. "Well, I can't wait to hear this story, and I believe that it should be totally accurate, based on what I read on the internet."

By ten, everyone was present. After all introductions took place, the questions and answers started rolling very fast. The group told Melissa all about the ordeals that the prisoners endured from the time they visited Doctor Sayahagain, until the trial was over and they were all free to go home again. They also spoke about the lawsuit, which never went to trial. Gene even let her listen to and see some of the recorded material that they had collected during the preparations for the trial and the lawsuit.

After several hours of questions, answers and viewing the material, Melissa was convinced that Doctor Telsdetrooth told her the absolute truth. She felt like a fool for having believed what the other doctors had told her before she met Doctor Telsdetrooth. Shortly after that, Gene told Melissa that they had told and shown her everything that they had, and she gratefully thanked them all.

She then concluded her interview, which she found to be extremely crucial to the writing of her journal, "I am totally shocked to have heard and seen such horrendous events! I am indebted to every one of you, as well as Doctor Telsdetrooth and Doctor Molergryndar, for opening my eyes. I was about to publish the journal with nothing but good things to say about all the doctors that I interviewed before I met Doctor Telsdetrooth, not knowing that every one of them was so malicious and dishonest. I guess I have enough now to publish the truth. Thank you all once again."

After Melissa concluded her statement, they ended the meeting, and she went home and decided to believe everything that Doctor Molergryndar had told her, because everything that Doctor Telsdetrooth told her was proven to be the truth, and the two doctors were friends. Besides, Doctor Molergryndar signed an affidavit that was notarized, in which everything that he told her was stated. Most importantly, she also followed Doctor Molergryndar's advice and went to two dentists for a checkup. They did exactly as Doctor Molergryndar suspected that they would do – they both found numerous hidden cavities, but all on different teeth. Of course, she also followed his advice and didn't have any work done by either dentist. She then took her test a little further and went to a third dentist, who told her that she had no cavities. She was then thoroughly convinced that Doctor Molergryndar told her the truth. She finally decided to become a regular patient at the third dentist's office. Melissa actually became much wiser from that point on – it was a lesson well-learned. The entire process was fully stated in her journal.

Published

DURING SEVERAL WEEKS OF going over her material and putting it in order, Melissa made sure that she emphasized that all the good things that the doctors had told her were not proven, and that they seemed to have been all lies, based on the confessions of Doctor Telsdetrooth, as well as the evidence that Gene Lissenzwel showed her. She mentioned that she had heard and seen enough evidence to believe that everything that Doctor Telsdetrooth had told her was true. She was given written and notarized permission by everyone associated with Gene Lissenzwel to quote them on everything that they had said, because they had proof, which was recorded and archived. Melissa also stated everything that she heard and saw on the recordings and videos when she had the meeting with Gene's group. She stated in the journal that everything that Doctor Molergryndar told her seemed to have been the truth because he signed a copy of his entire confessions, which was notarized. She also stated her own experiences when she followed his advice and visited two different dentists who claimed that they found cavities on different teeth. She further stated her experiences when she went to a third dentist.

Melissa finally sent the journal to be proofread, and after it was cleaned of all errors, she had it ready to be published. A couple of months later, the journal was published. Before releasing it, Melissa wanted to show it to Doctor Telsdetrooth, Doctor Molergryndar, Doctor Ryppemuff and Gene Lissenzwel, as a matter of courtesy. First, she planned to go to Doctor Ryppemuff's office to drop off a copy to him, but then she realized that she may have been in danger there, at Deprivayshun Psychiatric Hospital, so she decided to mail him a copy instead. Secondly, she went to see Doctor Telsdetrooth and gave him a copy for himself and another copy so he could give it to his friend, Doctor Molergryndar. Finally, she went to see Gene Lissenzwel and left him a copy of the journal.

A week later, after reading the journal, Doctor Telsdetrooth called her and told her that it was very well-written, and that it was the absolute truth. Coincidentally, Doctor Molergryndar called her the same day, and told her a very similar story. She never heard from Doctor Ryppemuff ever again. Upon reading the journal, Gene phoned her immediately and said, "Melissa, your journal was superbly written, and I think it's a very truthful and valuable publication. If you ever need a job, let me know. I can use someone with the talents that you have."

"Well, thank you Gene," she replied, "I'll keep your offer in mind, but I have a job right now."

They following day, Melissa presented the journal to her superiors. After reading it, they thought that it was a practically worthless book, based on its contents. They said that the story was too ridiculous to be true. They suspected that she didn't do any research at all, and decided to make up a story, and they concluded that she made it all up. They decided to put the journal to sleep, and not to do anything else about it. Of course it was published at tax payers' expense. The journal was not read by millions of people, as Melissa, Doctor Telsdetrooth and Doctor Molergryndar had hoped. The confessions made by both doctors were kept a secret from most people forever – giving such doctors as the bad ones mentioned in this story, and many others like them, the opportunity to keep practicing their malicious deeds.

Shortly after the journal was published, and its examination by Melissa's superiors, she was fired for having wasted government money on a poorly researched publication. Melissa was totally devastated.

After spending so much time and effort, the work that she thought was great was discarded as worthless.

After several weeks of unemployment and interview rejections, Melissa was starting to get depressed. She thought that she wouldn't be able to find a job after being fired for the reasons that her superiors had stated. She was thinking of several options – one of which was to move out of New York and try elsewhere, but then she realized that her records would follow her no matter where she went. Therefore, she decided to stick it out a little longer and continue looking for employment where she was.

After a few more weeks of rejection after rejection, Melissa was on the verge of total desperation. Her funds were running critically low. She had very little time before being completely penniless. The next day, late in the afternoon, it finally occurred to Melissa that Gene Lissenzwel had offered her a job. Among all people, she thought that he would understand her situation and realize that she was unjustly fired. She wasted no time before calling him. She was hoping that he'd still be in his office. She dialed his number, with both hope and fear of rejection at the same time. Gene was again alone in his office and getting ready to go home when his phone rang. "Gene Lissenzwel," he answered.

"Ah, Gene," she said, "this is Melissa Jernolrytar, how are you? Do you remember who I am?"

"I'm fine, thank you, Melissa," he replied. "Yes, of course, I definitely remember you. How are you? And how did it go with your journal?"

"I'm fine, thank you, Gene," she answered, "but I have bad news about the journal. I was wondering if I could come over to your office and tell you all about it."

"By all means, Melissa, I'm looking forward to it. Would tomorrow at nine be convenient for you?" he asked.

"Yes, great! I'll be there. Good night, Gene," she concluded.

"I'll be waiting for you, Melissa. Okay, good night," he also concluded.

The following morning, Melissa arrived at Gene's office before he was there. His assistant, Maria Jannytarboz, was already there. She welcomed Melissa and made her feel comfortable. Gene arrived a few minutes later and said, "Good morning, Melissa, nice to see you again."

"Good morning, Gene, thank you, and it's nice to see you, too," she replied.

"Have you had your breakfast yet?" he asked.

"No, not yet, and I'm starving." she answered.

"Great! I haven't eaten either," Gene added. "What are we waiting for? Would you like to go to my favorite place, Gudphood Diner, so we can use one of their private booths, and have breakfast and talk?"

"Yes," Melissa replied, "that'll be great! That happens to be my favorite place also. Besides, as I said, I'm starving, so let's go."

A short while later, they arrived at Gudphood Diner for that much-needed breakfast. As soon as they sat at the table, the waitress took their orders. They started talking as soon as the waitress walked away. After a few minutes, Melissa had told Gene everything that happened to her about the journal.

"Wow!" Gene exclaimed, "I'm surprised to hear that such a talented woman was fired for doing such a magnificent and accurate job. I can't believe that anyone would fire someone with so much talent. Would you be interested in working for me, Melissa?"

"Oh my God!" Melissa exclaimed. "I have to be honest with you, Gene, actually that was the reason why I wanted to talk to you. I ran out of options, and it was only yesterday that it finally occurred to me to call you."

"Well, Melissa," Gene went on, "I need someone who can create and put legal documents together. After you wrote that journal, there's no doubt on my mind that you can do a great job here. Would you be interested?"

"Oh, would I!" Melissa responded. "This is God-sent! I'm running out of money. I certainly need a job."

"What was your salary with the government, Melissa?" he asked. Melissa told him her previous salary, and Gene thought that she deserved twice that amount, and that's exactly what he offered her. "Are you satisfied with my offer, Melissa?" he asked.

"I'm completely overwhelmed!" she answered. "That's far more than I expected. I was actually going to ask you for an amount that was lower than what I was earning with the government. Okay, when can I start?"

"Well, now! I shouldn't have made you an offer then! I should have let you ask me for a starting salary, based on what you had on your mind!" said Gene as he laughed. He then said, "Don't worry! I'm just joking. You can start as soon as you're ready. When can you start?"

"Will tomorrow be too soon, Gene?" she desperately asked.

"Not at all. Oops, here's our breakfast," he said.

As they started eating, they continued talking, and within a few minutes, the deal was finalized. Melissa was hired on the spot. She would start the following day. She was extremely relieved and happy that she had finally found a job. She never really expected that the outcome of that telephone call to Gene would turn out to be as fantastic as it did. "Gene," She said, "I have to be honest with you. I tried to find employment all over. I was rejected by several potential employers because I had been fired for wasting taxpayers' money, as my superiors stated, and I am just about penniless. As I said before, it was only yesterday that it finally occurred to me to call you. I am indebted to you for hiring me."

"Well, Melissa," Gene continued, "I'll have to be honest with you, as well. I also tried to hire someone before, to do what you're going to do here, but I couldn't find anyone good enough to do it. I'm glad that no one hired you, and you decided to call me. I feel that I'm the one who has a lot to gain by you working for me. I also think that it was a good thing that I didn't hire anyone else, because I believe that you will do a better job than everyone that I interviewed, and I'm sure that your contribution to this firm will be extremely significant. By the way, you said that you're just about penniless – do you need a salary advance at this time?"

"No thank you, Gene," she answered. "I appreciate it, but I can manage until I get paid." Following that, they finished their breakfast and their conversation, and went their separate ways.

The following morning, Melissa reported to work at Lissenzwel & Associates. From that point on, her life completely turned around for the better. Her contribution did make a positive and significant impact on Gene's law firm.

Shortly after Melissa joined the firm, she learned from Gene that Doctor Honnastt was indeed a good doctor, and that she was his doctor, and that all his relatives were her patients as well. Melissa then took Doctor Telsdetrooth's advice and decided to become Doctor Honnastt's regular patient. The first thing that she did was to have her cholesterol checked, for which she paid a very reasonable amount. Doctor Honnastt gave her a detailed report, on which it was disclosed that her cholesterol was slightly high. Melissa followed the doctor's instructions, and she brought her cholesterol count to a safe level, without taking any medication.

Melissa was a very caring and compassionate person, so she kept in touch with Doctor Telsdetrooth and Doctor Molergryndar after she interviewed them. She even visited them at their homes, and occasionally did errands for them, and they appreciated it a great deal. In time, the two doctors even started loving her as the daughter that they never had.

Since Melissa's journal was never published, Doctor Telsdetrooth and Doctor Molergryndar continued their friendships and get-togethers with all the other bad doctors. However, they refrained from any malicious practices or conversations with the other doctors – they only spoke about good things, which the other doctors weren't too happy with, but they accepted whatever they talked about. Doctor Telsdetrooth and

Doctor Molergryndar also stopped going to Kuttemopen Hospital for their treatments. Doctor Telsdetrooth eventually went to Gud Hospital to get his cancer treatments, and Doctor Innaddayze did not retaliate against him for his past evil actions. Shortly after Doctor Telsdetrooth started his treatments at Gud Hospital, Doctor Molergryndar also became a patient there. Although their cancer stages were both terminal, Doctor Honnastt and Doctor Innaddayze reduced their suffering a great deal.

The two doctors had become even closer friends during their final days of their lives. One day, late in the afternoon, Doctor Telsdetrooth called Doctor Molergryndar and told him that he had a great idea. They spoke on the phone for a long time, and then they decided to go pay a visit to Gene Lissenzwel. Doctor Telsdetrooth phoned Gene, who agreed to wait for them after everyone else had already left the law firm. In about half an hour, the two doctors arrived at Lissenzwel & Associates, and Gene spent over three hours with them. After they finished whatever business they had, the two doctors left Gene's office and went to their respective homes. Gene then called Rebecca Fynedzowt and gave her another assignment.

Gastritis

A MAN NAMED ANDRE Hartbern had been complaining about his sour stomach for a long time – many years, to be exact. He felt the sourness right up to his throat. He was unable to eat or drink many of his favorite foods and beverages because almost everything aggravated his condition. Some things were more effective than others at making him feel miserable. Andre was a regular patient at a local hospital where his primary care physician was Doctor Laizee. One day, Andre went to the hospital for his routine visit. As soon as he walked into the examining room, Doctor Laizee looked at the computer monitor and then turned towards Andre and asked, "Do you have any pain?"

Andre imagined that the doctor asked him that question because it was part of his usual routine. "No," he answered, "I don't feel anything, except the problem with my stomach."

"What's the matter with your stomach?" asked the doctor. Although Andre had mentioned it to him during previous visits, the doctor didn't seem to know about it.

Andre answered, hoping that the doctor would do something about it, "It's burning so badly that almost everything I eat and drink makes me feel worse."

"That's caused by anxiety," said the doctor. "Would you like me to schedule an appointment for you to go see a psychiatrist?"

"No, I don't want to go see a psychiatrist," Andre replied.

"Mr. Hartbern, come back in six months," said the doctor. "Have your blood drawn a week before you come back to see me." Doctor

Laizee then gave Andre the necessary papers so he could go to the check-out desk to schedule his appointment.

Andre didn't feel like saying another word to Doctor Laizee, so he took the papers and went to the appointment desk. The receptionist scheduled his next appointment and gave him some papers for his blood work, and Andre walked out very disappointed. On his way home, Andre decided never to go back to the hospital. He also started thinking that he shouldn't bother going to any other doctor at all, after his experience with Doctor Laizee. He actually decided that that was his last visit to a doctor for the rest of his life.

As the days passed, the date for the appointment was getting closer and closer. Two weeks before the appointment, Andre thought that perhaps he should continue going to the doctor because, after all, he was getting his blood checked, as well as other routine checks that the hospital was providing for him. A week later, Andre finally changed his mind and decided to go have his blood drawn. The week after that, he left his home to go see the doctor again. On his way to the hospital, he decided not to say a word to the doctor, other than simply answering his questions as quickly as he could. Of course, he expected to be advised about the results of his blood test.

Andre arrived at the hospital and reported to the check-in desk. After waiting for a few minutes, he was called by a nurse. After the usual checks and questions from the nurse, he was told to have a seat in the waiting room and wait for the doctor to call him. After about half an hour, Andre was called by a doctor, but he was surprised because a different doctor called him – it was a woman. As soon as Andre walked into the examining room, she introduced herself, "I am Norma Sheekairs, and I am not a doctor – I am a nurse practitioner. How are you, Mr. Hartbern?"

"Fine, thank you," Andre answered. "What happened to Doctor Laizee?"

"Doctor Laizee is no longer working here," Nurse Sheekairs answered. "If you feel more comfortable with a doctor, let me know, and I'll cancel this appointment and reschedule you with a doctor."

"No, it's okay – I was just curious to know," Andre replied.

Nurse Sheekairs went over Andre's records and gave him the results of his blood test, which were all favorable. "Mr. Hartbern," she asked, "do you have any pain or anything else that's bothering you?"

Andre wasn't sure that he wanted to bother telling her about his stomach, but after a few seconds, he told her all about it, "Well, I've been having a problem with my stomach for a long time. Almost everything I eat…" Andre told her everything that he had told Doctor Laizee. He then waited for a comment from Nurse Sheekairs.

"Let me tell you what you probably have," the nurse responded. "It sounds like a very common problem called 'Acid Reflux.' Many people suffer from it. Let me show you an idea of what it is." Nurse Sheekairs even took the time out to draw a diagram of the entire gastric system, containing the stomach, esophagus, intestines, etc. She showed Andre where and how acid travels from the stomach to the esophagus, causing that burning sensation. After about half an hour, the nurse concluded her consultation by prescribing a medication called "Omeprazole," which is an acid-reducing medication. Andre was thrilled that someone finally listened to him and paid attention to his problem – he didn't care that she wasn't a doctor at all.

When Andre got his medicine, he started taking it immediately. After a few days, he noticed that it helped him tremendously, but it didn't cure the problem. As time passed, the medication wasn't helping him anymore.

Andre finally went back to the hospital for his next appointment. When he arrived, he found out that Nurse Sheekairs was no longer in the picture because she had moved elsewhere. Andre was assigned to a different doctor named Doctor Heesbadd. When Andre was called to see the doctor, he spent several minutes insisting that he had a problem with his stomach. Doctor Heesbadd spent the same amount of time ignoring what Andre was saying, and trying to convince him that it was all in his mind. After a few more minutes, Andre gave up, due to the fact that Doctor Heesbadd ignored him completely. The doctor then told him that he should go see a psychiatrist. Andre felt very frustrated, but maintained his calmness. After the doctor exhausted his futile attempts to have Andre committed, he called his boss – another doctor. The boss questioned Andre for about a minute, and he then decided to at least try to do something about Andre's stomach. He told the incompetent doctor to double Andre's dosage of medication and have him try it for a month to see if it helped.

Doubling the dosage did help Andre slightly, but not as much he had hoped. About a month later, Andre went back for his follow-up appointment. He was ready to have a verbal fight with the incompetent doctor if he started any nonsense about a psychiatrist. He was planning to open the door to the examining room and start a loud verbal confrontation with him, making sure that everyone in the waiting room heard everything. After about twenty minutes of waiting, instead of the quack calling him, to Andre's pleasant surprise, a new doctor called his name. His name was Doctor Guddok. Andre didn't need the confrontation that he expected to have with the quack. He was really glad because he wasn't really looking forward to it, and also because he needed attention regarding his sour stomach. After listening to Andre for less than a minute, Doctor Guddok asked him if he ever had an endoscopy done. "No, never," Andre answered.

"Never? Why not?" asked the doctor.

"No one ever mentioned it to me before," Andre replied. "Some doctors wanted to send me to a psychiatrist when I told them about this problem."

"Many doctors here are just passing through," Doctor Guddok added, "and they don't stay very long at this hospital. Sometimes some of them don't do what they should do. What you probably have is a bug in your stomach that, hopefully, can be treated with antibiotics."

The comment made by the doctor made Andre realize that no matter what the issue is, whether you get good service or not, depends on who you see. In the medical profession, however, your life could be at stake. Doctor Guddok sent Andre through the proper path. He sent him to a specialist named Doctor Gasstrodok in the Gastro Clinic in the same hospital, and Andre had an endoscopy done. The specialist, of course, took a tissue sample, a biopsy, to test for any malignancy.

Over a month later, Andre went back for the results. Well, at least, Doctor Gasstrodok told him that he didn't have cancer. The doctor told him that he had gastritis, caused by a bug, or bacterium, called "Helicobacter Pylori." Andre even asked the doctor to write down the name of the bacterium, and Doctor Gasstrodok had no objections. Andre was prescribed two different antibiotics that he had to take for two weeks – they were called "Amoxicillin" and "Clarithromycin." Andre knew that the bad news was that that wasn't a guarantee – it was only a hope that the antibiotics would cure him. The reason why Andre felt that way was because he was very inquisitive and asked many questions during his consultation. Doctor Gasstrodok told him that there have been cases when the antibiotics didn't help at all, but there were more cases when it did help and cured the problem.

After Andre Hartbern finished taking the antibiotics, he felt like a new man. However, Doctor Guddok told him to continue taking the Omeprazole to keep his acid reflux in check, because that was a very common, problem and it shouldn't be ignored.

Shortly after the gastritis incident, Doctor Guddok left the hospital and opened his own private practice. Eventually, when Andre went back to the hospital for his next appointment, he found out that Doctor Guddok was no longer there. Andre later learned where Doctor Guddok opened his office and became his regular patient at his private practice.

Nosebleeds

SHORTLY AFTER ANDRE HARTBERN'S gastritis incident, in the same part of town, a young girl named Lisa Poargurl was sitting at home eating dinner with her parents. Lisa was six years old, but she was very tall for her age. Her mother, Theresa, was a very nice woman of average height and weight, and always with a smile on her face. Her father, Pancho, was a huge man – about the same height as Sam Towhertz, but much broader.

About an hour after they finished eating, Lisa's nose started bleeding very profusely. She also started getting a headache. Pancho and Theresa did what they could to try to stop Lisa's nosebleed and make her headache go away. Among many things they tried, they gave Lisa a baby aspirin and told her to sit in a chair with put her head back, while facing the ceiling. After a while, Lisa was able to put her head down again, and the bleeding stopped. Shortly after that, her headache went away.

The next day, they sat at the dinner table and finished the leftovers from the night before. Shortly after they finished, Lisa's nose started bleeding again, accompanied by a severe headache. Her parents became very concerned about the situation. They repeated the same treatment that they gave her the night before, and after a while, everything was seemingly okay.

Several weeks passed, and Lisa's nose didn't bleed, and her headaches didn't come back. However, another evening, right after they ate their dinner, Lisa's nose started bleeding once again, and that time she had an even more severe headache.

The following day, they took Lisa to see Doctor Sayahagain. As soon as Lisa was called to go into the examining room, Theresa and Pancho got up and started walking with her. The receptionist, Betty Whilling, told them that they couldn't go inside because only the patient was allowed to go to the examining room. Theresa and Pancho disagreed with the receptionist, and after she spoke with the doctor, they were allowed to go inside.

Once inside, the doctor immediately started his "Ah" routine. After he finished, he turned on the microphone and told them to go see his receptionist and pay the bill. He also told them that his receptionist would give them the prescription for Lisa's medication. Pancho asked the doctor what the medication was for. The doctor looked at the form for the first time just to see the name. "Are you a doctor, Mr. Poargurl?" he asked.

"No," Pancho answered, "but what does that have to do with me asking you what the medication is for?"

"Mr. Poargurl!" Doctor Sayahagain yelled. "If you're not a doctor, then stop telling me how to treat my patients. Just take your daughter home and give her the medication, and you'll see that she'll be much better immediately."

Pancho didn't argue anymore because he thought that maybe the doctor had found something wrong with Lisa, and he prescribed the medicine that would take care of it. They left the examining room and paid the receptionist for an incredibly high bill. Then they went to the pharmacy across the street from the doctor's office to get Lisa's medicine. After that, they went home.

When they got home, they immediately gave Lisa her medicine. After a while, they sat at the table to eat leftovers from the night before. Shortly after they ate, Lisa's nose started bleeding, and of course, another severe headache set in once again. Her parents became almost devastated because of the sequence of events that had taken place. They gave Lisa another dosage of the medicine, but it didn't help her at all. Then they had to do what they did before when she had the same problem. After a while, Lisa was back to normal, but they planned to return to the doctor's office the next day.

The following day, Pancho stayed home from work, and they brought Lisa back to see the cruel doctor. Betty Whilling gave them another form to fill out. Pancho and Theresa were amazed, because the receptionist acted as though they had never been there before. Pancho then told her that they had already filled one out the day before. Betty looked it up and told Lisa to go see the doctor. The receptionist gave them a hard time again as Pancho and Theresa attempted to follow Lisa to the examining room, but after Betty spoke with the doctor, they were allowed to go inside. After Doctor Sayahagain put Lisa through his "Ah" routine, he turned on the microphone and told them to go see the receptionist and pay the bill, and that the receptionist would give them the prescription for Lisa's medication.

"Doctor Sayahagain," said Pancho, "you haven't even asked us why we're here, and most importantly, you seem to have forgotten that we were here yesterday. You also didn't bother to look at the paper that's right in front of you. Otherwise you would say and do something that makes sense. We're here because the medication that you prescribed for my daughter yesterday didn't work at all. She had another headache, and her nose was bleeding again, right after she took the medicine last night."

Doctor Sayahagain looked at the paper for the first time to see Pancho's name, "Mr. Poargurl," he said, "so you're the loud-mouth who told me how to be a doctor yesterday, and now you're telling me the same thing again. I don't know where you got your medical degree! I have no choice but to send your daughter to a psychiatrist named Doctor Louzi, because she's suffering from Bleadosis and Aikosis. Doctor Louzi specializes exclusively in the treatment of Bleadosis, and he'll probably send her to another psychiatrist named Doctor Louziar who specializes exclusively in the treatment of Aikosis. Consider yourself a lucky man because your bill is only $8,965, plus expenses plus other charges. Go see the receptionist. She'll take the money from you and give you details for the psychiatrist. Good bye. Next!"

"No, Doctor!" Pancho yelled. "YOU consider yourself a lucky man!" Betty Whilling didn't call the next patient because she heard Pancho yelling. Pancho then stood up and put his face only a few inches away from Doctor Sayahagain's face, "Let me tell you something, Doctor Quack!" he yelled again. "I'm not going to tear you apart because I have a wife and a daughter. Otherwise you wouldn't be alive right now. I'm taking my family out of here without paying your ridiculous bill, and if you try to do something about it, I will DEFINITELY forget that I have a wife and a daughter." Doctor Sayahagain literally trembled when Pancho faced him and spoke to him in such a threatening manner. Pancho then took Lisa by her hand and said, "Let's go home to see if we can find a real doctor – this is not a doctor; he's just an idiot and a thief." Pancho and his family walked out, and the doctor and Betty were speechless. Doctor Sayahagain didn't want to pursue the matter because he was actually intimidated by a patient for the first time during his long practice as a cruel rip-off doctor.

When they got home, Theresa said, "You know, Pancho, I read all about that famous case where there was a big trial. A woman doctor named Martha Innaddayze was held in a mental institution because she didn't want to be a butcher doctor at Kuttemopen Hospital. Instead, she wanted to cure people. Well, she's now working under the supervision of the doctor who rehabilitated her at Gud Hospital. Why don't we go there tomorrow to see if she can do something for Lisa?"

"That's a good idea," Pancho replied.

The following day, Pancho stayed home from work again, and they brought Lisa to Doctor Innaddayze. As soon as they walked into the examining room, the doctor asked, "Mr. and Mrs. Poargurl, have you taken Lisa to another doctor about her nosebleeds and her headaches?"

"Oh, God!" Pancho exclaimed. "We don't even want to talk about it!"

"Oh, oh!" Doctor Innaddayze exclaimed. "Don't tell me that you took Lisa to Doctor Sayahagain!"

"I read all about you, Doctor Innaddayze," Theresa interjected, "and it seems like you know Doctor Sayahagain very well, and also that he should change his name to Doctor Nightmare!"

"Well," the doctor replied, "I don't want to make any comments, but you're lucky to be here with Lisa, safe and sound, if you actually did take her to see Doctor Sayahagain. Anyway, let's get started. I'm going to examine Lisa now to see if I can find the problem." After a few minutes, Doctor Innaddayze finished giving Lisa a brief examination. "Mr. and Mrs. Poargurl," she said, "I can't find anything wrong with her without conducting any tests. You stated in the application that Lisa had four nosebleeds recently, accompanied by headaches. When did her problem start?"

"Only a few weeks ago," Pancho answered.

"She never had it before?" asked the doctor.

"No," Theresa answered.

"When and at what time of the day did the headaches and nosebleeds start?" the doctor asked.

"The other night," Pancho answered, "a while after we ate our dinner."

"What did she eat?" asked the doctor.

"Wonton soup, chow mein and white rice from a Chinese restaurant," Theresa answered.

"Was that the first time that Lisa ate Chinese food?" the doctor asked.

"Yes," Pancho answered, "Theresa had it before we were married and she loves it, but we didn't have a Chinese restaurant near us until a couple of months ago. Lisa and I finally had a chance to try it, and we also love it now."

"And when did it happen again – when she had the same problem?" asked the doctor.

"The following night," Pancho answered, "also a while after we ate."

"And what did she eat that night?" asked the doctor.

"The same thing," said Theresa, "we finished the leftovers."

"It says here that she had it four times," said the doctor as she looked at the form. "Tell me when and how she had it the third and fourth times."

"Come to think of it," said Pancho, "it happened a few weeks later, when we ate Chinese food again, but not the same thing. We had low mein, spare ribs, egg rolls and egg drop soup, and we ate the same thing the following night. Both nights, she had the same problem. Is it the Chinese food that caused it, Doctor Innaddayze?"

"I doubt it very much," the doctor answered, "but I'm almost one hundred percent sure that it was the MSG in it that caused it."

"What's MSG?" asked Pancho.

"It's a flavor enhancer that brings a fantastic taste out of almost any food. It's actually an organic salt, and Chinese people use it very extensively. It stands for 'Monosodium Glutamate,' and it causes severe side effects on many people," she answered.

"Wow!" said Theresa. "So, if we stop eating Chinese food, then Lisa should be okay. Is that right, Doctor Innaddayze?"

"Well," the doctor answered, "we don't know for sure if that's the problem, but I'm almost sure. We can find out once and for all by doing a simple test. I know it sounds cruel, but I think we should do it. Here's my plan – which I have already recommended to numerous other patients who came here suffering from similar side effects – after you leave here, go to the same Chinese restaurant and order the same thing that you ate the last time. After they give you the food, tell them that you want to order the same identical food again, but tell them not to use MSG on the second order. Make sure that they mark the order that has no MSG, and keep it separated from the one that has MSG. When you go home, give Lisa a very small amount of the food that has MSG – about one quarter of the amount that she usually eats, and then let her have all she wants of the MSG-free food. If my hunch is correct, she should get a slight nosebleed and a slight headache. If that happens, then you know that the MSG causes it, and she can continue enjoying as much MSG-free Chinese food as she wants. I happen to be a Chinese food lover myself, and even though MSG doesn't cause any noticeable side effects on me, I refuse to eat it because I do know that it causes many problems on many people. Besides, not every side effect is noticeable, so, even if I don't notice anything, something could happen to me if I eat MSG."

"That's very interesting," said Theresa. "I'll remember all that."

"Well," Doctor Innaddayze continued, "there's more – a doctor that I know told me that he suspects that MSG causes your sugar level to go up, causing diabetes, but he hasn't done any research on that yet. His hunch might be right, but I don't know. Anyway, with all this said, go home and try my plan. By all means, if this doesn't work, come back to me, and we'll do some tests to get to the bottom of Lisa's problems. If it does work, please call me and tell me all about it."

"Okay, Doctor," said Pancho, "we'll try it right away. How much do we owe you, Doctor Innaddayze?"

"The cost of medical care has gone astronomically high," the doctor went on. "Especially since that famous case that made headlines all over the world. Medical insurance premiums skyrocketed after the companies had to pay hundreds of millions of dollars to settle the case. I'm sorry that I have to present you with a bill, which is very high, but the cost of running this hospital has also skyrocketed. I actually feel bad about your bill because all I did was to give you advice and a physical examination to Lisa, without any tests – I didn't do anything else, and I didn't prescribe any medication. I also only spent about fifteen minutes with you, but I am compelled by the hospital to charge you for my services, according to what I did and the time I spent with you, which I have to account for. As I said before, your bill is rather high, but it's the best that I could do for you – it comes to a grand total of $175."

"Whew!" Pancho exclaimed. "For a minute there, I thought the bill was going to be high – $175 is nothing. Doctor Sayahagain told us that his bill was $8,965, plus expenses plus other charges, after doing nothing at all for Lisa. He wanted to send her to a psychiatrist, and he only spent about twenty minutes with us."

"Oh, my God!" the doctor exclaimed. "$8,965! That's outrageous! Well, as I said before, I won't make any comments."

Following that, the Poargurl family left the doctor's office very hopefully. When they got home, they did exactly as Doctor Innaddayze had instructed them to do. Indeed, they found out that it was the MSG that was causing Lisa's headaches and nosebleeds. When they fully tested Doctor Innaddayze's plan, and were satisfied that she was right, Pancho called her to tell her all about it. She was delighted to hear the good news. "By the way," she said, "I forgot to tell you before – MSG is also used on many packed foods. If Lisa ever gets the same problems, after eating something that you bought that was ready to eat, check the ingredients to see if it contains MSG, or Monosodium Glutamate. Sometimes they use different names, so, if she gets the same problems, and you don't see MSG, then I suggest that you check all the ingredients. Look them up on the internet, one by one, and see which one is MSG."

Theresa, Pancho and Lisa Poargurl started reading the ingredients of all prepared foods that they bought, and they started avoiding MSG from that moment on. They continue enjoying MSG-free Chinese food to this day.

Headaches

NOT TOO LONG AFTER Lisa Poargurl's nosebleeds, there was a woman named Kate Smhartd. She lived in the same neighborhood. She was at her home, getting ready to go to the store with her little boy. Kate was a single mother and had a son named Dominic, who was five years old. Kate was a career woman of average size and looks – one thing for sure is that she was very smart. They stepped out of their home, and when they started walking on the sidewalk, Dominic bumped into a parking meter. He hit his head on the pole of the meter, and Kate instantly tended to his needs. He wasn't complaining about any pain, and she couldn't see anything at all, where Dominic's head hit the pole. She concluded that it wasn't anything serious, and they continued walking to the store.

A few minutes later, they arrived at their destination and started shopping. After a while, they had bought everything that they needed and left the store. They started walking back home. Along the way they met Kate's friend, Miriam Pheelswel. She also had a little boy about Dominic's age, whose name was Robby. The two mothers talked as they walked, and the two boys started doing what little boys do when they get together. After a while, Kate and Dominic arrived at their home. They invited their friends to have lunch with them, but Miriam told Kate that she'd take a rain check because she was in a hurry.

Two days later, Dominic told his mother that he had a headache. It was a good thing that Kate always kept fresh baby aspirins at home for just such an occasion. She then gave him one aspirin. Shortly after that, the headache went away, and they continued their activities. Kate didn't know why Dominic had gotten a headache, because he never did before, but she was happy that it went away.

The next day, Dominic told his mother that he had another headache. Kate gave him another baby aspirin, and as the day before, the headache went away almost immediately. By that time, Kate was getting very concerned about Dominic's headaches. Later on that day, Dominic had still another headache. Kate gave him another baby aspirin, but she decided to take him to the doctor. Her usual doctor was on vacation, so she had to find a different doctor for Dominic's problem. Kate then remembered seeing a doctor's office, a few days before, on her way to the store. She decided to take Dominic there.

A few minutes later, they arrived at Doctor Sayahagain's office. Kate approached the receptionist's desk, and was given a form to fill out. After she completed the form, she was told to have a seat and wait. After a while, Dominic was called in. Kate stood up to accompany him to the examining room, but the receptionist abruptly intervened and said, "Lady, no one other than the patient is allowed to go into the examining room."

"No way!" Kate replied in a rather loud voice. "My son will not see the doctor alone. I have to go with him."

"I don't understand why you have to give me such a hard time," Betty Whilling complained as she stood up. "Rules are rules. Well, just a minute then, I'm going to tell the doctor. I'll be right back." She then started walking towards the examining room. As soon as she arrived, she leaned towards the doctor. "That stupid woman doesn't want her brat to come in alone," she whispered into the doctor's ear because his door was open.

"Okay, make an exception this time," Doctor Sayahagain replied, also in a whisper. "Let her come in. I'll take care of her."

Betty went back to tell them to go inside, and Kate and Dominic went into the examining room together. As soon as they arrived, the doctor told Betty to bring another chair from the waiting room, and then he told Dominic to have a seat. When Betty returned with another chair, Kate sat in it, and the doctor started his "Ah" routine as soon as Kate sat down, "Open your mouth and say, 'Ah,' Sonny." Dominic did as the doctor told him, and Doctor Sayahagain told him to say, "Ah" again. Dominic obeyed the doctor for the second time, and the doctor then went on with his usual routine to get rid of them as quickly as possible, "That'll be $100 plus expenses plus other charges. Go see my receptionist, so she can tell you what the total of your bill is. She'll also give you a prescription for your medicine. Good bye. Next!"

As soon as Kate noticed that the doctor was trying to get rid of them, she was very concerned about the outcome of her visit. "Doctor Sayahagain," she said, "the reason why we're here is because my son gets frequent headaches. You didn't even bother to do anything about it, even though it's written down on my application. Why did I bother to fill it out then, if you don't even trouble yourself to look at it? And what is that prescription that you mentioned for?" Betty heard Kate talking, so she waited before calling the next patient.

The doctor became very obnoxious when Kate questioned him. He looked at the form, simply to see what her name was. "Who's the doctor here, Miss Smhartd, you or me?" he asked.

"I'm not claiming to be a doctor," Kate answered. "That's why I brought my son to see you, because you're the doctor. At least, I think you are."

"Well then, let me do my job," the doctor went on. "Don't you know, Miss Smhartd, that when a child tells you that he has a headache, he's only doing it to get attention?"

Dominic was also extremely bright, and he interjected before Kate had a chance to answer the doctor's question, "No, Mr. Doctor Sayahagain, I'm not trying to get attention. I do have a headache."

Kate was quite capable of handling a verbal confrontation with the doctor, so she said, "Don't worry, Dominic, I believe you. Well, Doctor

Sayahagain, if that's the case – that he doesn't really have a headache – then why did you prescribe medication for him if he doesn't need it, because as you said, there's nothing wrong with him?"

"I didn't want to tell you this," the doctor went on, "but your son needs to see a psychiatrist." He then looked at the form again, to see what Dominic was complaining about. "He's suffering from Aikosis," he said, "and if you continue your persistence, then I suggest that you, too, should go to the psychiatrist."

"Why does he have to go see a psychiatrist?" asked Kate.

"Miss Smhartd," the doctor asked, "who are you going to believe, a great doctor, or a three-year-old boy?"

"No, Mr. Doctor Sayahagain," Dominic interjected, "I'm not three. I'm five."

"Three or five," said the doctor, "what's the difference, and what do you know about anything anyway, Kid?"

"The difference is two," Dominic responded, "and I know plenty, because I know how to read and write, and add and subtract numbers – my mommy taught me."

"Enough!" the doctor shouted. "That's a bunch of nonsense. Now, let's send you to a psychiatrist, Sonny."

By that time, Kate was totally irate, but she decided to hear what the doctor had to add. "Okay, Doctor Sayahagain," she said, "let me tell you something – if I have to choose who to believe between you and my son, I'd believe him anytime. Anyway, what is the procedure to take Dominic to a psychiatrist?"

"Your bill is now $355, plus expenses plus other charges," Doctor Sayahagain responded. "Go see my receptionist, so she can total it up. She'll give you the information for an emergency appointment with the psychiatrist. His name is Doctor Louzi, and he specializes exclusively in curing Aikosis. Good bye. Next!"

"Okay, Doctor, good bye," said Kate as she decided to proceed with those instructions, to see if maybe the psychiatrist would look into her son's headache problems. Following that, Kate paid her tremendously inflated bill and walked out. As soon as they left, Doctor Sayahagain called Doctor Louzi to tell him about the phony diagnosis.

Shortly after Kate and Dominic left, Dominic complained about still another headache, but that time it was very severe. While they walked to the psychiatrist's office, she had to give him two baby aspirins before the headache went away. By then, she was beginning to get very worried about his problem.

In about twenty minutes, Kate and Dominic arrived at Doctor Louzi's Office. She rushed to the receptionist's desk, and was given a form to fill out. After Kate completed the form, the receptionist told Dominic to go see the doctor. Kate started following Dominic to the examining room, but the receptionist quickly interfered and said, "Excuse me, Miss Smhartd, only the patient is allowed to go see the doctor."

"No! No way!" Kate yelled. "I have to go with him. My son won't go all by himself."

"Those are the rules," said the receptionist. "I'm sorry, you can't go in."

"Well, okay," said Kate as she stopped walking, "in that case, we'll go home. Good bye! Come back, Dominic – we're leaving." Dominic returned to where Kate was standing, and they started walking towards the exit door.

"Okay, just a minute then," the receptionist intervened as she started walking away. "Let me tell the doctor." Kate and Dominic stopped just before they reached the exit door. In a few seconds, the receptionist was by the doctor's side and whispered into his ear, "That woman doesn't want her son to come in alone. She wanted to go home when I told her that he had to come in by himself."

"Okay," the doctor replied, "let her come in – that's okay this time." The receptionist then went back and told Kate to go in with Dominic. When they finally walked in to see the doctor, he told Dominic to lie down on the sofa, and Kate sat in a chair next to him. "Hey, Kid, my name is Doctor Louzi," he said. "You're a great-looking young man. I hope you're a good patient as well. What is your name?"

"Dominic, Mr. Doctor Louzi," he answered after he looked at his mother, "but Mommy wrote my name down on that paper that's in front of you. I know that, because I already know how to read, and I saw her write it down. Why didn't you look at it, Mr. Doctor Louzi?"

The doctor was temporarily speechless, and Kate said, "Okay, Doctor Louzi, I'm very worried about Dominic's severe headaches. They only started a couple of days ago, and he never had them before in his entire life."

When Kate said that, the doctor completely ignored her, and started his usual garbage – he didn't even hear what Kate told him about Dominic's headaches. "Now, Dominic, can you see in the dark?" he asked.

"No, Mr. Doctor Louzi, I'm not a bat," Dominic answered.

The doctor looked at the form for the first time, just to see Kate's name and also what Dominic was complaining about. "Okay, just as I thought," said the doctor. "It was several months ago when I had a patient here suffering from a very common mental problem exactly like your son's, Miss Smhartd. The condition is called 'Aikosis,' which is a very severely debilitating mental illness. Your son urgently needs the attention of a very highly respected specialist who specializes exclusively in the treatment of Aikosis. His name is Doctor Louziar. He works wonders, but he costs more than I do. Are you willing to spend that extra money for your son's life, Miss Smhartd?"

Kate was actually very scared because she thought that the doctor had found something extremely wrong with Dominic. She answered with a sad face when she heard the doctor make that statement about her son's life. "Of course, Doctor," she answered, "money is no object when it comes to my son's life."

"Okay, go pay my fee," the doctor concluded, "and my receptionist will make an emergency appointment for your son to see Doctor Louziar. Good bye."

Kate and Dominic walked out of the examining room and went to see the receptionist, who wrote some numbers on a piece of paper and totaled them up. The amount was $1,275. She collected the money from Kate and called Doctor Louziar right there and then to make an appointment for Dominic, which was made for the next half hour. The receptionist then gave Kate instructions for Dominic's appointment with Doctor Louziar. Kate left Doctor Louzi's office, hoping that Doctor Louziar would look into Dominic's headaches. As soon as Kate and Dominic left, Doctor Louzi phoned Doctor Louziar and said, "Hey, Louziar, Louzi here. How's it going?"

"Okay. What's up?" Doctor Louziar replied.

"I'm sending you another victim," Doctor Louzi responded. "His name is Dominic Smhartd, and he's five years old. Make sure you tell his mother that he's suffering from Aikosis."

"Yeah, I know," Doctor Louziar continued, "your receptionist just called me. Okay, you've sent me quite a few Aikosis victims in the past few months. Don't worry, I'll tell her that her son is suffering from Aikosis."

"Louziar," Doctor Louzi went on, "let his mother go in with Dominic when you talk to him, because she was going to walk out of my office when my receptionist told her that her son had to see me without her."

"Okay, I'll remember that," Doctor Louziar replied, "better yet, I'll tell my receptionist right now to make a note of that, and also that he's suffering from Aikosis."

A little later, Kate and Dominic arrived at Doctor Louziar's office. After Kate filled out a form, the receptionist looked at it and noticed that Kate was the woman who had to go in to see the doctor with her son. The receptionist then went inside and informed the doctor that

Kate and Dominic were there, but because she wrote it down on the paper, she didn't say anything about the bogus illness or the fact that Kate had to go in with Dominic. She left him the papers and walked back to her desk. Kate and Dominic waited about ten minutes before they were called in to see the doctor. As soon as they walked in, Doctor Louziar noticed that Kate was there, so he was very confused because he knew that only the patient was allowed to be in the examining room. Because he didn't look at the papers his secretary brought him, he didn't read that Dominic was the patient Doctor Louzi called him about, and he didn't know that Kate was the woman he should allow into the examining room. Doctor Louziar then asked, "Which one of you two is the patient, or are both patients here?"

"I am, Mr. Doctor Louziar," Dominic answered before Kate was able to reply.

"You have to step outside then, Lady. Only the patient is allowed to be here in the examining room," said the doctor.

"Here we go again!" Kate yelled. "Let's go home, Dominic." Kate took Dominic's hand and started walking out.

"Now, just a minute," said the doctor. Kate and Dominic then stopped, while Doctor Louziar looked at the form for the first time, just to see what the patient's name and problem were. He then saw that the receptionist had made a notation disclosing that Dominic was the Aikosis victim that he had told her to make a note of, and also that his mother had to come in with him. Then he finally realized why Kate was there. He also saw Kate's name and said, "Dominic, my name is Doctor Louziar. Please sit in this chair next to me. Please, Miss Smhartd, sit here next to him. He then started his massive and expensive dose of rigmarole, "Let me tell you that I am not cheap, but I am good – I hope you understand that. As a psychiatrist, my fee is…" The doctor spent several minutes telling Kate what the inflated price of his absurdly costly cruelty was.

Kate was then beginning to believe that she was being maliciously ripped off without any regards to her son's condition. She pretended that she was paying attention to what the doctor was saying, but she didn't think that she had any intention of complying with his demands. Doctor Louziar went on and on for several more minutes. By the time he finished his last sentence, Kate was totally amazed, shocked and annoyed, but she maintained a sense of serenity.

After a slight pause, the doctor decided to talk about his bill again, "So far, your bill is $13,850, Miss Smhartd. Our automated system figures it all out. Here, take a look." The doctor showed Kate a small monitor screen on his desk. After Kate looked at the monitor, the doctor went on, "Now, let us continue. Dominic, can you see in the dark?"

"Of course not Mr. Doctor Louziar," Dominic replied, "I'm not a bat, and I already told that to Mr. Doctor Louzi."

"Doctor Louziar," asked Kate, "what does that have to do with his headaches?"

The doctor totally ignored what Kate asked him about Dominic's headaches. He then went on with his nonsense. After a while, he decided to get rid of Dominic and collect a huge fortune from Kate. "Miss Smhartd," he said, "your son's condition is far worse than I thought. He's suffering from a very common mental illness called 'Aikosis.' We have to hospitalize him immediately. Your bill here comes to $17,655. Go see my receptionist. She will collect the money from you and make an emergency appointment for your son to be admitted to Kuttemopen Hospital for an immediate evaluation."

Kate couldn't stand it anymore, so she yelled again, "DOCTOR LOUZIAR, if you think that I'm going to pay that ridiculously inflated bill, you're CRAZY, and if you think that I'm going to take my son to that hospital that you mentioned, you're even CRAZIER than I thought! As a matter of fact, I think that YOU are totally INSANE! YOU are the one who needs a psychiatrist! You didn't do anything for my son, and what's more, you didn't say anything constructive whatsoever. All you said was a load of nonsense that was intended to

Roy Manganelli

impress me – well, you did just the opposite, because you made me see very clearly that you're a complete QUACK and..."

Doctor Louziar interrupted Kate to prevent the patients in the waiting room from hearing any more of her verbal attacks on him. Even though the door to the examining room was closed, they heard plenty, because Kate was yelling very loudly. "Miss Smhartd," He said, "there are laws against not paying your bills. I'll sue you if you refuse to pay me. What's more, I'll sue you for my court expenses, as well as whatever I lose from my practice while I'm in court. What's better, to pay $17,655 now, or pay hundreds of thousands of dollars after you waste a lot of our time in court?"

Kate wasn't afraid of the doctor, and she yelled at him even harder as she continued bombarding him with the truth, "Sue me if you want to, DOCTOR QUACK! There's no court in the world that will render a verdict in your favor! You may have been ripping off a lot of unsuspecting people all your years as a QUACK, but this is where you met your match. I dare you to sue me, so we can both see what'll happen to you. What's more, DOCTOR QUACK, I'm sure that Doctor Louzi called you when I was on my way here, to tell you to tell me that Dominic is suffering from that stupid and childish name that he made up for the phony diagnosis. I don't believe that you're smart enough to come up with a stupid name like that all by yourself."

Kate's voice had been so loud, that everyone in the waiting room heard everything. Some people left with the intention of never returning to Doctor Louziar's office again. They made sure, by making a commotion to make everyone notice that they were leaving. The doctor then did some yelling of his own, "NOW, LOOK AT WHAT YOU HAVE DONE! Some of my patients have left! That'll be added to the lawsuit against you!"

"GOOD!" said Kate as she challenged the doctor even further. "The more you demand, the less you'll get! You have my name and address, and I'll be waiting for notification of the lawsuit against

450

me!" She then stood up and grabbed Dominic by his hand, and they walked out of the examining room. She was in a rage as she walked past the receptionist's desk and went into the waiting room to exit the building.

When she walked through the waiting room, she was applauded by the rest of the patients, and another woman made a remark, "That's my girl! There's no way that I'm ever coming back to this doctor again, but I didn't leave before because I wanted to hear the end. All these people here felt the same way when you started yelling at the QUACK!" As soon as the woman said that, Kate walked out, and all the other patients got up and walked out as well, without even seeing the doctor.

Kate didn't know how lucky she was that she stopped the path that would eventually have led Dominic right into Doctor Ryppemuff's hands at Deprivayshun Psychiatric Hospital, where his life would have been totally ruined. If that had happened, providing that Dominic would have survived the ordeal, Kate probably would have also been imprisoned to stop her from getting Dominic out of Deprivayshun Psychiatric hospital.

As soon as Kate left, Doctor Louziar called his attorney to start a lawsuit against her. His attorney told him to explain the entire incident. After several minutes of questions and answers, the attorney told the doctor that it would be a very difficult case to win, and that he'd rather not handle it.

The doctor lost all the patients that he had for the rest of the day. Therefore, he had plenty of time on his hands. He started calling all his friends to see if anyone had a lawyer that they would recommend. As the day passed, Doctor Louziar was given several names, and he started calling them. One by one, they all told him that it would be futile to attempt to bring the case to court. They also told him that he'd be ridiculed in court, and that he'd be losing a great deal of time and money for nothing. As the hours went by, the doctor persisted with his attempt to find someone who'd handle his case. After talking to different attorneys, he decided to accept his losses and continue ripping off other victims with his expensive rigmarole.

When Kate arrived at her home, she was totally frustrated about what happened in Doctor Louziar's office. She was also completely devastated about not being able to do anything about Dominic's headaches. She wasn't sure about what she was going to do at that moment, but she knew that she had to try to find a real doctor who'd do something about her son's problem. That same evening, Dominic got another severe headache that took three aspirins to make it go away. After supper, Kate phoned her friend, Miriam, to see if she wanted to bring her son, Robby, for lunch the next day, so he could play with Dominic. Both Kate and Miriam were self-employed and worked at home doing business on the internet, so they were able to come and go as they pleased.

Miriam had no plans for the next day. "Sure, Kate," she replied, "I'll be glad to accept your invitation. Do you need anything for me to bring you?"

"No, thank you, Miriam," Kate answered. "I only need your company and moral support. Just be here, please. I have a morbid story to tell you about."

"Okay, Kate," Miriam replied, "we'll be there. Good night."

"Thanks," said Kate. "I'm pleased to hear that you'll be here. I'll see you tomorrow. Good night, Miriam."

The next morning, as soon as Dominic got up, he told his mother that he had another headache. She had to give him two more aspirins. After a while, the headache went away, and they ate their breakfast. Shortly after that, Miriam and Robby arrived at Kate's house. The two boys started playing right away. Kate and Miriam started talking about old times in college. A little after Miriam and Robby arrived, Dominic went running to Kate saying that he had another headache. Kate gave him another aspirin, and his headache went away. It was then that Kate started telling Miriam the whole story about the three doctors who had done absolutely nothing about Dominic's headaches. "And here we are,"

Kate concluded, "and he still has those terrible headaches. I hope that the quack takes me to court. I'd like to see everyone's reactions when I say a few things about him there. As a matter of fact, if he sues me, I'll represent myself and counter sue him."

"Oh my God!" Miriam exclaimed. "Those were terrible doctors! Why don't you bring Dominic to my doctor? He was my physician at a local hospital, where Robby was born. He just opened his own private practice a few months ago, and he's very good."

"Sure, what's his name?" asked Kate.

"Doctor Guddok – he's not far from here," Miriam replied.

Kate became all excited and asked, "Can I bring him in the morning?"

Miriam became equally excited and said, "I'll tell you what, let me call him right now. He should still be in his office. Give me your phone book." Kate gave Miriam the phone directory, and Miriam looked through the listings until she found the doctor's name and number, which she dialed immediately.

The doctor was alone in his office, getting ready to go home, when he picked up the phone on the first ring, "Doctor Guddok."

"Hello, Doctor, this is Miriam Pheelswel. I'm happy to hear that you're still in your office, and I'm sorry to bother you at this time. How are you?" she asked.

"Hello, Miss Pheelswel. I'm fine, thank you, and how can I help you?" he asked.

"I have a friend who has a little five-year-old son," Miriam went on. "He's getting severe headaches very frequently, and he had one a few minutes ago. His mother is very worried. Can she go to your office first thing in the morning?"

"Yes, of course she can bring him in the morning," the doctor answered, "but I think that I'd like to speak with her, so I can ask her a few questions. If you give me her name and number, I'll phone her right now."

"Thank you, Doctor," Miriam replied, "but I think I can do better than that – I can put her on the phone right now. She's right here with me. I'm calling you from her house."

"Wonderful!" he exclaimed. "Please put her on."

Miriam handed the phone to Kate. "Hello," said Kate.

"Hello, Miss, I'm Doctor Guddok. What's your name?" he asked.

"My name is Kate Smhartd, and thank you for talking to me," she replied.

"I'm glad to speak to you, Miss Smhartd," he said. "I understand that your son has been getting frequent headaches."

Kate was happy to hear that a doctor was concerned about Dominic's headaches, and she finally felt that someone was actually helping with the situation. "Yes, Doctor," she happily responded, "and they only started a few days ago. He never had a headache in his entire life before these headaches started. Doctor Guddok, I know that if my friend, Miriam, recommends you, then you must be a good doctor. When can I bring my son to see you?"

"Thank you for the compliment, Miss Smhartd. Does he have any allergies?" he asked.

"Ah, no, at least not that I know," she answered.

"Has he suffered a blow to his head recently?" the doctor asked.

"No, I don't think so," Kate answered. "Just a minute please, Doctor Guddok, let me ask my son." Kate then turned towards Dominic and asked him, "Have you hit you head recently?"

"Of course, Mommy," Dominic answered. "Don't you remember when I ran into the parking meter the other day?"

Kate made a facial expression, which showed confusion and said, "Thank you, Honey. I'm sorry, Doctor Guddok, it was stupid of me not to remember, but it must be because I'm so worried about his headaches. The other day he walked into a parking meter and bumped his head on the pole."

Doctor Guddok raised his voice slightly and went on, "Miss Smhartd, I strongly suggest that you bring him to your regular doctor immediately! This could be a very serious problem, and it should be looked into very urgently."

"Yes, I know, Doctor," she replied, "but my doctor is on vacation, and I already went to see three other doctors, and they didn't even bother to examine my boy. The first doctor told me that my son was only pretending to have a headache to get attention. Then he sent him to a psychiatrist, and the psychiatrist sent him to another psychiatrist. None of the doctors did anything at all. Now his headaches are getting worse." Of course, Kate didn't mention the scandal that she caused at Doctor Louziar's office.

Doctor Guddok decided to make a sacrifice and said, "I'll tell you what, Miss Smhartd, I was just getting ready to go home, but I think that this is a very serious matter. If you're willing to, you can bring your son to my office right now, so we can try to find the cause of his headaches, and treat it."

"Thank you, Doctor Guddok!" Kate very enthusiastically replied. "That's wonderful! We'll leave right now, and we'll be there shortly."

The doctor then added, "It's probably nothing serious, but we can't take any changes. Bye, Miss Smhartd, I'll be waiting."

"Bye, Doctor," she replied. As soon as Kate hung up the phone, she asked Miriam if she could accompany her to the doctor's office. Miriam was happy to go so they could continue talking, and she could find out what the doctor would do about Dominic's headaches. It was also a chance for their two kids to continue being with each other.

A few minutes later, they arrived at Doctor Guddok's office. He was a very handsome man, extremely neat and seemingly well-organized. As soon as they walked into the waiting room, being a single and free woman, Kate immediately noticed his overall good appearance. The doctor devoted all his attention to Dominic and said, "Good evening, I am Doctor Guddok. You must be that smart young man that your mommy told me about. Miss Pheelswel and Robby, do you mind waiting here in the waiting room while I bring my patient and his mommy to the examining room?"

"No, wait a minute, Doctor Guddok," Kate intervened, "I don't mind if they come with us. Actually I want them to be there, if you don't mind."

"No, not at all," said the doctor. "Okay then, follow me Young Man, and we'll see how smart you really are. Please follow us, Miss Smhartd, and you, too, Miss Pheelswel. You, too, Robby." The doctor tried to make Dominic feel comfortable as they walked towards the examining room. "What is your name, Young Man?" he asked.

"My name is Dominic, Mr. Doctor Guddok," he answered with his usually interesting manners.

"That's a very nice name," the doctor added, "and you're a very respectful young man." As soon as they arrived at the examining room, the doctor went to work right away. "Where did Dominic hit his head, Miss Smhartd?" he asked.

"On his left side, right above his ear," Kate answered.

The doctor wasted no time, as he started giving Dominic's head a thorough examination. He examined it for several minutes, and after he finished, he turned towards Kate and said, "Miss Smhartd, I can't see anything at all visually." Just as soon as the doctor said that, Dominic told his mother that he was getting another headache. "This is very urgent," said the doctor. "I'll need Dominic's help to assist me with a machine that I have. Let us all go there, and I'll explain to Dominic what I need him to do for me." They started walking towards the x-ray machine. When they arrived, the doctor said, "Dominic, you have to be very smart to do this. Only YOU are allowed to remain there, to see if you can hear any sounds coming out of the machine. I want you to sit in this stool and put your head right against this thing you see here. Now, you have to be absolutely still while you listen. I'll tell you when to start listening and when you can move again." Dominic was all excited about being there, not knowing that he was going to have an x-ray taken. When Dominic did what Doctor Guddok told him, the doctor told the others to go to the safe area behind the door, where they could look through a glass wall. The doctor swiftly walked away from Dominic to join the others behind the wall. As soon as the doctor was inside, he said, "Dominic, be absolutely still until I tell you that you can move again. Okay, start listening right now, but don't move." He threw the switch on, and after a few seconds, he turned it off again and walked out from behind the wall with Kate, Miriam and Robby. When he was standing next to Dominic, he said, "Dominic, you can move now, and thank you. Did you hear anything?"

Dominic answered with a big smile on his face, "I heard some kind of clicking sounds, Mr. Doctor Guddok."

"Very good, Dominic," the doctor went on, "your mommy was right – you're very smart! You have been a great help. Now I can get my machine fixed, since you found the problem. Thank you again."

"You're welcome," Dominic replied.

The doctor immediately retrieved the x-ray from the machine and started examining it. After a few minutes of going over the x-ray very thoroughly, he turned towards Kate and said, "Miss Smhartd, I can't see anything at all wrong with your son's head. That doesn't mean that there's nothing wrong – it simply means that the x-ray didn't reveal it. I don't have an MRI machine here. I always send any patient who needs an MRI to Doctor Honnastt at Gud Hospital – she's the best I know. I strongly recommend that you take Dominic there, because this could turn out to be something very serious. Please don't think that I'm trying to scare you – I simply mean that something has to be done very fast before something does happen."

"Okay, Doctor Guddok," Kate replied, "I'll do anything to take care of his problem. When can I bring Dominic to Doctor Honnastt at Gud Hospital?"

The doctor answered, as he reached for the phone and started dialing, "I wouldn't waste any time. I know Doctor Honnastt personally. I know that she wouldn't mind if I call her right now, to see if she can see Dominic right away. She's only fifteen minutes away from here. I hope she hasn't left yet."

"Gud Hospital," the operator answered.

"This is Doctor Guddok. I'd like to speak with Doctor Honnastt, please. Is she still there?" he asked.

"Just a minute please, let me find out," the operator answered.

While the doctor waited, he asked, "How's your headache, Dominic."

Dominic looked up, smiled and said, "Not as bad as before, but I still have it."

"Yes, Doctor Guddok," said the operator, "Doctor Honnastt is still here. I'll connect you."

"Thank you, Operator," said the doctor.

"Doctor Honnastt," she answered.

The doctor was relieved to hear her voice. "Hi, Doctor Honnastt," he said. "This is Doctor Guddok. I'm glad that you're still there. I need a big favor from you."

"Oh, oh!" Doctor Honnastt exclaimed. "There you go again, with your big favors. Oh, well, what is it this time?"

"I have a very smart young man here, who's five years old," Doctor Guddok replied. "His name is Dominic, and he gets severe headaches very frequently. In fact, he has one right now. He was a big help for me when he found the problem with my x-ray machine. I understand that you're having some noises coming out of your MRI machine. I'm sure that Dominic can help you to identify those noises, so you can fix the machine right away in case you need to use it again. When can you see him?"

"Geez!" Doctor Honnastt exclaimed, "I'm sure that you want me to see him right now! Okay, I was just getting ready to go home, but if he's only five, and has a headache right now, send him over."

"You're as wonderful as always," said Doctor Guddok, "thank you Doctor Honnastt. He'll be over with his mommy in about fifteen to twenty minutes. Bye."

"Bye. I'll be waiting," she said. The doctor then turned towards Kate.

"You're also wonderful, Doctor Guddok," she said. "How much do I owe you?"

"I'll tell you what, Miss Smhartd," the doctor replied, "it was a pleasure meeting you and Dominic – that makes us even. However, I do want you to keep me informed regarding Dominic's headaches, because sometimes Doctor Honnastt forgets to tell me about the patients that I send her."

"Oh, no Doctor!" said Kate, in a rather loud voice. "I can't accept..."

The doctor interrupted her and said, "Go, Miss Smhartd! Doctor Honnastt is waiting, and she wants to go home. Besides, Dominic found the problem with my machine, and now I can get it fixed – that's enough payment for me. Bye."

"Okay, Doctor, thank you," said Kate. "I'll call you. Bye."

After they left the doctor's office, Kate thanked Miriam for having referred her to such a wonderful doctor. She told Miriam that Doctor Guddok would be her doctor from then on. Miriam told Kate that she would go with her to Gud Hospital, but it was getting late, and she had many errands to do before going to bed. Miriam also told Kate that Gud Hospital is where her son, Robby, was born, and that it was a good hospital.

About twenty five minutes later, Kate and Dominic arrived at Gud Hospital. As soon as they entered the main lobby, the guard at the door greeted them with a big smile and a great deal of courteousness. He looked at Kate and said, "Good evening, Miss." He then looked at Dominic and asked, "Are you Mr. Dominic, Sir?"

Dominic looked straight up at the guard's face and smiled, as he usually did. He, once again, very vividly displayed his respectful manners and said, "Yes Sir, Mr. Guard." The guard then laughed out loud.

A woman, who was standing nearby, heard the guard laughing and looked towards him. She saw Kate and Dominic standing next to the guard, who made a signal to her that indicated that Dominic was the patient that she was waiting for. She then started walking towards them. When she approached them, she said, "Well, now, you're a very handsome young man. My name is Doctor Honnastt, and what is your name?"

"Dominic, Mrs. Doctor Honnastt," he answered.

As soon as Kate saw Doctor Honnastt, she wondered if she was in any way related to Doctor Guddok, because Kate found her to be very beautiful and attractive, and similar in appearance to him. She thought that the two doctors would make a nice couple, if they weren't related.

"Well, come on, we have to hurry," the doctor went on. She then started walking away very fast, and Dominic followed her. "Dominic, I need you to listen to my machine immediately. Please follow us Miss – oops, I'm sorry, I don't know your name."

"Kate Smhartd," she said.

The doctor continued talking as they headed towards the MRI room, "Glad to meet you, Miss Smhartd. Let's hurry up, so Dominic can listen to my machine. Do you still have a headache, Dominic?"

"A little bit," he answered.

When they arrived, the doctor asked Kate if Dominic was Claustrophobic – afraid of enclosed places. Kate told her that he wasn't. Then she instantly went to work on Dominic's problem, "Dominic, here's the machine I want you to listen to. It has been making some sounds lately. Now, listen to me very carefully, Dominic. Only the person listening to the sounds can go inside. When I open the door, I want you to go inside and lie down facing up. As soon as you lie down, stay absolutely quiet and still. After I close the door, the sounds will begin. I don't want you to move or say anything until all the sounds stop and I open the door. Do you think you can do it?"

"Sure, that's a piece of cake for me." he replied.

"Very good, Dominic," the doctor added, "I knew you were a smart boy, because Doctor Guddok told me." When Dominic was securely placed inside of the MRI machine, with the door closed, Doctor Honnastt turned on the switch, and the sounds started. She made sure that the procedure wouldn't take too long – she was only doing his head. After a few moments, it was all over, and Doctor Honnastt stopped the machine and opened the door. She then said, "Dominic, please come out now and tell me what the noises sounded like."

"That was easy!" Dominic replied as he came out of the machine. "The noises sounded like one of those machines that they use on the street to break the cement, but the sounds were a lot lower."

"Oh my God!" the doctor exclaimed. "That was great! No one before you was able to identify the noises. Now I can have a repairman come in and fix the machine for me. I'll be right back. Don't go away yet." Doctor Honnastt took the information from the MRI machine and went to the technician's desk for an immediate reading. When she arrived, she handed the readout to the technician and said, "Please, study this very carefully, Joe. The patient is having frequent headaches, and he's only five years old."

Joe went to work on it immediately and said, "Okay, Doctor Honnastt, I'll bring it back to you when I'm done."

In less than a minute, Doctor Honnastt went back to join Kate and Dominic. "Miss Smhartd," she said, "Joe Besttek is our best technician when it comes to reading MRI reports. He was kind enough to stay here late tonight to help me with Dominic's MRI. He won't take long reading the results. If there's a problem with Dominic's head, Joe will find it."

"Okay, Doctor Honnastt. I hope so," Kate replied.

"Let's go into my examining room," said the doctor. "It's more comfortable in there." They then started walking away from the MRI room.

Just as they were about to enter Doctor Honnastt's examining room, Joe also started walking towards them with the MRI sheet in his hands – he moved very slowly. When he arrived, he said, also with a very slow tone of voice, "Doctor Honnastt, I'm sorry, but I was unable to find anything wrong with Dominic's head – everything seems normal. I can't imagine why he's getting headaches. However, I haven't given up yet – I only came into your examining room so we can both look at it and see if we can find something unusual – four eyes are better than two. Here, let me put it up next to this light, so we can both study it."

Doctor Honnastt and Joe Besttek spent several minutes studying the MRI, and they were unable to come up with anything abnormal. The doctor agreed with Joe and said, "You're absolutely right, Joe, everything looks normal. She then wondered how Dominic's headaches started. She turned towards Kate and asked, "Miss Smhartd, do you have any idea what has been causing his headaches?"

"Yes," Kate answered, "he hit his head against a pole the other day, but he wasn't in any pain, and there wasn't even a mark on his head where he hit it."

"Oh!" Doctor Honnastt exclaimed. "Now we have something to go by! No one mentioned that to me before. I guess it's as much my fault for not asking you, but I thought that the headaches came for no obvious reason. What part of his head was hit?"

"On his left side, right above his ear," Kate answered as she touched Dominic's head, "right here."

The doctor started physically examining Dominic's head where it was hit. After a minute or two, she turned towards Kate again and said, "Miss Smhartd, I can't see anything wrong, but…"

"I'm sorry, Doctor Honnastt," Joe abruptly interrupted the doctor, before she was able to complete her sentence, "I didn't mean to cut you off, but as soon as Miss Smhartd mentioned the location of the impact, I started studying that part of the MRI, and there seems to be a very small dot that doesn't look normal. I had to use a magnifying glass to see it. Here, take a look." Joe handed the magnifying glass to Doctor Honnastt.

After looking at the sheet for only a few seconds, she agreed with him, "You're absolutely right, Joe, it's not normal, but it's so tiny that it can't be seen with the naked eye. Even with the magnifying glass, it's hard to see it." She then turned towards Kate and asked, "Did I tell you that Joe's the best we have, Miss Smhartd?"

"You certainly did, Doctor Honnastt," Kate answered. "Thank you Mr. Besttek. You're the best." Joe made a gesture, acknowledging what Kate said.

"Now that I think we have something," the doctor continued, "let's take it a little further. I'd like to use Joe's magnifying glass and look at Dominic's head again." Joe handed the magnifying glass to Doctor Honnastt, and she started parting Dominic's hair at several places to see his scalp. After a few seconds of not finding anything, she turned towards Joe again, "Joe, can you tell me approximately where that tiny dot is in relation to Dominic's ear?"

Joe studied the printout again and calculated where the dot was. After a few seconds, he replied, "Well, let me see. According to the MRI, it should be exactly a half inch right above the center of his ear."

The doctor put her index finger on Dominic's head and asked, "Right about here?"

Joe looked at the doctor's finger and answered, "That looks about right. If it's not there, then, it should be nearby."

"Aha!" The doctor exclaimed with a very loud voice, after looking through Dominic's hair. "Oh my God! Here it is! It's so tiny, that

I had to use the magnifying glass to see it. Even with it, it's difficult to see it clearly, but it's there for sure." Doctor Honnastt showed the dot to Joe, because he had been such a big help in finding the problem – actually, he was the one who found it. She then handed the glass to Joe and said, "Take a look, Joe, and you, too, Miss Smhartd, after Joe looks at it."

After Joe saw the dot, he handed the glass to Kate, who also looked at it. After everyone agreed that there was definitely a tiny dot on Dominic's head, the next step was for the doctor to investigate further, to get to the bottom of Dominic's headaches. Joe's help wasn't needed anymore, but he wanted to remain there, so he asked, "Doctor Honnastt, do you mind if I stay here, while you find out what it is?"

"Not at all, Joe," Doctor Honnastt replied. "Actually, I wouldn't have it any other way, but you must ask Miss Smhartd if she minds, and of course you must ask Mr. Dominic also."

"I don't mind," Kate and Dominic answered almost simultaneously, before Joe had a chance to ask them.

"As a matter of fact," Kate added, "I wouldn't have it any other way either."

"Me neither," said Dominic.

"Thank you, all three of you," Joe replied.

The doctor then opened a drawer and took out a much more powerful gadget that she put on her right eye to take another look at the dot. After she looked at it, she said, "I can see it clearly now, and it seems like the blow against the pipe caused a hair to grow backwards into a small blood vessel, causing it to swell a tiny amount, but enough to restrict the flow of blood. I think we can fix this right away." Doctor Honnastt removed the gadget from her eye, took a jar of anesthetic out of the drawer and said, "Now, Dominic, I'm going to get something that looks like clear gelatin out of this jar. I'm going to put a tiny amount on your head. You won't feel a thing. Is that okay with you?"

"Sure, that'll be fun," Dominic replied. "My mommy never lets me put stuff on my hair!" Everyone laughed very loudly when Dominic said that, and Dominic was totally thrilled at the thought of having something put on his hair.

"Okay, then," Doctor Honnastt continued, "here we go, Dominic." The doctor applied some of the ointment on the ingrown hair. After about a minute, she took out a very thin instrument from the drawer and put her gadget on her right eye again. She then said, "Okay, Dominic, I'm going to move some of your hairs around a little bit. Let me know if it hurts at anytime, is that ok?"

"It's okay with me, and it won't hurt me at all – you'll see," he answered.

The doctor used the instrument, with the intention of removing the defective hair, with root and all. She tugged on it a little bit to see if Dominic felt any pain. "Does this hurt?" she asked.

Dominic looked up at the doctor and answered, "No, Mrs. Doctor Honnastt, I told you that it wouldn't hurt me at all."

It was then that the doctor abruptly pulled on it and removed it completely. After finishing, she turned towards Dominic and asked, "Did you feel any pain at all, Dominic?"

"No, of course not," he replied, "I told you that it wouldn't hurt me." As soon as Dominic answered Doctor Honnastt's question, he suddenly turned towards his mother and said, in a very loud voice, "Hey, Mommy! My headache just went away!"

Immediately after Dominic told Kate that his headache was gone, she burst into tears, hugged the doctor as well as Joe and said, "Thank you, Doctor Honnastt and Mr. Besttek, you're two angels in disguise. Doctor Guddok was right about you, Doctor Honnastt, and you were right about Mr. Besttek. How much do I owe both of you?"

"Miss Smhartd," said the doctor, "since you were sent here by Doctor Guddok, this one is on the house, but I don't know about Joe's fee, and also the hospital's fee."

"As far as my fee is concerned," Joe interjected, "it's on the house also. Besides, I was already paid by a big hug from Miss Smhartd."

"My God!" Kate exclaimed very loudly, while still in tears. "Doctor Guddok didn't charge me anything either! The three of you are so unlike the first three doctors that I visited. They didn't even do anything to help, and you have done wonders. I think that I'd be taking advantage of you two if I don't pay you anything, so I…"

"Don't worry, Miss Smhartd," the doctor abruptly interrupted her, "both Joe and I have learned a lot tonight. I'm going to fully document this historic operation into the hospital's journals. I'm sure that Joe will also find some way to improve his techniques, as a result of what happened here tonight."

"Miss Smhartd," Joe added, "Doctor Honnastt and I are not charging you anything for this visit, but we both have to account for what we did here tonight. The hospital may send you a small bill – if they do, it shouldn't be much."

The reason why Doctor Honnastt and Joe Besttek did not bill Kate for their services was because they were there past their work hours. They weren't getting paid by the hospital for their time, but they did have to account for the use of the hospital's rooms, equipment and tools. It was something very unusual, but they did it anyway.

"Okay," said Kate, "thank you both again. "I am totally overwhelmed by your kindness. After visiting the other three doctors, I was beginning to think that I'd never step into a doctor's office again. I guess there are angels in this world. I know the two of you are angels for sure, as well as Doctor Guddok."

"Now, Miss Smhartd," said Doctor Honnastt as she decided to call it a night, "I don't think it's necessary for Dominic to come back, but I want you to keep me informed about his condition. Here's my card. Please feel free to call me anytime. We're finished now."

"And here's my card also, Miss Smhartd," said Joe, "in case you want to call me for any reason."

"I'm really speechless at this point," said Kate, "and it's so late that it's way past Dominic's bedtime. I really must go. Good night, angels, and may God reward you for your actions. Dominic, say, 'Good night' to these two angels."

"Good night, Angels," said Dominic as he looked at Doctor Honnastt and Joe Besttek.

Everyone laughed very loudly when Dominic replied, and Doctor Honnastt concluded for the night by saying, "Good night, Miss Smhartd. I am extremely tired. Joe and I are leaving also. Don't forget to call me. Good night, Mr. Dominic, and thank you for listening to my machine."

"Good night, Miss Smhartd and Mr. Dominic," Joe added. "By the way, Dominic, you have a very beautiful and smart mommy." Dominic looked at Kate, and they both smiled and left.

The following day, Kate phoned both Doctor Guddok and Doctor Honnastt to report to them, as they had asked her to. They were extremely happy to hear that Dominic's headaches were totally gone. Kate also called Joe Besttek to tell him the good news. He was also delighted to hear it.

A few days later, when fully recovered from her ordeal, Kate wanted to do something for the three people that she referred to as "Angels." She invited them to an expensive restaurant near her home. They gladly accepted and agreed to meet the following Saturday. Kate also invited her best friend, Miriam Pheelswel, and her boyfriend, Robby's father. Of course, Robby was also invited.

On Saturday, everyone met at the restaurant. As soon as they sat at the table, they started talking about the headache incident. When the headache conversation was concluded, they started talking about many other subjects. It was then revealed that the only ones in the group who had relationships with someone were Miriam and her boyfriend. Everyone else was free as a bird. During their dinner and conversation, they had put all formalities aside and started calling each other by their first names.

Before long, a very strong relationship was beginning to develop between Kate and Joe. Doctor Guddok and Doctor Honnastt were also looking at each other as they never had done before. Several hours later, they decided to end their get-together, but promised to continue their relationship. They planned to get together again. Following that plan, Kate paid for their dinner, and everyone went home for the night.

After that wonderful time that they had at the restaurant, it didn't take long for Joe and Kate to begin dating. Doctor Guddok and Doctor Honnastt also started dating shortly after Joe and Kate did.

Many months after the headache incident, Kate still hadn't received the bill from Gud Hospital for the services provided, and Dominic's headaches never returned.

Sometime later, Kate Smhartd finally married Joe Besttek, and they have two children in addition to Kate's son, Dominic. Joe loves and treats Dominic as his own son, and Kate and Dominic adore him.

Miriam Pheelswel finally married her boyfriend, Robby's father, and they have three additional children. They still maintain a close relationship with the others.

Doctor Honnastt and Doctor Guddok finally got married, and they have three children. A few years after they were married, they jointly opened a brand new hospital, which they decided to call "Last Hope Hospital." They gave it that name because it was the last hope that some patients had after being diagnosed with certain ailments that other doctors or medical institutions were unable or unwilling to treat. After they opened Last Hope Hospital, Doctor Honnastt and Doctor Guddok maintained a very close and significant relationship with Gud Hospital. All of Doctor Guddok's patients from his private practice followed him to be his loyal patients at his new location – Last Hope Hospital. Doctor Honnastt and Doctor Guddok still run Last Hope Hospital today, with honesty and efficiency.

Doctor Innaddayze was thoroughly trained while Doctor Honnastt was making preparations to open her own hospital with her husband,

Doctor Guddok. Before Doctor Honnastt left Gud Hospital, Doctor Innaddayze took over as Head Physician of the hospital. To this day, Doctor Innaddayze still practices there with a great deal of compassion, honesty, respect and dignity.

Joe Besttek is still the best technician that Doctor Honnastt and Doctor Guddok had ever known, so they asked him if he wanted to work for them when they opened Last Hope Hospital. He was delighted, so he told Doctor Innaddayze that he would train someone else thoroughly before leaving Gud Hospital. Doctor Innaddayze agreed and told him that he would always be welcome to return if anything ever went wrong. After Joe trained someone else, he left and never returned to work there again. However, he did maintain a close relationship with the hospital. The technician who took his place was trained by Joe, so he also turned out to be extremely good.

The Surprise

SOMETIME LATER, ON A Monday morning, Gene Lissenzwel sent letters to several people and informed them that he wanted to have an urgent meeting with them, which was to take place at ten in the morning the following Monday.

A week later, everyone met where indicated, and Gene began talking about his hidden motive for inviting all these people to the meeting, "Some of us here know who Doctor Telsdetrooth and Doctor Molergryndar are, "but most of you don't. Let me talk about these two doctors, for the benefit of those of you who don't know who they are…" Gene spent a few minutes talking about them. He then went on with his explanation as to why he invited everyone to the meeting, "Doctor Telsdetrooth passed away several months ago, and all his worldly possessions went to Doctor Molergryndar, as it was indicated in their wills that the survivor would inherit the decedent's possessions. Doctor Molergryndar recently passed away also. I have to reluctantly say that they were two very malicious doctors until the last days of their lives. The reason why I am insulting them in this manner is because they made it conditional that I should say exactly what I said, in order for their wills to be valid. They also admitted it themselves that they were malicious, and they wanted me to say it at this point, so everyone knows it. Doctor Telsdetrooth and Doctor Molergryndar came to my office one day after everyone else had gone home. They asked me to draw wills for them. They named all the employees of my law firm when the lawsuit against the nine doctors and the two hospitals was settled – which at that point were only Melissa

Jernolrytar, Maria Jannytarboz and myself. They also named Doctor Honnastt, Doctor Innaddayze, Elizabeth Syckcolun, all the ex-prisoners and Francesca Rooindteath. I had to hire Rebecca Fynedzowt to locate Francesca. Because she has a different last name now, Rebecca had a difficult time finding her, but here she is, all grown up into a fine lady, with her husband and two beautiful children. Anyway, the two doctors named each and every one of us, by name, in their wills. It was their wish that I should not mention anything about this to anyone until after their deaths. In spite of the fact that they had been very wicked during their careers, they honestly had a change of heart when they were approaching their ends. They thought, for some reason, that we all deserve their money. They were able to accumulate almost two hundred million dollars between the two, and their last wish was for us to have it all. Although they had separate wills drawn, they didn't want the wills to be read to you until they both passed away, because there is a clause in both wills stating that the survivor was to receive the decedent's money. Of course, Doctor Telsdetrooth's will was already read in order to transfer his money to Doctor Molergryndar's account, and that's where all the money is now, waiting for his will to be read. They both named Melissa Jernolrytar as the recipient of ten percent of their fortune. The rest is to be divided equally among everyone else. Let me read the entire will now, and after I finish reading it, anyone who wishes to read it, may do so. Before I read the will, are there any questions?"

Following Gene's opening statement, all the heirs, except Gene, of course, were totally shocked to hear the news. Almost everyone had several questions to ask. After a while, all the questions had been asked and answered. Following the questions-and-answers session, Gene proceeded with the reading of the will. After the reading, there were again many questions and answers. When the day passed, everything pertaining to the doctors' wills was done, and the meeting ended.

Almost all the heirs were already very well-off, financially, due to the original trial, the lawsuit and their original fortunes. They didn't need any more money, but they eventually received their shares of the doctors' fortune.

Sometime after receiving his share of the inheritance, Sam Towhertz came up with a brilliant idea – he wanted to help people who weren't as fortunate as he had been. In time, with the help of Gene Lissenzwel, he founded "Towhertz Philanthropical Society." Since he was such a wealthy man, he set aside his entire inheritance plus a great amount of his original money to fund the society. He told some of his wealthy colleagues that if they wanted to contribute to the society, they were welcome to do it. Many of the wealthy people that he knew pitched in very generously, including many of the people who were at the reading of the will. Sam was very careful in donating the society's funds – he made sure that the money went to people who really needed it. After all the swindles that he had heard of, he made sure that no fraudulent claims were made against the society's money.

As time passed, the society was responsible for saving the lives of many starving people throughout the world. The society was also providing shelter, medical care, etc. for millions of people. Donations into the society were endless, and so were the society's activities.

Epilogue

REVEREND STOOMAYKAR IS STILL making soup and stew from the bodies of deceased old people. The members of his congregation love it so much that the attendance doubled in the last few years, just because of the deliciously flavorful soup that the reverend makes. He had to double his order of corpses from Doctor Oargandeelar, who is now supplying Reverend Stoomaykar with two bodies every month, and some months even three bodies. The minister is now more selective – he told the organ dealer to send him only bodies of people who are eighty and up. The dealer still has no problems filling his orders in time for every congregation meeting. The reverend has to boil the flesh even longer now, because the age requirement for his corpses went up. He also had to raise the price of every meal, but the members don't mind at all paying the extra amount because they find the unique taste of his soup and stew to be worth whatever he asks for it. It is still not known whether or not the members of the congregation know that they're eating human flesh, because Doctor Oargandeelar never asked the reverend.

Maria Jannytarboz remained as a devoted employee of Gene Lissenzwel & Associates as Gene's secretary and administrative assistant, until he decided to change that – he knew that she was extremely bright, and because she had already graduated from college with honors, he offered her the opportunity to go to law school at his expense. The offer was so good that she couldn't refuse it. Gene hired an assistant, so Maria could train her before starting law school. Eventually, Maria passed her bar and became an associate attorney with the firm.

Elizabeth Syckcolun is still living today, several years after being wrongly diagnosed with advanced colon cancer. She's living a normal life without any pain whatsoever – and most importantly, without ever really having contracted cancer at all. She was definitely lucky when she was wrongly diagnosed, because she never went to see Doctor Sayahagain. If she had gone, she probably would have ended up as a prisoner at Deprivayshun Psychiatric Hospital, after getting unnecessary surgery at Kuttemopen Hospital. She never went to visit Reverend Stoomaykar's congregation either. If she had gone and joined the group, she would be eating soup and stew made from the deceased bodies of old people. She decided to continue having annual checkups, but she's now more cautious about what the doctors tell her. She was smart enough to look for another hospital, and finally ended up as a regular patient at Gud Hospital under Doctor Martha Innaddayze's care. If Elizabeth had gone for the operation at Kuttemopen Hospital, would she still be alive today? Well, we won't know the answer to that question because it never happened, but look at what happened to her husband, James! One thing for certain is that she would have less money in the bank, if any at all, if she had gone for the operation.

After Melissa Jernolrytar's interview with Doctor Telsdetrooth, she realized that Elizabeth and James had been victims of the cruelties dished out by Kuttemopen Hospital. As soon as she started working for Gene Lissenzwel, she asked Rebecca Fynedzowt to help her locate Elizabeth Syckcolun. With Rebecca's great abilities, Melissa had all the information that she needed about Elizabeth in less than an hour. Melissa gave Elizabeth a copy of the journal that she wrote about all the doctors and hospitals involved. Elizabeth read the journal and eventually found out about the cigarette ashes in the urn on her mantelpiece. After Elizabeth read the journal, she contacted Gene Lissenzwel to represent her. He started another lawsuit against Doctor Butchar and Kuttemopen Hospital. With Gene's great abilities and expertise, again, the case was settled out of court. After the settlement,

Elizabeth threw out the urn with the cigarette ashes inside. Elizabeth Syckcolun was already very wealthy when she inherited her share of Doctor Telsdetrooth's and Doctor Molergryndar's fortune. She is now even wealthier, due to the new settlement, and enjoying good health. She still maintains that youthful look that she always enjoyed.

Sam Towhertz eventually had a talk with the employee who dropped the sledgehammer on his toe. August Hahmerdrawpper was very apologetic. Sam told him that he knew that it was an accident, because the incident took place after a very cold night. There was a frozen puddle on the ground that caused August to slip and fall, dropping the sledgehammer on Sam's foot. After his conversation with Sam, August Hahmerdrawpper remained as one of Sam Towhertz's numerous loyal employees.

To this day, Doctor Butchar has never sent Rebecca Fynedzowt her check for the investigative work that she did at Kuttemopen Hospital. She didn't bother to pursue the matter because she had accomplished far more than she had expected and imagined during that investigation. Besides, she didn't have any proof of ever working there, and she felt that Doctor Butchar never kept any records at all of her employment at the hospital.

Doctor Theeph, Doctor Krooll, Doctor Dredfall, Doctor Malishuss and Doctor Wykkedd are still under the government program to do research in an attempt to find the cure for cancer. They still haven't reported the discovery of the cure to the government, nor will they ever. The cure for cancer remains a secret forever. They heard rumors that other research organizations have also found the cure for cancer and are also keeping it a secret. The five doctors are also continuing doing bogus studies on hundreds of different products to keep increasing their bank accounts as they invest in the stock market. As long as they continue receiving the grant money, they'll keep their operation going. The doctors still make frequent trips to The Bahamas, as well as to many other recreational paradises – it's all in the name of research. They're making sure, with the help of Wallace Koropted, that the media keeps track of their activities, so their donations keep pouring in. Their routine will probably last for many more years. Some of their children have grown up, and the doctors are hiring them to work at Ghetrychkwik Cancer Research Center, with the intention of keeping the operation going, generation after generation. The doctors' salaries are now a whopping $44,500,000 annually each, from the grant money alone. The five doctors are all billionaires now, due to their bogus product studies. They have also heard rumors that similar studies are being conducted by other organizations for the sake of making money.

Is it true that other research organizations have found the cure for cancer, and are keeping it a secret? Maybe so, or maybe not, but how can it be possible that some have been in existence more that fifty years, collecting donations, and haven't found it yet? That's certainly hard to believe!

Doctor Sayahagain, Doctor Louzi, Doctor Louziar, Doctor Byggliar, Doctor Sharlottan, Doctor Butchar, Doctor Manypewlatar, Doctor Oargandeelar, Doctor Ryppemuff, Kuttemopen Hospital, Deprivayshun Psychiatric Hospital and Diebroak Senior Citizens Home are still in business today. They got away with everything that they did, and are still committing their usually cruel deeds. They had to double all their fees in order to make up for the losses that they incurred during and after the trials and all the lawsuits against them. That's why the cost of medical services is so high today – not to mention the cost of medical insurance. The doctors and hospitals who were fined in this story, and others like them, are the cause of it all.

Don't forget, if it is absolutely necessary for you to go to a doctor or hospital, make sure that you tell someone that you went there to seek medical services, and also, make sure that you go to a good doctor. By all means, try to avoid visiting any of the bad doctors and hospitals mentioned in this story – you may or may not be surprised if you find others like them somewhere in your own neighborhoods.

Make sure to choose the right doctor, but don't choose one based on recommendations – remember that Doctor Sayahagain, Doctor Louzi, Doctor Louziar, Doctor Byggliar and Doctor Sharlottan were all very highly recommended professionals, and they were the worst of doctors. How do you go about choosing the right doctor? – I DON'T KNOW, but remember, BEWARE OF DOCTORS AND HOSPITALS. The end.

About the Author

AFTER MANY YEARS OF telling stories, I have decided to write several books about the many tales that I told my children at bedtime when they were small. They enjoyed every one of my stories, even when they were growing into adolescence. They wanted to hear a different story every night before they went to sleep.

This is one story that I never told my children, but I did tell it to a group of adults during a convention. The president of a major corporation advised me that I should write a book about it. Well, that was a couple of decades ago, but here I am, and I just finished writing it now. Of course, I added a few things to the story to make it conform more adequately today.

"The Clock of Peaceville" and "King Generous and King Selfish" were the first two books that I published. "Beware of Doctors and Hospitals" is my third book. I am writing many other books, which will be published in the near future.

I have a Computer Science degree from NYCC. I have done many things in my life, but I am now a retired real estate broker. I am a divorced father of two grown children. I love the outdoors, but what I enjoy the most is fishing on the ocean, and I can't seem to get enough of it. When I'm not fishing, I am writing stories.

Anyone wishing to communicate with the author, for any reason, may do so at P.O. Box 150366, Brooklyn, N.Y. 11215.

www.ingramcontent.com/pod-product-compliance
Lightning Source LLC
Chambersburg PA
CBHW031813170526
45157CB00001B/39